Infectious Diseases in Pediatric Otolaryngology

Tulio A. Valdez • Jesus G. Vallejo
Editors

Infectious Diseases in Pediatric Otolaryngology

A Practical Guide

Springer

Editors
Tulio A. Valdez
Department of Pediatric Otolaryngology
Connecticut Children's Medical Center
Hartford, CT, USA

Jesus G. Vallejo
Department of Pediatrics
Section of Infectious Diseases
Baylor College of Medicine
Texas Children's Hospital
Houston, TX, USA

ISBN 978-3-319-21743-7 ISBN 978-3-319-21744-4 (eBook)
DOI 10.1007/978-3-319-21744-4

Library of Congress Control Number: 2015945018

Springer Cham Heidelberg New York Dordrecht London

Printed on acid-free paper

Springer International Publishing AG Switzerland is part of Springer Science+Business Media (www.springer.com)

Preface

The practice of medicine requires constant teamwork among various disciplines to achieve the best results in patient care. In this textbook *Infectious Diseases in Pediatric Otolaryngology*, we set up to provide an easy to use guide for the management of infectious conditions in the head and neck using the same collaborative model that we use in the everyday management of patients. Each chapter compiles the expert opinions and recommendations of pediatric otolaryngologist and pediatric infectious disease specialists to provide a comprehensive approach to the management of these conditions.

Infectious diseases constitute a large portion of the practice of pediatric otolaryngology. It is also important for pediatric practitioners to identify conditions that may require surgical management. We have tried not to standardize therapy, but rather have chosen to preserve the differences among the recommendations of the authors in order to illustrate that a variety of approaches to treatment may be available.

Finally, we would like to thank the many contributors for their excellent and timely chapters and the editorial staff at Springer for their wonderful assistance. We hope that students, pediatric and otolaryngology residents, and practicing physicians find the guidelines outlined in this book useful and readily accessible.

We would like to specially thank our wives Carole and Karen and our children Isaac, Cristian, and Eric for their unwavering support during this project.

Hartford, CT, USA — Tulio A. Valdez
Houston, TX, USA — Jesus G. Vallejo

Contents

Contributors

Nicholas J. Bennett, M.B.B.Chir., Ph.D. Division of Infectious Diseases and Immunology, Connecticut Children's Medical Center, Hartford, CT, USA

Claire Bocchini, M.D. Department of Pediatrics, Section of Infectious Diseases, Baylor College of Medicine, Houston, TX, USA

Texas Children's Hospital, Houston, TX, USA

Judith R. Campbell, M.D. Department of Pediatrics, Section of Infectious Diseases, Baylor College of Medicine, Houston, TX, USA

Texas Children's Hospital, Houston, TX, USA

Luis A. Castagnini, M.D., M.P.H. Department of Pediatrics, Baylor College of Medicine, San Antonio, TX, USA

Daniel C. Chelius, M.D., F.A.A.P. Department of Otolaryngology—Head and Neck Surgery, Baylor College of Medicine, Houston, TX, USA

Texas Children's Hospital, Houston, TX, USA

Melanie S. Collins, M.D. Department of Pediatric Pulmonary Medicine, Connecticut Children's Medical Center, Hartford, CT, USA

University of Connecticut School of Medicine, Farmington, CT, USA

Armando G. Correa, M.D. Department of Pediatrics, Baylor College of Medicine, Houston, TX, USA

Texas Children's Hospital, Houston, TX, USA

Valerie Cote, M.D., C.M., F.A.A.P., F.R.C.S.C. Division of Pediatric Otolaryngology, University of Connecticut School of Medicine, Hartford, CT, USA

Connecticut Children's Medical Center, Hartford, CT, USA

Jonathan D. Crews, M.D., M.S. Department of Pediatrics, Section of Infectious Diseases, Baylor College of Medicine, Children's Hospital of San Antonio, San Antonio, TX, USA

Andrea T. Cruz, M.D., M.P.H. Department of Pediatrics, Baylor College of Medicine, Houston, TX, USA

Jennifer Dang, M.D. Department of Otolaryngology, Baylor College of Medicine, Houston, TX, USA

Henry M. Feder Jr., M.D. Department of Pediatrics and Family Medicine, University of Connecticut Medical Center, Farmington, CT, USA

Marisol Fernandez, M.D. Department of Pediatric Infectious Diseases, Dell Children's Medical Center, Seton Healthcare Family, Austin, TX, USA

Carla M. Giannoni, M.D. Department of Pediatric Otolaryngology, Baylor College of Medicine, Houston, TX, USA

Texas Children's Hospital, Houston, TX, USA

Meha Goyal, B.B.A. Department of Otolaryngology - Head and Neck Surgery, Baylor College of Medicine, Houston, TX, USA

Christopher R. Grindle, M.D. Division of Otolaryngology—Head and Neck Surgery, University of Connecticut School of Medicine, Connecticut Children's Medical Center, Hartford, CT, USA

Amy L. Hughes, M.D. Department of Otolaryngology and Communication Disorders, Boston Children's Hospital, Boston, MA, USA

Amal Isaiah, M.D., D.Phil. (Oxon.) Department of Otorhinolaryngology—Head and Neck Surgery, University of Maryland School of Medicine, Baltimore, MD, USA

Kyle Johnson, M.D. Department of Otolaryngology, University of Connecticut School of Health Sciences, Farmington, CT, USA

Nicholas Karter, M.D. Department of Otolaryngology, University of Connecticut, Farmington, CT, USA

Katherine R. Kavanagh, M.D. Department of Otolaryngology, Connecticut Children's Medical Center, Hartford, CT, USA

Deidre R. Larrier, M.D. Bobby Alford Department of Otolaryngology Head and Neck Surgery, Baylor College of Medicine, Houston, TX, USA

Lucila Marquez, M.D., M.P.H. Department of Pediatrics, Sections of Pediatric Infectious Diseases and Pediatric Hospital Medicine, Baylor College of Medicine, Houston, TX, USA

J. Chase McNeil, M.D. Department of Pediatrics, Section of Infectious Diseases, Baylor College of Medicine, Houston, TX, USA

Thomas S. Murray, M.D., Ph.D. Department of Medical Sciences, Frank H. Netter MD School of Medicine at Quinnipiac University, Hamden, CT, USA

Department of Pediatric Infectious Disease, Connecticut Children's Medical Center, Hartford, CT, USA

Mary F. Musso, D.O. Department of Pediatric Otolaryngology, Baylor College of Medicine, Houston, TX, USA

Texas Children's Hospital, Houston, TX, USA

Julina Ongkasuwan, M.D. Department of Otolaryngology—Head and Neck Surgery, Baylor College of Medicine, Houston, TX, USA

Alexander J. Osborn, M.D., Ph.D. The Voice Clinic, Toronto, ON, Canada

Kevin D. Pereira, M.D., M.S. Department of Otorhinolaryngology—Head and Neck Surgery, University of Maryland School of Medicine, Baltimore, MD, USA

Department of Pediatric Otolaryngology, University of Maryland School of Medicine, Baltimore, MD, USA

Mark D. Rizzi, M.D. Department of Otolaryngology, The Children's Hospital of Philadelphia, Philadelphia, PA, USA

Corrie E. Roehm, M.D. Department of Pediatric Otolaryngology, Dell Children's Hospital, Austin, TX, USA

Scott R. Schoem, M.D. Department of Otolaryngology, Connecticut Children's Medical Center, Hartford, CT, USA

Matthew Sitton, M.D. Department of Otolaryngology, Baylor College of Medicine, Houston, TX, USA

Texas Children's Hospital, Houston, TX, USA

Douglas S. Swanson, M.D. Department of Pediatrics, Children's Mercy Hospital, Kansas City, MO, USA

University of Missouri, Kansas City, MO, USA

Yamilet Tirado, M.D. Department of Otolaryngology, Miami Children's Hospital, Miami, FL, USA

Brandon H. Tran, M.D. Neuroradiology Section, Baylor College of Medicine, Houston, TX, USA

Luis D. Vilchez-Madrigal, M.D. Department of Otolaryngology—Head and Neck Surgery, National Children's Hospital, San Jose, CR, USA

Ronald J. Vilela, M.D. Department of Pediatric Otolaryngology—Head and Neck Surgery, Baylor College of Medicine, Houston, TX, USA

Texas Children's Hospital, Houston, TX, USA

Part I
Ears

Chapter 1
Management of the Child with Otorrhea

Luis D. Vilchez-Madrigal and Alexander J. Osborn

Abbreviations

AOM	Acute otitis media
CN	Cranial nerve
CSF	Cerebral spine fluid
CT	CAT scan
ENT	Ear nose and throat
MEE	Middle ear effusion
MRI	Magnetic resonance imaging
MRSA	Methicillin resistant *Staphylococcus aureus*
OME	Otitis media with effusion
TM	Tympanic membrane
TOM	Tuberculous otitis media
TT	Tympanostomy tube

Otitis Externa

Pathophysiology and Etiology

The ear possesses two primary defense mechanisms to protect it from the development of otitis externa [1]. The most important mechanism is the slightly acidic and hydrophobic cerumen barrier. The acidity of the cerumen, as well as a mild lysozyme contained therein, presents an inhospitable environment for fungal and bacterial pathogens. Furthermore, the hydrophobic barrier imparted by cerumen

L.D. Vilchez-Madrigal, M.D. (✉)
Department of Otolaryngology—Head and Neck Surgery, National Children's Hospital, San Jose, Costa Rica, USA
e-mail: lvilchezm@hnn.sa.cr

A.J. Osborn, M.D., Ph.D.
The Voice Clinic, Toronto, ON, Canada

T.A. Valdez, J.G. Vallejo (eds.), *Infectious Diseases in Pediatric Otolaryngology*,
DOI 10.1007/978-3-319-21744-4_1

protects the very thin squamous epithelium of the ear canal. The second, albeit less potent, mechanism is the migratory pattern of this epithelium. There is a constant lateral migration of the epithelial layer away from the tympanic membrane towards the canal meatus. Desquamated elements are thus amalgamated into the cerumen and expunged from the ear canal. Infectious otitis externa arises when the above-mentioned defense mechanisms are compromised. Breakdown of the cerumen barrier, for example through physical disruption or extended exposure to water, grants the pathogen access to the epithelium. Such actions that break down the barrier are also likely to cause maceration of the skin, providing a portal of entry for the microbial pathogens and initiating inflammatory processes.

Bacterial infection is the most common cause of otitis externa [2]. The most common pathogens are *Pseudomonas aeruginosa* and *Staphylococcus* species. Other species such as *Coryneform* and *Bacteroides* are found in a significant minority of patients (10–20 %) [3]. Fungal infections, usually with *Candida* or *Aspergillus* species, tend to be rare in published series. Fungal otitis externa tends not to be a primary infection, but rather a secondary infection that arises if the environment of the external auditory canal is disrupted with topical antibiotics or steroids. Hearing aid users can often demonstrate a benign-appearing, asymptomatic, superficial colonization of the external auditory canal with *Candida*.

Clinical Presentation

Otitis externa secondary to either bacterial or fungal pathogens typically results in itching or pain localized to the external auditory canal. Patients will often complain of otorrhea or residue left on the pillow after a night's sleep. Often debris composed of squamous elements, bacterial or fungal cells, and purulence will accumulate in the external auditory canal, resulting in decreased hearing and a sense of blockage in the affected ear.

On exam, the ear may be tender to manipulation of the auricle or tragus (Fig. 1.1). The ear canal may be edematous, erythematous, or both and edema may obscure the view of the tympanic

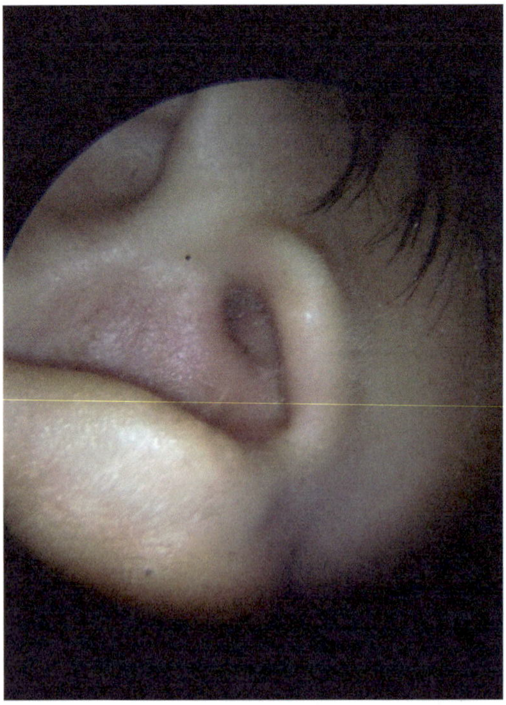

Fig. 1.1 Acute otitis externa. Edema and erythema of the pinna and the ear canal can be noted

membrane. Such cases require a good deal of care on the part of the clinician as increased edema often correlates with exquisite tenderness. The fluid or debris in the ear canal itself is variable and its character gives the clinician a clue as to the nature of the offending pathogen. Thin, slightly cloudy fluid is often present in early bacterial otitis externa, while a thicker, creamy, pale yellow accumulation of debris is present in more established cases. Fungal otitis externa secondary to *Aspergillus* typically presents with chunky white debris with black clumps, giving rise to the classic description of wet newspaper seen in otolaryngology textbooks [1].

Treatment

The primary treatment for infectious otitis externa is the application of topical antiseptic or antibiotic agents; however, adjuvant therapies are both important and often overlooked. Careful debridement of the ear canal is important in order to provide access of topical agents to the bacteria or fungi that would otherwise be protected within or behind debris. Furthermore, some topical agents are ototoxic or highly irritating to the middle ear, and thus an assessment of whether the tympanic membrane is perforated or not helps guide the practitioner in the choice of agents. In addition to debridement, maintenance of dry ear precautions promotes resolution of the infection. Affected individuals should be encouraged to use a swimmer's ear plug or a cotton ball saturated with petroleum jelly to occlude the ear canal when there is any chance of water entering the ear, such as with swimming, bathing, showering, or washing hair. Other measures to avoid the accumulation of moisture within the ear canal should also be taken such as avoiding the use of headphones, hearing aids, occlusive ear buds, or ear plugs other than for brief periods as described above.

Treatment of otitis externa rarely requires systemic antibiotics. Topical treatments fall into three categories: (1) drying and acidifying agents, (2) antimicrobial agents, and (3) steroids [4]. These treatment options are discussed in detail in Chap. 2.

Drying and acidifying agents. A number of acidifying preparations containing acetic acid (combined with isopropyl alcohol, aluminum acetate, or propylene glycol) are available, and can be used for both bacterial and fungal otitis externa. These agents have the potential to be highly irritating to an inflamed or macerated canal epithelium. Furthermore, these agents cannot be used in the presence of a tympanic membrane perforation due to the sensitive nature of the middle ear mucosa. Because of these two reasons, these agents are rarely used to treat acute infection; however they can be used as part of a maintenance routine in individuals with an intact tympanic membrane and a propensity towards otitis externa. The application of such agents (after showering or swimming, for example) can prevent or reduce the frequency of otitis externa.

Antimicrobial agents. Antibiotic drops are the most commonly used therapeutic option for otitis externa. Prior to the introduction of fluoroquinolone topical antibiotics, the mainstay of treatment was a mixture of neomycin, polymyxin, and hydrocortisone (Cortisporin). This preparation had the advantage of being inexpensive as well as helping to reduce inflammation with the presence of steroids. Concerns over the potential ototoxic effects of neomycin (an aminoglycoside) and polymyxin limit the use of these antibiotics to cases without a tympanic membrane perforation [5]. Because general practitioners often initiate therapy in the absence of a clear view of the eardrum, this preparation is seldom first-line therapy.

In cases of fungal otitis externa antifungal agents are required [6]. Miconazole, nystatin, tolnaftate, and ciclopirox olamine are all available in solution form and thus have the advantage of being able to be prescribed by the general practitioner and administered by the patient; however, debridement is an essential aspect of otomycosis therapy.

Steroids. Hydrocortisone and dexamethasone are often included in antibiotic preparations, or may be delivered separately if combination agents are not available. The benefit in symptom resolution provided by the addition of steroids is 0.8 days [5].

Follow Up

Topical treatment of bacterial otitis externa should be carried out for a minimum of 7 days. If a wick was place, it should be removed at the end of the antibiotic course. Dry ear precautions should be maintained until the patient returns for their follow-up appointment, typically in 2–3 weeks. In patients prone to recurrent infections, the application of drying or acidifying drops are used in any maintenance regimen should be avoided until the ear canal is entirely healed and residual signs of inflammation have resolved. Repeat otoscopy must be performed to evaluate for a residual tympanic membrane perforation. Perforation is a rare sequella of otitis externa, except in cases of *Aspergillus* [7].

Malignant Otitis Externa

Malignant otitis externa, or necrotizing otitis externa, occurs when bacterial or fungal otitis externa spreads beyond the ear canal and affects the temporal bone [8]. In children, this is rare but is seen in immunocompromised individuals. *P. aeruginosa* and *S. aureus* are the most common pathogens leading to malignant otitis externa. Clinically, these patients present with longstanding otalgia, which may be out of proportion to the findings on physical exam. Infection may spread from the temporal bone along the skull base and result in cranial nerve paralysis, most commonly of CN VII. In the absence of cranial nerve palsy, the diagnosis of malignant otitis externa requires a high index of suspicion.

Keratosis Obturans and Canal Cholesteatoma

Both of these entities present as an external auditory canal filled with squamous debris. There is often a secondary bacterial infection in both cases resulting in pain or otorrhea; however, on close examination, the two processes represent different etiologies [9]. Keratosis obturans arises from a circumferential accumulation of squamous debris. Debridement will not demonstrate any focal abnormality and the entire canal may be inflamed or irritated. Treatment consists of regular debridement and treatment with topical antibiotics and steroids to reduce inflammation when it occurs. Keratosis obturans is rare in children. Canal cholesteatoma, on the other hand, can be seen in children and typically arises from a focal invasion of the osseous canal by squamous elements. This forms a pocket of keratin debris, which provides a favorable environment for infection. Conservative treatment with topical antibiotics and frequent debridement may allow the canal epithelium to heal, but surgery is often required.

Dermatitis

Allergic, contact, and systemic dermatitis can all affect the external ear. Typically the inflammation associated with these conditions produces a serous otorrhea; however, excoriation of the canal skin by the patient due to itching may sometimes provide a portal of entry for bacteria and see a fulminant bacterial otitis externa as described previously. Treatment of allergic or contact dermatitis is removal of the offending agents. Common offenders are neomycin, shampoo, hairspray, or hearing aid molds. Less commonly steroids can cause hypersensitivity. Systemic dermatitis such as psoriasis or seborrhea can affect the ear and are often treated with topical steroids.

CSF Otorrhea

Spontaneous CSF otorrhea is seldom seen in children, but should be considered in the setting of temporal bone trauma. A ruptured tympanic membrane or tympanostomy tube is required for the fluid to escape the middle ear space. The fluid can be collected and tested for β-transferrin to confirm the nature of the otorrhea. Fluid may be collected at home and kept refrigerated for at least 24 h before being submitted to the laboratory, thus facilitating this testing. Leaks may spontaneously resolve with bed rest and a lumbar drain, but frequently require surgical repair.

Middle Ear

Otorrhea secondary to middle ear pathology is seen when there is a tympanic membrane (TM) perforation. It can have an acute onset in the presence of acute infection or as a complication of an acute process. Longstanding ear discharge results from chronic ear infections.

Acute Otitis Media

Pathophysiology of Otorrhea in AOM

Acute otorrhea in AOM occurs secondary to a perforation of the tympanic membrane. Following transient hearing loss perforation is the second most common intratemporal complication [10]. The purulent fluid within the middle ear is responsible for the TM bulging found in cases of AOM. The non-compliant bony walls of the middle ear associated with acute inflammatory process and mucosal edema creates a high-pressure environment. The compliant tympanic membrane starts to bulge to relieve the pressure. A perforation is seen when permanent pressure over the weakest point of the tympanic membrane creates a breach that will allow the fluid to come out as otorrhea.

Once perforation has happen spontaneous healing may occur and usually the tympanic membrane will close after the suppurative process ends. If the membrane does not heal for longer than 3 months it is considered a chronic perforation. The presence of otorrhea in a chronic perforation is known as chronic otitis media. Suppurative complications of otitis media may happen in the presence of acute or chronic tympanic membrane perforation [11].

Clinical Presentation

The child with AOM often presents with fever, irritability, and ear pain. These symptoms can vary depending on the age of the patient; for example small non-verbal children usually point towards the problematic ear by pulling, tugging or rubbing the affected ear. Gastrointestinal symptoms can also be associated. Older children who are verbal can identify the affected ear.

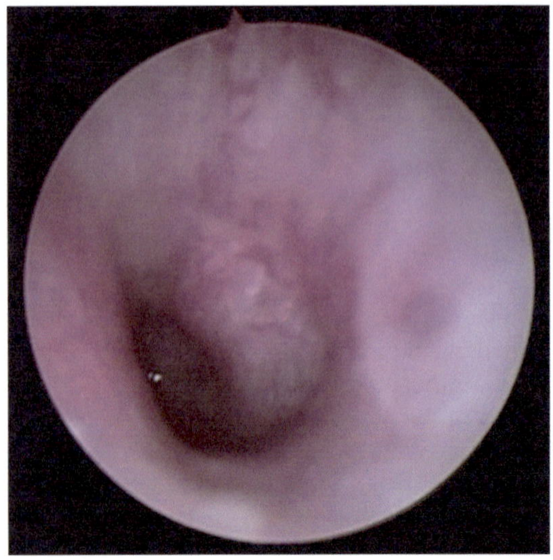

Fig. 1.2 Acute otitis media. TM with severe bulging

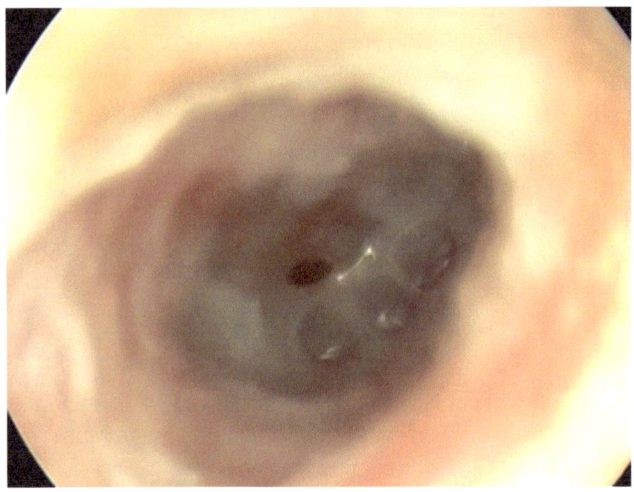

Fig. 1.3 Acute suppurative otitis media. Otorrhea through central perforation of the TM, air-fluid level is noted

On physical examination, AOM is diagnosed with moderate to severe bulging of the tympanic membrane or new-onset of otorrhea not due to Acute Otitis Externa. It can also be diagnosed with mild bulging of the TM and recent (less than 48 h) onset of ear pain or intense erythema of the TM with presence of middle ear effusion (Fig. 1.2). Unilateral or bilateral ear compromise should be determined [12]. Interestingly acute otorrhea correlates with a transient relief of otalgia due to sudden decrease of pressure in the middle ear. The presence of otorrhea is easily identified in the ear canal as wetness or abundant discharge from the middle ear through a tympanic membrane perforation (Fig. 1.3).

Severe cases of AOM often presents as a toxic appearing child, with persistent otalgia for more than 48 h with temperature above 39 °C (102.2 °F) in the previous 48 h.

Treatment

Goals of treatment of AOM are to decrease severity and duration of symptoms and to prevent complications. In order to achieve these, patients are treated with analgesics, antibiotics and in cases of recurrent AOM or suppurative complications with tympanostomy tubes.

Initial observation without antibiotics can be offered to children with new onset and uncomplicated mild AOM. Nonetheless, parent/caregiver should be committed to follow-up and be able to begin antibiotics if the child worsens or fails to improve within 48–72 h of AOM onset. In terms of analgesia, it should be used in all cases, whether antibiotics were prescribed or not. Usually oral acetaminophen and ibuprofen are given alone or in combination to treat AOM. Topical analgesic drops are not recommended because there is insufficient evidence about their efficacy in AOM [13].

Antibiotics should be used in patients with severe symptoms, young children (<6 months of age), children with bilateral AOM and all cases that present otorrhea. The treatment of AOM is discussed in Chap. 3.

Follow Up

The follow-up of a child who was managed with initial observation should include a rescue prescription of antibiotics, parent information to fill the prescription if the child fails to improve within 48–72 h after the initial encounter or if symptoms worsen during the illness. On the other hand, if initial antibiotic therapy was chosen the parent should be instructed to assess the evolution of symptoms. Improvement usually happens within 48–72 h of therapy. If no clinical improvement happens parents are instructed to return for a new assessment and possible change of antibiotic.

Once AOM is successfully treated, middle ear effusion (MEE) can persist for 3 months in 10 % of the patients after the initial episode. Otitis Media with Effusion is defined as the presence of MEE without clinical symptoms. The decision on when to reassess the patient should be in discretion of the treating physician keeping in mind the possibility of residual tympanic membrane perforation.

Chronic Otitis Media

Chronic Otitis Media is defined as a tympanic membrane perforation associated with intermittent or persistent otorrhea for more than 3 months [1]. It can be further categorized as chronic suppurative otitis media (tympanic membrane perforation without cholesteatoma) and cholesteatomatous otitis media (tympanic membrane perforation with cholesteatoma).

Chronic suppurative processes are the result of either an unhealed acute infection that persists over time or chronic Eustachian tube dysfunction with subsequent tympanic membrane perforation. Associated changes in the mucosa such as granulation tissue or hypertrophy of the middle ear lining are often seen. On physical examination, chronic suppurative otitis media usually shows a central tympanic membrane perforation, middle ear mucosa often reveals edema, erythema, and sometimes-even granulation tissue can be found (Fig. 1.4).

Cholesteatoma is seen as a keratin cyst lodged in the middle ear with the potential to erode the ossicles and adjacent bony structures [1]. Primary acquired cholesteatoma is the result of chronic Eustachian tube dysfunction that induces a tympanic membrane retraction pocket with subsequent perforation. Secondary acquired cholesteatoma is seen either by migration or implantation of tympanic membrane squamous layer into the middle ear. The otoscopic appearance of cholesteatoma varies. It can be seen either as keratin debris in a retraction pocket or as white pearly lesion through a marginal tympanic membrane perforation (Fig. 1.5).

Otorrhea in chronic otitis media is precipitated by offending factors such as water exposure, upper respiratory tract infection or in cholesteatoma due to keratin infection. The most commonly encountered germs responsible for persistent otorrhea are *Pseudomonas aeruginosa*, *Proteus mirabilis* and *Staphylococcus aureus* [14].

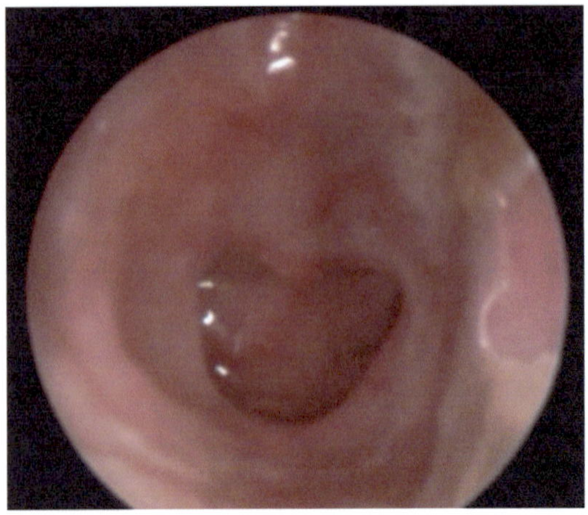

Fig. 1.4 Chronic suppurative otitis media. Central perforation of the TM. Edema and erythema over the promontory. No evidence of cholesteatoma

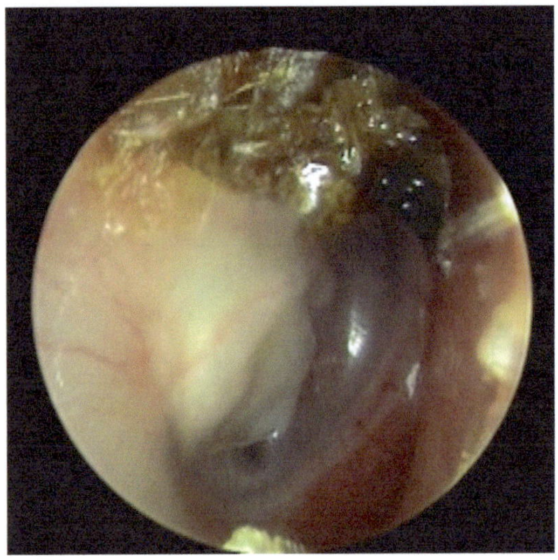

Fig. 1.5 Cholesteatoma. White mass behind the TM. Debris on the superior quadrant of the TM

Children with congenital cholesteatoma usually presents with an intact tympanic membrane, and no history of surgical procedures to the eardrum or middle ear. Otorrhea is rare. In these cases diagnosis is made as an incidental finding during physical examination or due to unilateral hearing loss.

In all cases audiological tests should be obtained to determine the degree of hearing loss. Imaging with CT scan is also granted. Extension of the disease is assessed for further surgical planning.

Management of chronic otitis media is challenging and usually requires a stepwise approach. The main goal is to obtain a safe, dry ear; it is of utmost importance to properly identify the presence of cholesteatoma. Generally, water precautions, aural toilet followed by topical antibiotic drops with or without oral antibiotics is given initially. There are various types of surgical procedures that are used to improve the patient's condition. Tympanoplasty can be used to seal the perforation and prevent further episodes of otorrhea. Mastoidectomy with or without tympanoplasty is used to clean the ear from cholesteatoma. Depending on the surgical technique performed the possibility of middle ear reconstruction to improve the hearing can be feasible.

Tympanostomy Tube Otorrhea

Tympanostomy tube otorrhea is defined as ear discharge in the presence of pressure equalizer tubes (Fig. 1.6). Indications for Tympanostomy Tubes (TT) include restoration of hearing in Chronic Otitis Media with Effusion (OME) and Recurrent Acute Otitis Media (RAOM). The most common complication of tympanostomy tubes is otorrhea (TTO). This complication is seen in approximately 16 % of children within 4 weeks of the procedure and 26 % overall at any time the tube is in place. Other possible complications are TT blockage, granulation tissue, displacement into the middle ear and premature extrusion of intubated ears. Long-term sequelae after extrusion can include: myringosclerosis, atelectasis and persistent perforation [15].

The common pathogens seen in TTO are *Haemophilus influenzae*, *Staphylococcus aureus*, *Pseudomonas aeruginosa*, *Streptococcus pneumoniae* and *Moraxella catarrhalis* [16]. Interestingly the presence of *Pseudomonas aeruginosa* and *Staphylococcus aureus* are seen more frequently in children with a history of submersion.

TTO can be categorized as early postoperative (within 4 weeks of TT placement), delayed otorrhea (4 or more weeks from TT placement), chronic otorrhea (persisting 3 months or longer) and recurrent otorrhea (3 or more discrete episodes).

The clinical symptoms of an uncomplicated episode of TTO are: low-grade fever (less than 38.5 °C/101.2 °F), absence of concomitant bacterial infection (sinusitis, pharyngitis or cellulitis of the pinna) and painless ear discharge. The latest meaning that the TT is patent and helping to evacuate the fluid that usually builds up in the middle ear.

In terms of treatment, topical antibiotics with steroids have proved to be more effective than oral antibiotics and watchful waiting. Persistent otorrhea at 2 weeks of initial treatment was found to be 5 %, 44 % and 55 %, respectively. The median duration of the initial episode of otorrhea was 4 days for topical antibiotics with steroids, 5 days for oral antibiotics and 12 days for watchful waiting [16]. Topical preparations approved for use with tympanostomy tubes (ofloxacin, ciprofloxacin-dexamethasone or ciprofloxacin-hydrocortisone) should be used for a maximum of 10 days.

In the case of persistent otorrhea despite adequate ear care (removal of obstructing debris in the ear canal or within the tympanostomy tube) and appropriate antibiotic treatment, granulation tissue around the TT, fungi, MRSA infection and the presence of biofilms [17] should be rule out as a probable cause. If no response is noted to the above mention measures the definitive treatment should be tube removal.

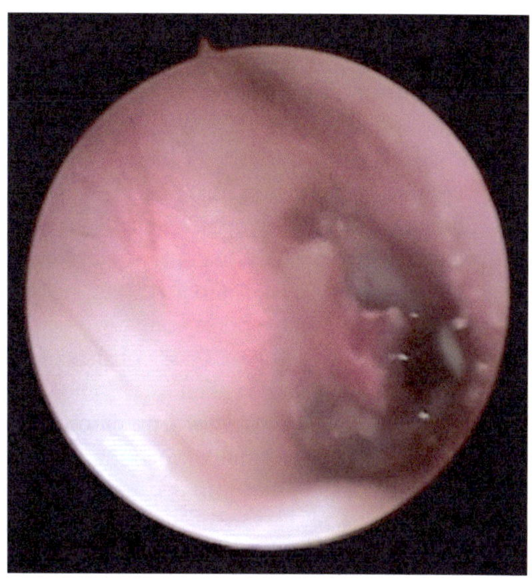

Fig. 1.6 Tympanostomy tube otorrhea. Pus coming out of the middle ear through the tympanostomy tube lumen

Of note children who presents with signs of severe infection (high fever, severe otalgia and toxic appearance), cellulitis of the pinna or adjacent skin, and concurrent bacterial infection (sinusitis, pharyngitis or pneumonia) can be treated with oral antibiotics with or without concurrent topical antibiotic therapy.

Gradenigo Syndrome

Gradenigo syndrome, or petrous apicitis presents as an intra-temporal complication of Acute Otitis Media. Although is rarely seen it is a life threatening condition that should be kept in mind.

Initially, the infection from middle ear cleft spreads through the air cells reaching the petrous apex of the temporal bone. The extradural inflammation and close proximity of the trigeminal ganglion and abducens nerve to the petrous apex are responsible for the cranial nerve deficits commonly encountered [18]. Since this condition is a complication of AOM the causative germs generally isolated are, *Streptococcus pneumoniae*, *Haemophilus influenzae*, and *Moraxella catarrhalis* nonetheless *Staphylococcus aureus* and *Pseudomonas aeruginosa* have also been implicated [19].

Clinically the classic triad of acute suppurative otitis media, deep facial pain in the distribution of the trigeminal nerve and sixth cranial nerve palsy is rarely seen completely, high variability in presentation is often seen, therefore a high index of suspicion is required for proper diagnosis. Imaging with CT scan is the first line investigation. Imaging usually shows soft tissue densities in the middle ear and mastoid with loss of cortical integrity of the petrous apex. The MRI usually shows evidence of dural enhancement and changes of intensity at the level of the petrous apex, allowing ruling out early intracranial complications.

The isolation of the causative organism is sometimes difficult. The initial treatment of petrous apicitis should include the use of broad-spectrum intravenous antibiotics as soon as possible, while further investigations are being completed. Topical otic antibiotics drops with steroid can be prescribed if there is a tympanic membrane perforation. Drops can also be prescribed if a myringotomy and tympanostomy tube has been placed for sampling and drainage of the middle ear. More aggressive approach consisting of mastoidectomy with petrous apex drainage can be considered in cases not responding to the conservative treatment.

Tuberculosis

Tuberculous otitis media (TOM) is a rare and infrequent cause of otorrhea in children. The importance to identify this entity as a cause is based in its potential for complications. *Mycobacterium tuberculosis* is the responsible microorganism in 95 % of the cases [20]. The infection can reach the middle ear by several pathways such as: hematogenous spread, inhalation with subsequent migration from the nasopharynx through the Eustachian tube to middle ear or by direct inoculation from the external ear canal. It is also important to take into account a history of traveling to endemic areas; positive contact with ill patients and immunosuppression.

The classic description of TOM consists of a triad of painless otorrhea, facial nerve palsy and hearing loss. Initially, it can be seen as chronic otorrhea that is not responding to the general treatment. Clinically the child will present with chronic otorrhea refractory to medical treatment. Cranial nerve deficits can be seen especially when the facial nerve is affected. The classic description of multiple tympanic membrane perforations is rarely noticed [21].

The diagnosis of TOM can be challenging and it is typically based on histological presence of granulomas and Langerhans giant cells with caseation necrosis, presence of acid fast bacilli on acid fast stain, growth of *Mycobacterium tuberculosis* in culture or if available positive PCR for

Mycobacterium tuberculosis. It should be noted that childhood tuberculosis (pulmonary and extrapulmonary) is a paucibacillary disease, with relatively lower culture yields than are seen in adults. Therefore, the diagnosis is often based upon a positive skin test, epidemiological risk factors and clinical presentation.

In general, TOM can be treated with the same regimens as used for pulmonary tuberculosis. A 6-month, 4-drug regimen consisting of isoniazid, rifampin, pyrazinamide, and ethambutol for the first 2 months and isoniazid and rifampin for the remaining 4 months is recommended for treatment of drug susceptible infection. In cases of multi-drug resistant infection, consultation with an expert in tuberculosis is recommended [22].

References

1. Flint PW, Haughey BH, Lund VJ, Niparko JK, Richardson MA, Robbins KT, Thomas JR, editors. Cummings otolaryngology—head and neck surgery. 5th ed. Philadelphia: Elsevier/Mosby; 2010.
2. Roland PS, Stroman DW. Microbiology of acute otitis externa. Laryngoscope. 2002;112(6):1166–77.
3. Osgusthorpe JD, Nielsen DR. Otitis externa: review and clinical update. Am Fam Physician. 2006;74(9):1510–6.
4. Rosenfeld RM, Singer M, Wasserman JM, Stinnett SS. Systematic review of topical antimicrobial therapy for acute otitis externa. Otolaryngol Head Neck Surg. 2006;134(4 Suppl):S24–48.
5. Rosenfeld RM, Schwartz SR, Cannon CR, Roland PS, Simon GR, Kumar KA, et al. Clinical practice guideline: acute otitis externa. Otolaryngol Head Neck Surg. 2014;150(1 Suppl):S1–24.
6. Ho T, Vrabec JT, Yoo D, Coker NJ. Otomycosis: clinical features and treatment implications. Otolaryngol Head Neck Surg. 2006;135(5):787–91.
7. Song JE, Haberkamp TJ, Patel R, Redleaf MI. Fungal otitis externa as a cause of tympanic membrane perforation: a case series. Ear Nose Throat J. 2014;93(8):332–6.
8. Franco-Vidal V, Blanchet H, Bebear C, Dutronc H, Darrouzet V. Necrotizing external otitis: a report of 46 cases. Otol Neurotol. 2007;28(6):771–3.
9. Persaud RA, Hajioff D, Thevasagayam MS, Wareing MJ, Wright A. Keratosis obturans and external ear canal cholesteatoma: how and why we should distinguish between these conditions. Clin Otolaryngol Allied Sci. 2004; 29(6):577–81.
10. Bluestone CD. Clinical course, complications and sequelae of acute otitis media. Pediatr Infect Dis J. 2000;19: S37–46.
11. Bluestone CD, Simons JP, Healy GB. Bluestone and Stool's pediatric otolaryngology, vol. 1. 5th ed. Shelton: People's Medical Publishing House; 2014. p. 761–847.
12. Lieberthal AS, Carroll AE, Chonmaitree T, et al. The diagnosis and management of acute otitis media. Pediatrics. 2013;131(3):964–99.
13. Foxlee R, Johansson A, Wejfal J, et al. Topical analgesia for acute otitis media. Cochrane Database Syst Rev. 2006;3, CD005657.
14. Madana J, Yolmo D, Kalaiarasi R, Gopalakrishnan S, Sujatha S. Microbiological profile with antibiotic sensitivity pattern of cholesteatomatous chronic suppurative otitis media among children. Int J Pediatr Otorhinolaryngol. 2011;75:1104–8.
15. Rosenfeld RM, Schartz SR, Pynnonen MA, Tunkel DE, et al. Clinical practice guideline: tympanostomy tubes in children. Otolaryngol Head Neck Surg. 2013;149(1 Suppl):S1–35.
16. van Dongen TMA, van der Heijden GJMG, Venekamp RP, Rovers MM, Schilder AGM. A trial of treatment for acute otorrhea in children with tympanostomy tubes. N Engl J Med. 2014;370:723–33.
17. Barakate M, Beckenham E, Curotta J, Da Cruz M. Bacterial biofilm, adherence to middle-ear ventilation tubes: scanning electron micrograph images and literature review. J Laryngol Otol. 2007;121:993–7.
18. Sherman SC, Buchana A. Gradenigo syndrome: a case report and review of a rare complication of otitis media. J Emerg Med. 2004;27(3):253–6.
19. Burston BJ, Pretorius P, Ramsden J. Gradenigo's syndrome: successful conservative treatment in adult and paediatric patients. J Laryngol Otol. 2005;119:325–9.
20. Nicolau Y, Northrop C, Eavey R. Tuberculosis otitis in infants: temporal bone histopathology and clinical extrapolation. Otol Neurotol. 2006;27:667–71.
21. Cho YS, Lee HS, Kim SW, et al. Tuberculous otitis media: a clinical and radiologic analysis of 52 patients. Laryngoscope. 2006;116:921–7.
22. Cruz AT, Starke JR. Treatment of tuberculosis in children. Expert Rev Anti Infect Ther. 2008;6(6):939–57.

Chapter 2
Infections of the External Ear

Mary F. Musso and Jonathan D. Crews

Abbreviations

AAO-HNSF	American Academy of Otolaryngology—Head and Neck Surgery Foundation
AOE	Acute otitis externa
EAC	External auditory canal
NOE	Necrotizing otitis externa
RHS	Ramsey-Hunt syndrome
RP	Relapsing polychondritis
VZV	Varicella-zoster virus

Anatomy of the External Ear

The components of the external ear include the auricle and the external auditory canal (EAC). Both contain elastic cartilage derived from mesoderm [1]. During gestation, the auricle is formed from six hillocks, derived from branchial arches I and II. As the mandible grows, the auricle ascends from the lateral commissure of the mouth to the temporal area [1]. Sebaceous glands and hair follicles line the subcutaneous layer of the auricle. Adipose tissue is mostly restricted to the lobule.

The EAC travels inward through the tympanic part of the temporal bone. The canal extends from the concha to the tympanic membrane and typically measures 2–3 cm in adults [2]. The anterior portion is approximately 6 mm longer than the posterior wall. Laterally to medially, the canal curves slightly superiorly and posteriorly, creating an S-shape. The outer third is cartilaginous, lined with

M.F. Musso, D.O.
Department of Pediatric Otolaryngology, Baylor College of Medicine, Houston, TX, USA

Texas Children's Hospital, 6701 Fannin Street, Suite 540, Houston, TX, USA
e-mail: mxmusso@texaschildrens.org

J.D. Crews, M.D., M.S. (✉)
Department of Pediatrics, Section of Infectious Diseases, Baylor College of Medicine, Children's Hospital of San Antonio, San Antonio, TX, USA
e-mail: crews@bcm.edu

T.A. Valdez, J.G. Vallejo (eds.), *Infectious Diseases in Pediatric Otolaryngology*,
DOI 10.1007/978-3-319-21744-4_2

skin, and the remaining inner two-thirds are osseous [2]. The isthmus, the narrowest part of the canal, connects the cartilaginous and bony segments. The skin lining the EAC consists of keratinizing stratified squamous epithelium. Sensory innervation of the EAC includes contributions from cranial nerves V, VII, IX, and X. This extensive sensory innervation is partly responsible for the otalgia clinically noted with otitis externa.

The external ear has multiple mechanisms to prevent infection. The tragus and antitragus, the cerumen coating the skin, and the isthmus of the canal all serve to protect the EAC [3]. The skin lining the cartilaginous canal contains hair cells, ceruminous glands, and sebaceous glands—these adnexal structures contribute to the pilosebaceous unit and provide an initial barrier against pathogens. The mildly acidic (pH 6.0–6.5) cerumen is formed by glandular secretions and sloughed epithelium. In general, cerumen migrates past the isthmus, laterally along the canal, and extrudes into the auricle, helping to keep the canal free of debris [1]. It serves as one of the primary barriers to infection of the canal and is composed of hydrophobic lipids, creating a waterproof layer on the canal. Its acidic nature discourages fungal and bacterial growth. Excessive cleaning or instrumentation of the canal can alter its primary protective barrier and subsequently lead to infection.

Infections within the EAC can spread to adjacent structures. The floor of the cartilaginous canal contains slits, known as the fissures of Santorini, which permit the spread of infection or neoplasms from the EAC to the parotid gland and surrounding tissues. Hematogenous extension to the mastoid segment of the temporal bone is facilitated by vessels that penetrate the tympanomastoid suture. Infections can also spread through lymphatic drainage from the canal. Anteriorly and superiorly, the canal drains to the preauricular lymphatics in the parotid gland and the superior deep cervical nodes. The inferior portion of the canal drains into the infra-auricular nodes and posteriorly, lymphatic drainage moves into the postauricular nodes and the superior deep cervical nodes [1].

Acute Otitis Externa

Acute otitis externa (AOE), commonly referred to as "swimmer's ear", is the most common infection of the external ear. It is an inflammatory condition of the EAC, typically caused by a bacterial pathogen, resulting in pain and variable degrees of swelling.

Otitis externa results in an estimated 2.4 million yearly US healthcare visits (8.1 visits per 1000 persons), costing $489 million in direct healthcare costs [4]. A seasonal peak occurs during the summer months due to elevated ambient humidity and increased participation in recreational water activities. The incidence of otitis externa is highest in children. For example, from 2003 to 2007, rates of US ambulatory visits for otitis externa were highest among children 5–9 years (18.6 visits per 1000 persons) and 10–14 years (15.8 visits per 1000 persons), compared to children 0–4 years (6.9 visits per 1000 persons) and 15–19 years (8.8 visits per 1000 persons) [4].

Pathogenesis

Disruption of the natural protective mechanisms of the external ear is necessary for the development of AOE. Cerumen, a hydrophobic substance composed of glandular secretions and sloughed squamous epithelium, supports a dry environment in the EAC. Additionally, the acidic nature of cerumen inhibits bacterial and fungal growth [5]. When water contaminates the ear canal, the excessive moisture promotes skin maceration, alters the local microbial flora, increases local pH, and changes the quality and quantity of cerumen [6]. Localized trauma, whether from aggressive cleaning or scratching, can injure the skin of the canal and thereby provide an entry point for pathogens.

The role of recreational swimming in the development of AOE is widely recognized. Outbreaks of AOE have been reported following exposure to swimming pools, hot tubs, and natural bodies of water [7, 8].

Poor water quality, as evidenced by inadequate chlorination and high counts of *Pseudomonas aeruginosa*, has been implicated in some, though not all, outbreaks associated with swimming pools [7]. Among swimmers in natural waters, factors associated with the development of ear disease include warmer ambient temperature, prolonged swimming, and head immersion [8, 9].

Various medical conditions increase the risk of developing AOE, including dermatologic conditions (atopic dermatitis, allergic dermatitis, psoriasis), diabetes mellitus, congenital or acquired immunodeficiency, or a history of radiation therapy. Additionally, devices that occlude the external canal (i.e. hearing aids, earphones) can predispose an individual to AOE.

Microbiology

The bacterial flora of the EAC is predominantly composed of gram-positive organisms. Coagulase-negative *Staphylococcus* (especially *Staphylococcus epidermidis* and *Staphylococcus auricularis*) and coryneform bacteria (diphtheroids) are the most frequent colonizing organisms of the ear canal in healthy individuals. Gram-negative organisms are less prevalent, isolated from <5 % of EAC specimens [10]. Following prolonged water exposure, however, the flora of the EAC changes, becoming dominated by gram-negative organisms [6].

Pseudomonas aeruginosa is the most frequent pathogen in AOE, identified in 22–62 % of cases in series on AOE (Table 2.1) [11–14]. *Staphylococcus aureus* (11–34 % of cases) is the most important gram-positive pathogen [11–14]. Various *Enterobacteriaceae* (*Escherichia coli*, *Klebsiella* species, *Enterobacter* species, and *Proteus mirabilis*) and non-fermentative gram-negative bacteria (*Acinetobacter* species and *Stenotrophomonas maltophilia*) have also been recovered from individuals with AOE, but at a much lower incidence [11, 12, 15]. The majority of patients have a single organism isolated on culture, with polymicrobial infections occurring in only one-third of patients [16]. Coagulase-negative *Staphylococcus* and diphtheroids, while frequently isolated from cultures of the ear canal, are normal constituents of the external ear and should be regarded as commensals. Anaerobes are rarely identified in uncomplicated AOE [12].

Diagnosis

Acute otitis externa is a clinical diagnosis consisting of the rapid onset of signs and symptoms of ear canal inflammation [17]. Otalgia is the most common symptom. Patients can experience itching or fullness within the ear canal, hearing loss, or pain with chewing. The characteristic finding of

Table 2.1 Microbiology of acute otitis externa

	Dibb WL, 1991 [11]	Clark WB, 1997 [12]	Jones, RN 1997 [13]	Drehobl M, 2008 [14]
Number of patients	226	23	433	627
Gram-positive organisms				
Staphylococcus aureus	34.1 %	30.4 %	11.8 %	10.8 %
Gram-negative organisms				
Pseudomonas aeruginosa	22.1 %	60.9 %	48.7 %	62.2 %
Proteus mirabilis	3.5 %	8.7 %	5.3 %	–
Enterobacter species	4.0 %	4.3 %	3.7 %	4.0 %
Klebsiella species	5.3 %	–	2.5 %	4.9 %
Escherichia coli	4.9 %	–	–	2.1 %

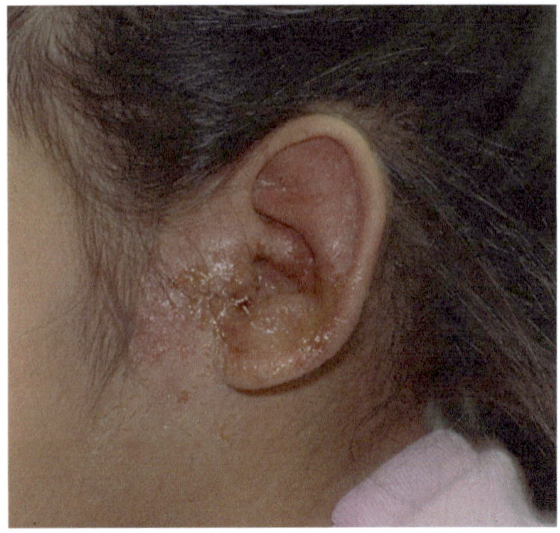

Fig. 2.1 Acute otitis externa. A severe case of acute otitis externa. There is profuse otorrhea with soft tissue swelling that extends beyond the canal, involving the pinna and the preauricular space (courtesy of Dr. Ellen Friedman)

exquisite tenderness with manipulation of the tragus or pinna is frequently observed in patients with diffuse canal swelling. On examination, one finds erythema and swelling of the EAC, often with purulent debris (Fig. 2.1). With severe disease, cellulitis of the pinna and regional lymphadenopathy can be present. Otoscopy with visualization of the tympanic membrane, while often difficult due to EAC swelling, should be performed in all patients as a nonintact tympanic membrane influences management decisions.

Clinicians should be careful to differentiate AOE from other conditions that cause otalgia and otorrhea. Otitis media with perforation, frequently confused with AOE, will present with a middle ear effusion and less severe tenderness with tragus pressure. Fungal otitis externa ("otomycosis") and chronic otitis media will have a more protracted duration of symptoms. When dermatologic conditions involve the ear canal, patients experience prolonged ear pain and less otorrhea than with AOE. Causes of ear pain unrelated to ear pathology include temporomandibular joint (TMJ) syndrome, tonsillitis or peritonsillar infections, and dental disorders.

Cultures of the ear canal are not necessary to diagnose AOE. For routine, uncomplicated AOE, cultures are unlikely to impact management decisions. However, for patients with severe disease or who have an inadequate response to treatment, cultures should be obtained.

Treatment

The management of uncomplicated AOE consists of topical antibiotics and pain control. In 2014, the American Academy of Otolaryngology—Head and Neck Surgery Foundation (AAO-HNSF) updated their evidence-based recommendations on the management of AOE [17].

Topical antibiotics are the cornerstone of treatment for uncomplicated AOE. Topical therapy allows for high concentrations of antimicrobials to be delivered to the site of infection while minimizing the risk of side effects [18]. In contrast, systemic antibiotics can promote selective pressure for resistant organisms, carry a greater risk of side effects, and achieve lower local drug concentrations [19]. The efficacy of topical therapy for AOE has been demonstrated in numerous randomized controlled trials [20–24]. Clinical cure rates up to 80 % can be achieved within 10 days of therapy with topical antibiotics [20]. Various preparations are approved for AOE, including antiseptics and antibiotics, with or without a corticosteroid (Table 2.2).

Table 2.2 Ototopical preparations for the treatment of acute otitis externa

Drug	Name	Bottle size (mL)	Cost	
			Trade	Generic
Acetic acid 2.0 % solution	Acetic acid otic (generic)	15.0	–	$
Acetic acid 2.0 %, hydrocortisone 1.0 %	Acetasol HC (generic)	10.0	–	$
Neomycin, polymyxin B, hydrocortisone	Cortisporin otic (trade)	10.0	$$	$
Ofloxacin 0.3 %	Floxin otic (trade)	5.0	$$	$
Ciprofloxacin 0.2 %, hydrocortisone 1.0 %	Cipro HC (trade)	10.0	$$$	–
Ciprofloxacin 0.3 %, dexamethasone 0.1 %	Ciprodex (trade)	7.5	$$$	–

Source: Modified from Otolaryngol Head Neck Surgery, Vol. 150(1 Suppl), Rosenfeld RM, Schwartz SR, Cannon CR, Roland PS, Simon GR, Kumar KA, et al., Clinical Practice Guideline: Acute Otitis Externa, pages S1–S24, Copyright (2014) with permission from American Academy of Otolaryngology—Head and Neck Surgery Foundation, Inc.

Antiseptic agents are used predominantly for the treatment of mild-moderate AOE or for the prevention of AOE in at-risk persons (i.e. swimmers). Acetic acid and alcohol are the most commonly utilized antiseptic agents, although other agents (boric acid, aluminum acetate, and silver nitrate) have also been used [17]. These agents work through various mechanisms, including acidifying the local environment, to make the ear canal less tolerable for bacteria. Due to their acidic nature, some patients experience pain and local irritation with administration [25]. While effective in most cases of AOE, a randomized controlled trial found acetic acid alone had a lower cure rate than either an acetic acid-steroid combination or an antibiotic-steroid combination at 2 and 3 week follow-up [22].

Topical antibiotics are the most commonly prescribed agents for AOE, and the most frequently prescribed antibiotic preparation is a combination of neomycin and polymyxin B with hydrocortisone [26, 27]. It is an inexpensive and effective preparation that has been available for over three decades. Polymyxin B is active against *P. aeruginosa* and other gram-negative organisms, while neomycin, an aminoglycoside, provides activity against *S. aureus*. Aminoglycoside ophthalmic preparations—tobramycin 0.3 % solution, tobramycin 0.3 % and dexamethasone 0.1 % suspension, and gentamicin 0.3 % solution—have also been used for the treatment of AOE. While not FDA-approved for this indication, several small trials have found that clinical cure rates for these agents are similar to other topical antibiotic preparations [23]. Several limitations, however, exist for preparations containing aminoglycosides—the dosing schedule, the risk of contact dermatitis, and the risk of ototoxicity in patients with nonintact tympanic membranes.

The fluoroquinolones ofloxacin and ciprofloxacin, were developed into topical formulations for ear infections in the late 1990s [25]. They have broad antimicrobial activity, including both gram-positive and gram-negative bacteria, and benefit from a convenient dosing regimen, an excellent safety profile, and the ability to be used in patients with nonintact tympanic membranes. Several studies have demonstrated that quinolone agents perform as well, or better, than non-quinolone preparations [20].

The clinical cure rates are similar between the various classes of ototopical agents used for AOE, according to a systematic review of randomized control trials [20]. In a multicenter, randomized clinical trial composed of 1072 adult and pediatric patients, ciprofloxacin-dexamethasone and neomycin-polymyxin B-hydrocortisone given for 7 days had similar cure rates after 3 days (14 % vs. 10 %), 8 days (75 % vs. 72 %), and 18 days (98 % vs. 97 %). The only significant difference was found in the time to cure, which was 0.6 days shorter for the ciprofloxacin-dexamethasone suspension [24].

Before selecting a topical agent for AOE, clinicians should determine whether the patient has a nonintact tympanic membrane due to tympanic membrane perforation or tympanostomy tube placement. In such patients, clinicians should avoid prescribing potential ototoxic topical agents. Animal models have demonstrated that application of ototoxic agents into the middle ear can damage the hair cells of the inner ear [28]. Products to avoid in patients with nonintact tympanic membranes include preparations with a low pH (most antiseptic agents), alcohol, or aminoglycosides [17]. Despite the concern for ototoxic injury, the risk from topical aminoglycosides in humans appears to be low.

A review of 500 children who received an aminoglycoside containing preparation following tympanostomy tube placement revealed no cases of cochlear toxicity [29]. In a 2004 systematic review of the published literature, only 54 cases of inner ear toxicity attributed to gentamicin and 13 cases attributed to neomycin were identified [30]. Although the risk for ototoxicity may be low, given the availability of a safe and effective alternative, we recommend the use of a quinolone agent for all patients with AOE with a nonintact tympanic membrane.

Additional considerations when selecting a topical agent for AOE include the cost, dosing schedule, and side effects. The twice-daily dosing schedule for the quinolone agents is convenient and likely results in the greatest degree of adherence to therapy. In a single open-label trial, once-daily dosing of ofloxacin achieved good clinical outcomes [31]. In contrast, the neomycin-polymyxin B-hydrocortisone preparation generally requires that drops are administered four times daily. The risk of contact dermatitis appears to be greatest from the aminoglycoside-containing topical preparations, particularly neomycin [32]. While rare following a single course of treatment, these localized reactions can develop in patients when there is prolonged use.

Clinicians should promote the effective administration of ototopical medications through patient education and, if necessary, adjunctive drug delivery methods. Aural toilet or otologic debridement should be considered in patients with severe otorrhea or EAC swelling. The AAO-HNSF guidelines recommend that another person (i.e. the child's parent or caregiver) administer drops with the patient lying down and the affected ear facing up. After instilling the drops in the ear canal, the patient should remain in this position for 3–5 min [17]. Debris in the EAC or severe swelling can interfere with the effective delivery of medication to the site of infection. For such patients, clinicians should consider performing aural toilet, otologic debridement, or inserting an ear wick. Additionally, as ear pain from AOE can be intense, the degree of pain should be assessed and a pain control strategy developed. Benzocaine-containing otic solutions are topical anesthetics that can provide pain temporary relief. These products, however, are currently not approved by the US Food and Drug Administration and may not be safe if used with a nonintact tympanic membrane. We recommend orally administered analgesics (i.e. acetaminophen, ibuprofen) for children with otalgia from otitis externa.

Systemic antibiotics, when combined with topical therapy, provide no additional benefit for uncomplicated AOE [17, 22]. However, systemic antibiotics should be considered for immunocompromised patients or those with severe disease extending beyond the pinna. Empiric antibiotic therapy should cover *P. aeruginosa* and *S. aureus*, while definitive therapy should be directed by culture results.

Prevention

Preventive measures should be considered for individuals with recurrent episodes of AOE, especially swimmers and individuals with predisposing dermatologic conditions. No randomized controlled trials have been performed to identify the most effective strategies. Potential preventive measures include wearing ear plugs, blow drying the ear following water exposure (using a low setting and keeping the hair dryer >12 in. from the ear), and using an antiseptic agent before and after water exposure to re-acidify the ear canal.

Necrotizing (Malignant) Otitis Externa

Necrotizing otitis externa (NOE), also called malignant otitis externa, is a rare and severe invasive infection of the external auditory canal that involves the periauricular soft tissue and skull base. This disorder, which typically affects elderly individuals with diabetes mellitus, has also been reported in immunocompromised children, including children with HIV, malignancy, malnutrition, chemotherapy-induced

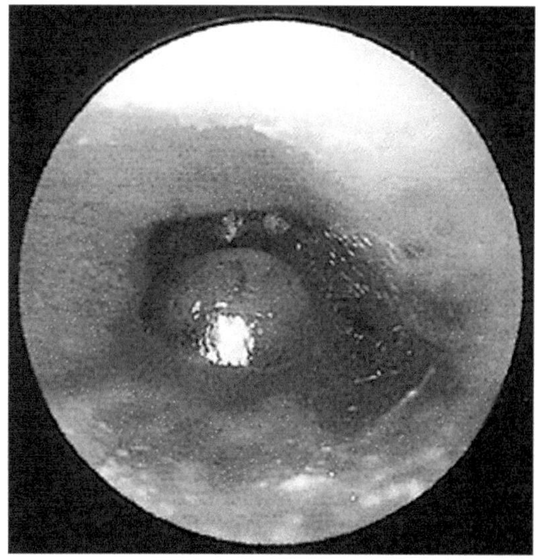

Fig. 2.2 Necrotizing otitis externa. Granulation tissue at the bony-cartilage junction (Reprinted with permission from [54]. Copyright Elsevier 2010)

neutropenia, aplastic anemia, and diabetes mellitus [33]. *Pseudomonas aeruginosa* is identified in >90 % of all cases of NOE in both adult and pediatric case series [33, 34]. Additional bacteria reported to cause NOE include *S. aureus*, *Klebsiella* species, and *P. mirabilis*. Rarely, fungal NOE has been reported, most often due to *Aspergillus fumigatus* [34].

Individuals present with exquisite otalgia and otorrhea, generally more severe than that found in uncomplicated otitis externa. While adult patients generally present with prolonged and progressive ear pain and otorrhea unresponsive to topical therapy, children tend to present more acutely. On examination, there is swelling of the pinna and periauricular soft tissue. Granulation tissue is frequently noted along the inferior portion of the EAC at the bony-cartilage junction (Fig. 2.2). Osteomyelitis of the skull base and cranial neuropathies develop with progression of the infection. Facial nerve palsy, which occurs at a higher rate in children than adults due to the proximity of the facial nerve to the ear canal, typically occurs early in the course of disease [33]. Additional complications, while rare, include meningitis, brain abscesses, and dural sinus thrombosis.

Necrotizing otitis externa is a diagnosis based on clinical, laboratory, and radiographic findings. Laboratory findings reveal an elevated erythrocyte sedimentation rate or C-reactive protein. While non-specific, markedly elevated levels of these inflammatory markers may suggest invasive disease. Controversy exists regarding the optimal imaging modality for the diagnosis and follow-up of NOE [34]. Historically, radionuclide (technetium-99 or gallium-67) scans, with or without single photon emission computerized tomography (SPECT) scanning, were preferred to detect and monitor disease from NOE [34]. Recent literature, however, has shown that magnetic resonance imaging (MRI), which can identify soft tissue changes and intracranial complications, is effective in following the course of disease in patients with NOE [35]. In comparison to radionuclide scans, MRI is more readily accessible and avoids exposure to radiation, a particularly important point in the pediatric population. Computed tomography (CT) imaging is able to detect early bone erosion; thus it may be the preferred technique to distinguish NOE from cases of uncomplicated, yet severe, external otitis.

Treatment for necrotizing otitis externa consists of prolonged systemic antibiotic therapy. The empiric antibiotic regimen should have activity against *P. aeruginosa*, with definitive therapy directed by culture results. Antipseudomonal beta-lactam agents (piperacillin-tazobactam, ticarcillin-clavulanate, ceftazidime, cefepime), fluoroquinolones, and carbapenems are agents with activity against *P. aeruginosa* that effectively penetrate bone tissue. The fluoroquinolones are frequently used for NOE in adults due to their safe side effect profile, excellent bone penetration, and availability in an oral formulation [34]. While fluoroquinolones are generally avoided in children due to the risk of injury to developing bones or joints, their use in NOE is justified when effective alternative agents are not available [36]. Prolonged antibiotic therapy for 6–8 weeks is generally recommended. Surgical intervention is limited to debridement of granulation tissue or to obtain biopsies for microbiologic and histologic specimens when there is diagnostic uncertainty. We recommend combination therapy (an antipseudomonal cephalosporin or a fluoroquinolone, plus an aminoglycoside) for initial gram-negative coverage to increase the likelihood of susceptibility in the event there is a drug-resistant organism. Following culture and susceptibility results, definitive therapy can be completed with a single agent (an antipseudomonal cephalosporin or fluoroquinolone) for a minimum of 6 weeks.

Fungal Otitis Externa (Otomycosis)

Otomycosis, also referred to as fungal otitis externa, is a fungal infection of the external ear canal. It is often superimposed on a chronic bacterial infection of the external canal or middle ear. The growth of fungi can be promoted with moisture, warmth, and darkness, features found in the external auditory canal [3]. *Aspergillus* species are the most common cause of otomycosis, particularly *A. niger. Aspergillus fumigatus* and *A. flavus* are associated with more invasive disease. Additional fungi reported to cause otomycosis include *Candida*, *Actinomyces*, and Zygomycetes; and less commonly *Fusarium*, *Scedosporium*, *Hendersonula*, *Rhodotorula*, and *Cryptococcus* [3, 37].

Predisposing factors for otomycosis include humid climate, cerumen impaction, ear instrumentation, immunodeficiencies, and use of ototopical antibiotics or broad-spectrum systemic antibiotics [38, 39]. Additional factors that can place patients at risk for otomycosis include: pregnancy, use of systemic steroids, presence of open mastoid cavities, hearing aids with occlusive molds, trauma, and bacterial infections [39]. Otomycosis should be considered in cases of otitis externa that have been refractory to antibacterial medications.

The symptoms commonly present at the time of diagnosis include pruritus, ear pain, aural fullness, persistent discharge, and increasing hearing loss [37]. The diagnosis is often made with otoscopy. Otologic examination shows one or more of the following signs: persistent white or colorless otorrhea, tympanic membrane perforation, edema, erythema of EAC and tympanic membrane, and whitish, cotton-like or greasy debris in the external auditory canal (Fig. 2.3) [37]. Microscopic exam

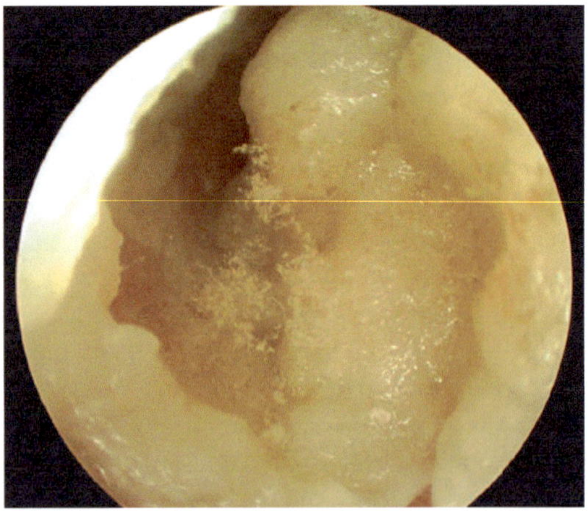

Fig. 2.3 Fungal otitis externa. Fungal filaments noted in the external ear canal (Reprinted from [55], with kind permission from Springer Science and Business Media)

facilitates visualization of the fungal elements. *Aspergillus niger* characteristically has black-headed conidiophores atop white filamentous hyphae, *A. fumigatus* has a pale blue-green appearance, and *Candida* is associated with a cream-colored discharge [40]. A fungal culture may be obtained to confirm the causative organism.

Treatment involves removing fungal debris under microscopy and drying the ear to discourage further fungal or bacterial growth. Topical acidifying solutions help inhibit bacterial and fungal growth. Acidifying agents commonly used for uncomplicated otomycosis include aluminum acetate otic drops (Burrow's solution), acetic acid (Domeboro), propylene glycol and acetic acid solution (VoSol), hydrocortisone 1 % propylene glycol acetic acid (VoSol HC), and boric acid solution. Alternative treatments include topical antifungals such as clotrimazole cream or solution (Lotrimin, Mycelex), ketoconazole, tolnaftate (Tinactin), nystatin, and ciclopirox olamine 0.77 %. When choosing a treatment modality it is important to determine if the tympanic membrane is intact. Antifungals can be ototoxic and clotrimazole, as well as the acidifying solutions, are painful when they enter the middle ear. A drying powder, such as boric acid or mycostatin, is a better option for non-intact tympanic membranes.

Multiple factors lead to recalcitrant infections. Effective management includes eliminating the factors precipitating the infection. For patients with generalized skin diseases, such as psoriasis or atopic dermatitis, fungal otitis externa can occur secondary to chronic treatment with topical steroids. These patients frequently complain of itching, have seborrheic dermatitis-like skin lesions, and have fungal elements that can be visualized in the epidermis [37]. A ventilation tube can act as a nidus for infection and should be removed in such cases. Patients with previous canal wall mastoid surgery requiring closed hearing aids tend to accumulate moisture. Ointments are not recommended in these patients. Chronic use of ototopical antibacterial and antifungal agents can perpetuate the problem by providing moisture for fungal growth. An acidifying or compounded powder is recommended in such cases. Compounded powders include Chloromycetin-sulfanilamide-Fungizone and Chloromycetin-sulfanilamide-Tinactin. Antiseptic agents including metacresylacetate (Cresylate), gentian violet, merbromin (Mercurochrome) and silver nitrate gel 1 % can also be tried for recalcitrant infections. Gentian violet is well tolerated in patients with mastoid cavities however it permanently stains skin and clothing, requiring careful application. Cresylate is a middle ear irritant and meticulous application is also advised.

Herpes Zoster Oticus

Herpes zoster oticus is a cutaneous disorder where herpetic lesions involve the external ear canal or pinna (Fig. 2.4). When accompanied by a peripheral facial palsy, it is called Ramsay-Hunt syndrome (RHS). Herpes zoster oticus and RHS are caused by reactivation of latent varicella-zoster virus (VZV) in the genticulate ganglion of the facial nerve. Both disorders can occur following a primary VZV infection (chickenpox) or immunization.

Conditions causing peripheral facial palsy in children include congenital anomalies, trauma, malignancy, otitis media, and various viruses (Epstein-Barr virus, cytomegalovirus, human herpes viruses 6 and 7, and measles) [41]. RHS causes approximately 16 % of peripheral facial palsies in children [42]. Its diagnosis is based on the history and physical exam findings. The clinical features of RHS in children are less severe than adults, with children experiencing less severe vestibulocochlear dysfunction (hearing loss, tinnitus, or vertigo) and often not developing the pathognomonic herpetic lesions until after the onset of facial palsy [42]. Occasionally, skin lesions will not appear in RHS despite VZV causing the facial palsy (*zoster sine herpete*).

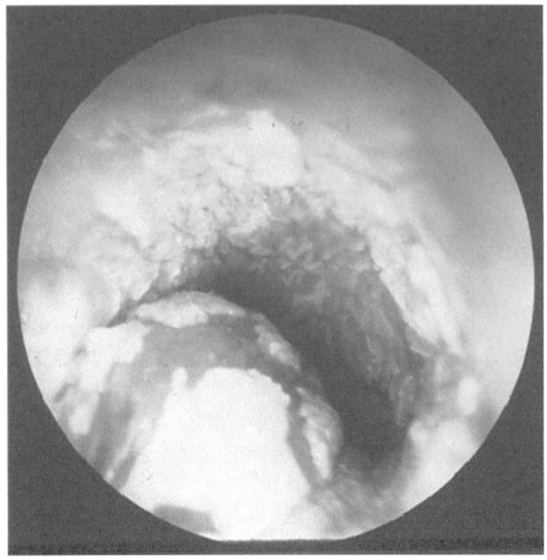

Fig. 2.4 Herpes zoster oticus. Multiple vesicles noted in the external auditory canal. (Reprinted with permission from [3]. Copyright Elsevier 2013)

The prognosis of herpes zoster oticus in children is excellent. Post-herpetic neuralgia is a rare complication. Children with RHS have a better recovery of facial nerve function than adults, with up to 79 % of children achieving full recovery [42].

Treatment for herpes zoster oticus typically consists of antiviral therapy. Both acyclovir and valacyclovir have activity against VZV and are well-tolerated by children. For children with Ramsay-Hunt syndrome, we recommend early initiation of a corticosteroid (prednisone 2 mg/kg/day divided in 2 doses—up to 80 mg per day) and acyclovir (80 mg/kg/day divided in 3 doses) for 1 week, to expedite recovery of facial nerve function. Eye care is important for patients with facial nerve palsy and ophthalmologic consultation should be obtained for patients with herpetic lesions involving the eye. For herpes zoster oticus, we recommend a 1 week course of acyclovir.

Furunculosis

A furuncle is a deep infection of the hair follicle in the cartilaginous portion of the EAC potentially progressing into an abscess with cellulitis. Furuncles appear as red, swollen, tender nodules and can have an overlying pustule (Fig. 2.5). When several hair follicles are infected the furuncles may merge to form a larger nodule, known as a carbuncle. The most common site of a furuncle involving the ear is at the junction of the concha and canal skin [1]. The most common infectious agent is *Staphylococcus aureus*. Cases of recurrent furunculosis are increasing in correlation to increased incidence of community-associated methicillin-resistant *S. aureus* [43].

Treatment includes drainage of infected material. For less complex lesions, spontaneous drainage can be encouraged with warm soaks. If this fails incision and drainage under local anesthesia is necessary to clear the canal obstruction. Empiric topical and oral antibiotics should cover *S. aureus*. Methicillin-resistant *S. aureus* ought to be considered for recurrent cases. Definitive therapy should be directed by culture results.

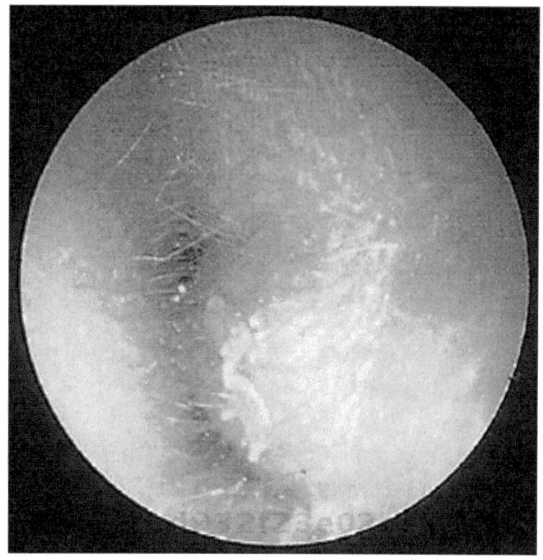

Fig. 2.5 Furunculosis. Localized swelling from a furuncle at the entrance of the ear canal. (Reprinted with permission from [54]. Copyright Elsevier 2010)

Differential Diagnosis of Non-infectious Conditions of the External Ear

Several noninfectious conditions present with ear pain, pruritus, and otorrhea mimicking otitis externa. These entities, which should be considered in the differential diagnosis of inflammatory conditions of the external ear, include relapsing polychondritis and dermatologic conditions.

Relapsing Polychondritis

Relapsing polychondritis (RP) is a rare disorder with characteristic episodic inflammation of cartilaginous structures. Cartilage of the ear, eustachian tubes, nose, trachea, larynx, ribs and joints may be affected. Recurrent episodes can lead to atrophy, scarring, and distortion of the involved cartilage. Otologic manifestations of RP are common and can involve the external, middle, and inner ear [44]. The most frequent presenting symptom is auricular chondritis [45].

Hearing loss, which can be either conductive or sensorineural, can occur in as many as 46 % of patients with RP, with vestibular dysfunction occurring in up to 6 % [44]. Closure of the EAC, serous otitis media and eustachian tube obstruction may lead to hearing impairment. Inflammation of the middle ear and vestibular structures and/or vasculitis of the internal auditory artery may cause sensorineural hearing loss and vestibular dysfunction with associated dizziness, ataxia, nausea, and vomiting [46]. A third of patients with RP have associated eustachian tube dysfunction [44]. Findings on examination include an erythematous or violaceous, tender, and edematous pinna. The noncartilaginous lobe is spared, distinguishing it from otitis externa.

The diagnosis is clinical. Patients frequently exhibit joint pain [45]. More than 30 % of patients with RP have a coexisting autoimmune, rheumatologic, or hematologic disorder [46]. Laboratory findings include anemia and an elevated erythrocyte sedimentation rate. Other laboratory markers that are nonspecific for RP but may help with categorizing the disease include anti-neutrophil cytoplasmic antibodies (ANCA), antinuclear antibodies, and rheumatoid factor [46].

Treatment of RP is focused on controlling symptoms. Mild cases of chondritis can be managed with non-steroidal anti-inflammatory drugs. The cornerstone of treatment is administration of systemic corticosteroids. A response of symptoms to corticosteroids is suggestive of a diagnosis of RP [45]. Patients unresponsive to steroids or intolerant of steroids can be treated with dapsone or immunosuppressive medications such as azathioprine, cyclophosphamide and methotrexate.

Dermatologic Conditions

Allergic and irritant contact dermatoses can mimic otitis externa. Allergic contact dermatitis is a delayed hypersensitivity reaction resulting from antigens such as poison ivy, metals, chemicals, rubber, and drugs. Nickel is the most common contact allergen. Nickel sensitivity can occur with earrings, causing inflammation at the site of the ear piercing that starts at the lobule and spreads toward the antihelix. Patients using hearing aids can develop a contact allergy to components of and chemicals used in the manufacture of hearing aid molds. Methyl methacrylate is the most common sensitizer [47]. The chronic use of ototopical agents used to treat otitis externa can cause a delayed hypersensitivity reaction. Numerous studies have shown neomycin as the leading topical medication causing sensitization [48–50]. Smith and colleagues concluded that benzalkonium chloride, a common preservative used in topical preparations to treat otitis externa, can also produce allergic reactions [51].

On physical exam, affected skin appears erythematous and weeping; at times vesicles are present. Scratching the overlying skin may lead to a secondary infection. Effective treatment begins with removing the causative agent. Patch skin testing is the gold standard to identify the agent causing allergic contact dermatitis [52]. Topical steroids and astringents help treat the surrounding skin, while systemic steroids should be considered only for severe reactions. Antibiotics may be used for secondary infections. When prescribing medications to patients with a history of allergic reactions, it should be kept in mind that ointment preparations tend to have fewer preservatives than creams and otic drops [53].

References

1. Linstrom C, Lucente F. Diseases of the external ear. In: Johnson JT, Rosen CA, editors. Bailey's head and neck surgery otolaryngology. Philadelphia: Lippincott Williams & Wilkins; 2014. p. 2333–57.
2. Moore KL, Dalley AF. Clinically oriented anatomy. 4th ed. Philadelphia: Lippincott Williams & Wilkins; 1999. p. 962.
3. Friedman E, Carrillo-Marquez M. Otitis externa. In: Cherry JD, Demmler-Harrison GJ, editors. Feigin and Cherry's textbook of pediatric infectious diseases. 7th ed. Philadelphia: Elsevier; 2014. p. 203–9.
4. Centers for Disease Control and Prevention (CDC). Estimated burden of acute otitis externa—United States, 2003–2007. MMWR Morb Mortal Wkly Rep. 2011;60(19):605–9.
5. Chai TJ, Chai TC. Bactericidal activity of cerumen. Antimicrob Agents Chemother. 1980;18(4):638–41.
6. Wright DN, Alexander JM. Effect of water on the bacterial flora of swimmers' ears. Arch Otolaryngol. 1974;99(1):15–8.
7. Reid TM, Porter IA. An outbreak of otitis externa in competitive swimmers due to *Pseudomonas aeruginosa*. J Hyg (Lond). 1981;86(3):357–62.
8. Van Asperen IA, de Rover CM, Schijven JF, Oetomo SB, Schellekens JF, van Leeuwen NJ, et al. Risk of otitis externa after swimming in recreational fresh water lakes containing *Pseudomonas aeruginosa*. BMJ. 1995;311(7017):1407–10.
9. Wade TJ, Sams EA, Beach MJ, Collier SA, Dufour AP. The incidence and health burden of earaches attributable to recreational swimming in natural waters: a prospective cohort study. Environ Health. 2013;12:67.
10. Stroman DW, Roland PS, Dohar J, Burt W. Microbiology of normal external auditory canal. Laryngoscope. 2001;111(11 Pt 1):2054–9.
11. Dibb WL. Microbial aetiology of otitis externa. J Infect. 1991;22(3):233–9.

12. Clark WB, Brook I, Bianki D, Thompson DH. Microbiology of otitis externa. Otolaryngol Head Neck Surg. 1997;116(1):23–5.
13. Jones RN, Milazzo J, Seidlin M. Ofloxacin otic solution for treatment of otitis externa in children and adults. Arch Otolaryngol Head Neck Surg. 1997;123(11):1193–200.
14. Drehobl M, Guerrero JL, Lacarte PR, Goldstein G, Mata FS, Luber S. Comparison of efficacy and safety of ciprofloxacin otic solution 0.2% versus polymyxin B-neomycin-hydrocortisone in the treatment of acute diffuse otitis externa. Curr Med Res Opin. 2008;24(12):3531–42.
15. Roland PS, Stroman DW. Microbiology of acute otitis externa. Laryngoscope. 2002;112(7 Pt 1):1166–77.
16. Brook I, Frazier EH, Thompson DH. Aerobic and anaerobic microbiology of external otitis. Clin Infect Dis. 1992;15(6):955–8.
17. Rosenfeld RM, Schwartz SR, Cannon CR, Roland PS, Simon GR, Kumar KA, et al. Clinical practice guideline: acute otitis externa. Otolaryngol Head Neck Surg. 2014;150(1 Suppl):S1–24.
18. Ohyama M, Furuta S, Ueno K, Katsuda K, Nobori T, Kiyota R, et al. Ofloxacin otic solution in patients with otitis media: an analysis of drug concentrations. Arch Otolaryngol Head Neck Surg. 1999;125(3):337–40.
19. Weber PC, Roland PS, Hannley M, Friedman R, Manolidis S, Matz G, et al. The development of antibiotic resistant organisms with the use of ototopical medications. Otolaryngol Head Neck Surg. 2004;130(3 Suppl):S89–94.
20. Rosenfeld RM, Singer M, Wasserman JM, Stinnett SS. Systematic review of topical antimicrobial therapy for acute otitis externa. Otolaryngol Head Neck Surg. 2006;134(4 Suppl):S24–48.
21. Van Balen FA, Smit WM, Zuithoff NP, Verheij TJ. Clinical efficacy of three common treatments in acute otitis externa in primary care: randomized controlled trial. BMJ. 2003;327(7425):1201–5.
22. Roland PS, Belcher BP, Bettis R, Makabale RL, Conroy PJ, Wall GM, et al. A single topical agent is clinically equivalent to the combination of topical and oral antibiotic treatment for otitis externa. Am J Otolaryngol. 2008;29(4):255–61.
23. Sabater F, Maristany M, Mensa J, Vaillar E, Traserra J. Prospective double-blind randomized study of the efficacy and tolerance of topical ciprofloxacin vs topical gentamicin in the treatment of simple chronic otitis media and diffuse external otitis. Acta Otorrinolaringol Esp. 1996;47(3):217–20.
24. Rahman A, Rizwan S, Waycaster C, Wall GM. Pooled analysis of two clinical trials comparing the clinical outcomes of topical ciprofloxacin/dexamethasone otic suspension and polymyxin B/neomycin/hydrocortisone otic suspension for the treatment of acute otitis externa in adults and children. Clin Ther. 2007;29(9):1950–6.
25. Dohar JE. Evolution of management approaches for otitis externa. Pediatr Infect Dis J. 2003;22(4):299–305.
26. Bhattacharyya N, Kepnes LJ. Initial impact of the acute otitis externa clinical practice guidelines on clinical care. Otolaryngol Head Neck Surg. 2011;145(3):414–7.
27. McCoy SI, Zell ER, Besser RE. Antimicrobial prescribing for otitis externa in children. Pediatr Infect Dis J. 2004;23(2):181–3.
28. Roland PS, Rybak L, Hannley M, Matz G, Stewart MG, Manolidis S, et al. Animal ototoxicity of topical antibiotics and the relevance to clinical treatment of human subjects. Otolaryngol Head Neck Surg. 2004;130(3 Suppl):S57–78.
29. Berenholz LP, Burkey JM, Farmer TL, Lippy WH. Topical otic antibiotics: clinical cochlear ototoxicity and cost consideration. Otolaryngol Head Neck Surg. 2006;135(2):291–4.
30. Matz G, Rybak L, Roland PS, Hannley M, Friedman R, Manolidis S, et al. Ototoxicity of ototopical antibiotic drops in humans. Otolaryngol Head Neck Surg. 2004;130(3 Suppl):S79–82.
31. Torum B, Block SL, Avila H, Montiel F, Oliva A, Quintanilla W. Efficacy of ofloxacin otic solution once daily for 7 days in the treatment of otitis externa: a multicenter, open-label, phase III trial. Clin Ther. 2004;26(7):1046–54.
32. Van Ginkel CJ, Bruintjes TD, Huizing EH. Allergy due to topical medications in chronic otitis externa and chronic otitis media. Clin Otolaryngol Allied Sci. 1995;20(4):326–8.
33. Rubin J, Yu VL, Stool SE. Malignant external otitis in children. J Pediatr. 1998;113(6):965–70.
34. Rubin Grandis J, Branstetter BF, Yu VL. The changing face of malignant (necrotizing) external otitis: clinical, radiological, and anatomic correlations. Lancet Infect Dis. 2004;4(1):34–9.
35. Lee JE, Song JJ, Oh SH, Chang SO, Kim CH, Lee JH. Prognostic value of extension patterns on follow-up magnetic resonance imaging in patients with necrotizing otitis externa. Arch Otolaryngol Head Neck Surg. 2011;137(7):688–93.
36. Bradley JS, Jackson MA. The use of systemic and topical fluoroquinolones. Pediatrics. 2011;128(4):e1034–45.
37. Vennewald I, Klemm E. Otomycosis: diagnosis and treatment. Clin Dermatol. 2010;28:202–11.
38. Ho T, Vrabec J, et al. Otomycosis: clinical features and treatment implications. Otolaryngo Head Neck Surg. 2006;135:787–91.
39. Munguia R, Daniek S. Ototopical antifungals and otomycosis: a review. Int J Pediatr Otorhinolaryngol. 2008;72:453–9.
40. Hirsch B. Infections of the external ear. Am J Otolaryngol. 1992;13(3):145–55.
41. Kansu L, Yilmaz I. Herpes zoster oticus (Ramsay Hunt syndrome) in children: case report and literature review. Int J Pediatr Otorhinolaryngol. 2012;76(6):772–6.
42. Hato N, Kisaki H, Honda N, Gyo K, Murakami S, Yanagihara N. Ramsay Hunt syndrome in children. Ann Neurol. 2000;48(2):254–6.

43. Demos M, McLeod MP. Recurrent furunculosis: a review of the literature. Br J Dermatol. 2012;167:725–32.
44. Cody DTR, Sones DA. Relapsing polychondritis: audiovestibular manifestations. Laryngoscope. 1971;81:1208–22.
45. Edgar B, Blevins N, et al. Otologic manifestations of relapsing polychondritis. Review of literature and report of nine cases. Auris Nasus Larynx. 2006;33:135–41.
46. Gergely P, Poor G. Relapsing polychondritis. Best Pract Res Clin Rheumatol. 2004;18(5):723–38.
47. Cockerill D. Allergies to ear molds. Br J Audiol. 1987;21:143–5.
48. Fraki JE, Kalimo K, et al. Contact allergy to various components of topical preparations for treatment of external otitis. Acta Otolaryngol. 1985;100:414–8.
49. Carruthers JA, Cronin E. Incidence of neomycin and framycetin sensitivity. Contact Dermatitis. 1976;2:269–70.
50. Parila V, Hirvonen ML, et al. The pattern of cross sensitivity to neomycin secondary sensitization to gentamycin. Dermatologica. 1986;136:321–4.
51. Smith IM, Keay DG, et al. Chronic hypersensitivity in patients with chronic otitis externa. Clin Otolaryngol. 1990;15:155–8.
52. Beltrani VS, Beltrani VP. Contact dermatitis. Ann Allergy Asthma Immunol. 1997;78:160–73.
53. Sood S, Strachan DR, et al. Allergic otitis externa. Clin Otolaryngol. 2002;27:233–6.
54. Guss J, Ruckenstein MJ. Infections of the external ear. In: Flint PW, Haughey BH, editors. Cummings otolaryngology head and neck surgery. Philadelphia: Mosby; 2010. p. 1944–59.
55. Onerci TM. Diagnosis in otorhinolaryngology. Berlin: Springer; 2009.

Chapter 3
Otitis Media

Christopher R. Grindle and Armando G. Correa

Abbreviations

ABR	Auditory brainstem response
AOM	Acute otitis media
AR	Acoustic reflectometry
EAC	External auditory canal
ELISA	Enzyme linked immunosorbent assay
HL	Hearing level
IPD	Invasive pneumococcal disease
MEE	Middle ear effusion
OAE	Otoacoustic emission
OME	Otitis media with effusion
PCR	Polymerase chain reaction
PCV	Pneumococcal conjugate vaccine
PNSP	Penicillin-nonsusceptible *S. pneumoniae*
RSV	Respiratory syncytial virus
TM	Tympanic membrane
WBR	Wideband reflectance

C.R. Grindle, M.D. (✉)
Division of Otolaryngology–Head and Neck Surgery, University of Connecticut School of Medicine, Connecticut Children's Medical Center, Hartford, CT, USA
e-mail: cgrindle@connecticutchildrens.org

A.G. Correa, M.D.
Department of Pediatrics, Baylor College of Medicine, Houston, TX, USA

Texas Children's Hospital, 6701 Fannin St, Suite 1540, Houston, TX, USA
e-mail: acorrea@bcm.edu

T.A. Valdez, J.G. Vallejo (eds.), *Infectious Diseases in Pediatric Otolaryngology*,
DOI 10.1007/978-3-319-21744-4_3

Introduction

Otitis media is the term used to indicate the presence of inflammation of the mucoperiosteal lining of the middle ear and is a catch all term encompassing acute otitis media and otitis media with effusion. It is the second most common illness diagnosed in children [1] and the most common reason for children to receive antibiotic therapy [2, 3]. Most children have experienced at least 1 episode of AOM by age 3 and by age 6 nearly 40 % have had 3 infections [4]. Nearly 20 % of all young, school-age children at any given time have middle ear effusion (MEE)—regardless of source. The onset and course can be acute, subacute, chronic, asymptomatic, or recurrent. The term *acute otitis media* (*AOM*) is used to indicate the rapid onset of signs and symptoms of infection within the middle ear. *Otitis media with effusion* (*OME*), is used to indicate the presence of inflammation and fluid in the middle ear with neither signs nor symptoms of acute infection. *Middle ear effusion* (*MEE*) denotes the presence of fluid in the middle ear without reference to etiology, pathogenesis, pathology, or duration [5]. Middle-ear effusions may be purulent, serous or mucoid. The presence of fluid in the middle ear may lead to hearing impairment, and the extension of the infection beyond the middle ear may be a rare cause of suppurative complications such as mastoiditis or intracranial abscess. Treatment for OME and AOM are predicated on accurate diagnosis. Increasing effort is being made to be certain of diagnosis of AOM before prescribing antibiotic therapy so as to reduce antibiotic burden and decrease healthcare expenditure. Despite this, there is no gold standard for the diagnosis of AOM or OME. It is a clinical diagnosis with evolving symptoms based on disease state and progression.

Epidemiology and Pathophysiology

Acute otitis media is the number one bacterial infection that pediatricians in the United States encounter in young children. It accounts for as many as 25 % of office visits (frequently resulting in an antibiotic prescription) in children younger than 3 years [6] and tympanostomy tube placement in over 650,000 children annually [7, 8]. In total, direct and indirect costs related to AOM are estimated to be $3 billion annually, nearly half of which is attributable to AOM in children aged 1–3 years [9].

The introduction of the pneumococcal 7-valent conjugate vaccine (PCV-7) in 2000, followed by a 13-valent conjugated vaccine (PCV-13) in 2010, appear to be driving not only a reduction in the rates of AOM, but also an important shift in the overall microbiology of AOM [9]. Two additional factors that have likely altered the incidence and epidemiology of AOM in the US are the establishment of a more strict criteria for diagnosis and treatment of AOM through the dissemination of management guidelines by national organizations such as the American Academy of Pediatrics (AAP) and educational campaigns by the Centers for Disease Control (CDC) and other professional organizations highlighting the importance of judicious use of antimicrobials.

Although otitis media remains the most common condition for which antibacterial agents are prescribed for children in the US [8–10], there has been an overall downward trend in otitis media-related health care use since 2001 [10, 11]. Grijalva et al [2], noted a decrease in clinician visit for otitis media from 950 per 1000 children in 1995–1996 to 634 per 1000 children in 2005–2006, which was accompanied by a proportional decrease in antibiotic prescriptions for otitis media from 760 per 1000 to 484 per 1000 in the same time periods. In a recent database analysis of a large, nationwide managed care plan that included over six million primary otitis media visits for an 11-year period during the post PCV-era, Marom and colleagues, found a substantial decrease in otitis media visit rates in children from birth to 6 years, particularly among children younger than 2 years in 2010–2011 [11]. During these years, there was also a larger decrease in recurrent otitis media rates.

The more recent decrease seems to coincide with the PCV-13 administration in this age group [11]. Along with the decrease in otitis media rates, these authors found a 19 % decrease in need for ventilation tube insertion from 2010 to 2011, and a substantial decrease in the rate of mastoiditis.

Numerous host and environmental factors have been identified as independent risk factors for severe or recurrent AOM. Predisposing host factors include: male gender, prematurity, ethnicity (Native Americans, Alaskan Eskimo), young age at onset of AOM, or the presence of certain anatomic or immunologic defects (such as cleft palate or immunoglobulin deficiency). Environmental factors include: lack of breast feeding, use of pacifier, daycare attendance, exposure to cigarette smoke and other pollutants, and sleeping in a prone position.

Otitis media is best considered a disease of Eustachian tube dysfunction. The bacteria trapped in the middle ear represent the nasopharyngeal flora. The clinical course, along with epidemiologic data, support an association between viral respiratory infections and the development of AOM [12]. Antibiotic treatment is aided by gradual and/or spontaneous improvement in Eustachian tube function during the natural history of the disease.

Microbiology

Compared with the pre-PCV era, the proportion of AOM cases caused by *Streptococcus pneumoniae* has decreased, with a commensurate increase in nontypeable *Haemophilus influenzae* and *Moraxella catarrhalis* [13, 14] The development of antibiotic-resistant strains, which play a role in treatment failures, appears to be changing as well, as we are witnessing reductions in penicillin-nonsusceptible *S. pneumoniae* (PNSP) and increases in proportions of β-lactamase–producing *H influenzae* [15].

Before the widespread use of pneumococcal conjugated vaccines, *S. pneumoniae* was the predominant causative pathogen in AOM, acute bacterial sinusitis, and bacteremic community-acquired pneumonia among children [8]. In 2000, PCV-7 became the first US Food and Drug Administration (FDA)-approved pneumococcal vaccine for immunization of infants and young children. PCV-7 contained protein-conjugated antigens against 7 serotypes (4, 6B, 9V, 14, 18C, 19F, and 23F) of *S. pneumoniae* that caused invasive disease and AOM. In February 2010, a new 13-valent product was licensed—PCV13—which added 6 new serotypes (1, 3, 5, 6A, 7F, and 19A). Together, these 13 serotypes account for the majority of invasive pneumococcal disease (IPD) in the U.S., including serotype 19A, which had become the most common IPD-causing serotype in young children after the introduction of PCV-7 [16]. These serotypes also account for most penicillin-nonsusceptible *S. pneumoniae* (PNSP) strains [16]. PCV-13 is routinely administered as a 4-dose series, given at ages 2, 4, and 6 months, and a booster dose at age 12–15 months. Two placebo-controlled clinical studies evaluated the impact of PCV-7 on the overall rates of AOM in two distinct geographic subpopulations before PCV-7 was routinely used. In a study of more than 37,000 children in northern California, a 4-dose series of PCV-7 reduced visits for AOM by 7.8 % and antibiotic prescriptions by 5.7 % [17]. Similarly, Eskola and colleagues demonstrated a 7 % reduction in AOM in a subpopulation of Finnish children who had received PCV-7, compared with a control group [18].

In contrast to the PCV-7 pre-licensure studies noted above, two separate US studies showed an overall reduction on AOM rates of nearly 20 % since the routine use of PCV-7 vaccination [19, 20]. Likewise, Casey and Pichichero observed a 24 % reduction in overall cases of persistent AOM in their practice among young children who had received PCV-7 [13]. These data suggest the possibility that herd immunity is occurring with community-wide use of PCV-7 [13].

Several studies have elucidated the effects of PCV-7 on the microbiology of AOM. Most of these studies have shown that nontypeable *H. influenzae* accounts for nearly twice as many cases of culture-positive persistent/recurrent otitis media (PROM) than did *S. pneumoniae* [13, 14].

For the last two decades, two primary pathogens—*S. pneumoniae* and *H. influenzae*—have accounted for most of the resistant strains recovered in AOM. The percentage of PNSP appears to have dropped slightly, accounting for 10 % and 19 % of all *S. pneumoniae* recovered in PROM from sites in Rochester, New York, and Kentucky, respectively [13, 14]. More importantly, both sites noted that high-level PNSP (penicillin MIC >1.0 μg/mL) was only 5–6 % in PCV-7–vaccinated children [13, 14]. Additionally, a study from St. Louis of 327 children aged younger than 7 years with acute respiratory infection demonstrated a decrease from 25 to 12 % in the prevalence of nasal colonization with penicillin-intermediate or resistant *S. pneumoniae* during the years since the implementation of PCV-7 [21]. It now appears that β-lactamase–positive *H. influenzae* accounts for more than half of the *H. influenzae* strains recovered among children who have received PCV-7, making in vitro activity against *H. influenzae* an important consideration when choosing antibiotic [22].

Following the implementation of PCV-7 vaccination, AOM due to PCV-7– specific *S. pneumoniae* serotypes decreased by 49–57 % in vaccinated children, with a commensurate increase in infection due to non-PCV-7–related serotypes of *S. pneumoniae* [14, 18]. Importantly, serotypes 6A and 19A (not included in the PCV-7 vaccine) increased from 8 to 32 % of all *S. pneumoniae* serotypes recovered in one study of AOM [14]. The effect of the addition of serotypes 6A and 19A in the newer 13-valent PCV vaccine has not been fully evaluated, but recent reports from Israel suggest a near-elimination of pneumococcal AOM due to serotypes contained in the vaccine [23].

Approximately 30 % of middle-ear cultures show no growth. This sometimes may be the result of a failure of the culture techniques to detect fastidious bacteria, small numbers of bacteria, bacteria no longer capable of replication because of antibiotic therapy, or disease from microorganisms other than bacteria. Occasionally the bacterial infection has been eradicated, although signs and symptoms of inflammation are still present [24]. Aerobic pathogens can be found in middle-ear fluid by polymerase chain reaction (PCR) in a high percentage of "sterile" effusions [25]. It is still not clear whether this means these patients will benefit from antibiotic therapy. This figure also suggests that in some cases, middle-ear fluid is sterile and not formed as a response to bacterial infection. It supports the concepts that Eustachian tube dysfunction is the basic mechanism of otitis media, and that not all cases of otitis media require therapy [24].

Gram-negative enteric bacteria and *S. aureus* were the bacteria most frequently recovered from the middle ear of premature or term neonates in some early studies and may have represented the nasopharyngeal flora of these infants [26], as subsequent studies have indicated that these bacteria are uncommon in infections [24]. Young infants occasionally have Group B streptococci recovered from the middle ear [27]. The recovery of *Neisseria* species or of *S. epidermidis*, which are not usually associated with disease, also suggests that some bacteria recovered from the middle ear are, in fact, normal flora of the nasopharynx that have reached the middle ear after eustachian tube dysfunction and are not the cause of the otitis media. If a young infant (less than 2 months of age) has otitis media and appears toxic, one must consider obtaining blood culture, lumbar puncture and tympanocentesis; hospitalization for administration of intravenous antibiotics may also be indicated. AOM with low-grade fever in a well-appearing young infant can usually be treated with oral antibiotics provided that close follow-up can be ensured [24].

It has now been well established that viruses can not only predispose to otitis media because of inflammation of the eustachian tubes, but they can also be etiologic agents of otitis media [28, 29] Respiratory syncytial virus (RSV), parainfluenza viruses, coxsackie viruses, and others have been recovered from middle-ear fluid by conventional cell culture [30]. Viral antigens and genetic material have also been found by ELISA and PCR [31]. Studies suggest that the concomitant presence of a viral pathogen and a bacterial pathogen in the middle-ear space signals a disease process that is more difficult to eradicate [32]. On occasion, a virus is the only pathogen recovered.

Any respiratory viral infection can serve as an inciting event for the development of AOM. It is often thought that RSV is the agent most likely to do so [33]; however, the most comprehensive study on this issue to date shows that the difference in the prevalence of otitis media in children with culture-proven RSV infection versus the prevalence in infection with other respiratory viruses is small [34].

Bullous myringitis (blister formation on the tympanic membrane or skin of the external auditory canal) occurs in some cases of experimental infection of human volunteers with *Mycoplasma pneumoniae* [35]. However, later studies documented that *Mycoplasma* is a rare cause of otitis media, even in the presence of bullous myringitis [36]. In fact, when tympanocentesis is performed in patients with bullous myringitis, the breakdown of pathogens mirrors that of AOM in the absence of bullae (i.e., *S. pneumoniae*, nontypable *H. influenzae*, and *M. catarrhalis*) [36]. These findings suggest bullous myringitis is a variant of AOM. As such, it should be treated with the same antibiotics one would select for uncomplicated AOM. There is no need to add erythromycin or a newer macrolide to the treatment of patients with bullous myringitis [24].

Diagnosis

Although seemingly obvious, to properly diagnose otitis media, one must get an adequate view of the middle ear. This is not always easy. In general, the largest speculum possible should be used to examine the ear. This permits the widest possible field of view. The speculum should fit comfortably in and be well seated in the outer, cartilaginous portion of the external auditory canal (EAC). Using a smaller speculum limits the field of view and it is far easier to over-insert the speculum which may result in contact with the bony EAC, which is exquisitely painful. The EAC is often tortuous and gentle posterior traction on the pinna can be used to straighten the EAC and allow for better insertion of the speculum. Additionally, the speculum and/or otoscope should be held in such a way so as to brace it against the patient's head. Thus, with any sudden movements, the speculum and otoscope will move with the patient's head. All of these positioning techniques are aimed at reducing any discomfort associated with the exam. This is especially important in children. It can be difficult to examine infants and young children, proper positioning and technique can help in achieving a successful exam.

The normal tympanic membrane is a three layered membrane with an outer layer of stratified squamous epithelium, a middle fibrous layer and an inner mucosal layer of cuboidal epithelium contiguous with the middle ear mucosa. It is adult size at birth though its orientation changes dramatically over the first few years of life. At birth it is a nearly horizontal orientation (34° from the horizontal plane) but changes as the skull base grows to a more vertical orientation (63° from the horizontal plane) in adults [37]. The normal tympanic membrane is translucent and pearly gray. The malleus (short process and manubrium) can easily be seen. Other landmarks in the middle ear are typically visible through the tympanic membrane (Fig. 3.1). The most common reasons for the tympanic membrane not to appear normal are OME and AOM. There are many possible findings when examining the tympanic membrane (Table 3.1) and good description of the exam findings helps with communication between clinicians.

In contrast to a normal tympanic membrane, the exam findings in otitis media are quite different. Otitis media with effusion (Fig. 3.2a) will often present with complaints of fullness and possibly decreased hearing. It may also be asymptomatic. Exam findings in serous OME are usually a yellow or amber tympanic membrane with normal or retracted position. Mobility is usually impaired and air bubbles may be seen in the fluid in the middle ear space. Mucoid OME has a yellow to white or creamy color with a bulging, normal or retracted position. Mobility is usually decreased (Fig. 3.3). The findings in OME contrast with the findings in AOM. Here the patient may or may not complain or ear pain. The tympanic membrane will show prominent vessels on exam. There will be purulent effusion in the middle ear space and the tympanic membrane will appear in a normal or bulging position. Mobility will be decreased (Fig. 3.4).

Of paramount importance is making the correct diagnosis for a patient with otitis media as the diagnosis will determine the treatment. The 2013 clinical practice guideline on the diagnosis and management of AOM from the AAP [10] built upon and further clarified diagnostic criteria set forth in the 2004 AAP guideline [38]. The earlier guideline used a 3 part definition of AOM with 1. Acute

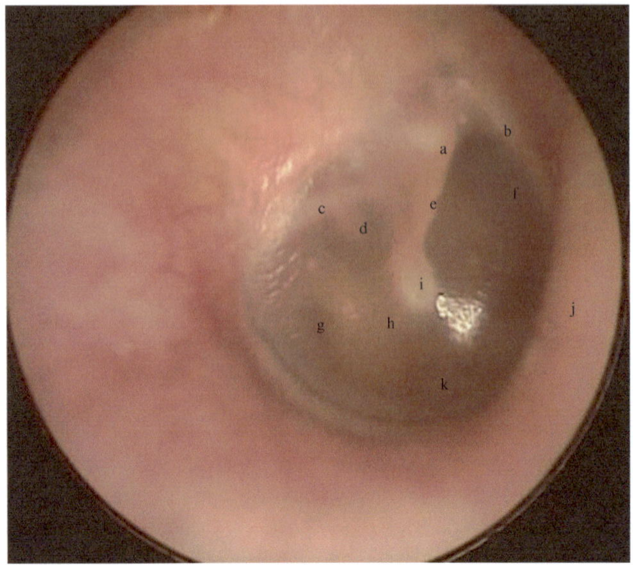

Fig. 3.1 A normal tympanic membrane and normal tympanic membrane with labels. (**a**) Lateral process of malleus (**b**) tympanic annulus (**c**) chorda tympani (**d**) incudostapedial joint (**e**) handle of malleus (**f**) shadow of Eustachian tube (**g**) shadow of round window niche (**h**) promontory (floor of middle ear) (**i**) umbo (**j**) bulge of anterior external auditory canal wall (**k**) hypotympanic air cells

Table 3.1 Findings on pneumatic otoscopy

Color	Position	Translucency	Mobility
Gray	Normal	Translucent	Normal
Yellow	Bulging	Semi opaque	Increased
Amber	Retracted	Opaque (dull)	Decreased
White			No movement
Red			
Blue			

onset of symptoms, 2. Presence of MEE, and 3. Signs of middle ear inflammation. Criticisms of these criteria were that they lacked precision to exclude OME and permitted the diagnosis of AOM in cases of acute onset of symptoms with otalgia and MEE but without other signs of inflammation on otoscopy. Additionally, the 2004 guideline included a category for "uncertain diagnosis" which may have permitted diagnosis of AOM without clear visualization of the tympanic membrane. The 2013 guidelines qualify these criteria and states that the diagnosis of AOM:

1. Should be made in children who present with moderate to severe bulging of the TM or new onset otorrhea not due to acute otitis externa.
2. Should be made in children who present with mild bulging of the TM AND recent onset (less than 48 h) of ear pain (holding, tugging, rubbing of the ear in a nonverbal child) or intense erythema of the TM.
3. Should NOT be made in children who do not have MEE (based on pneumatic otoscopy and/or tympanometry)

The new guidelines place great importance on the otoscopic exam of the patient to make the correct diagnosis. A study by Karma et al [39] looked at over 2900 children over the course of 2 years at 2 separate sites—totaling over 11,000 visits. Physical exam findings, the color, position and the mobility of the TM were recorded. AOM was diagnosed if the child had MEE and fever, earache, irritability, ear rubbing or tugging simultaneous other upper respiratory symptoms, vomiting or diarrhea.

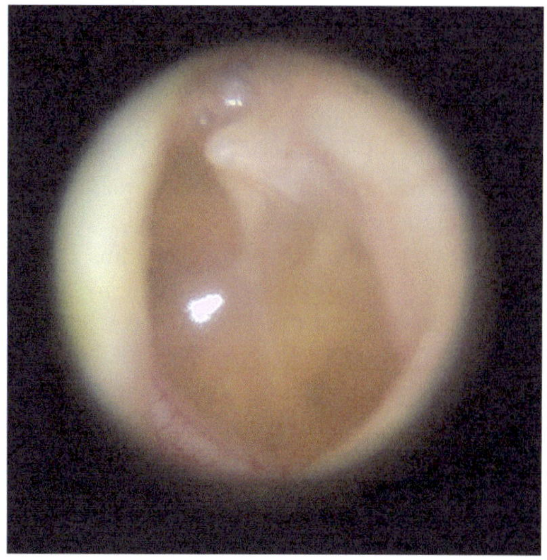

Fig. 3.2 Serous otitis media in left middle ear

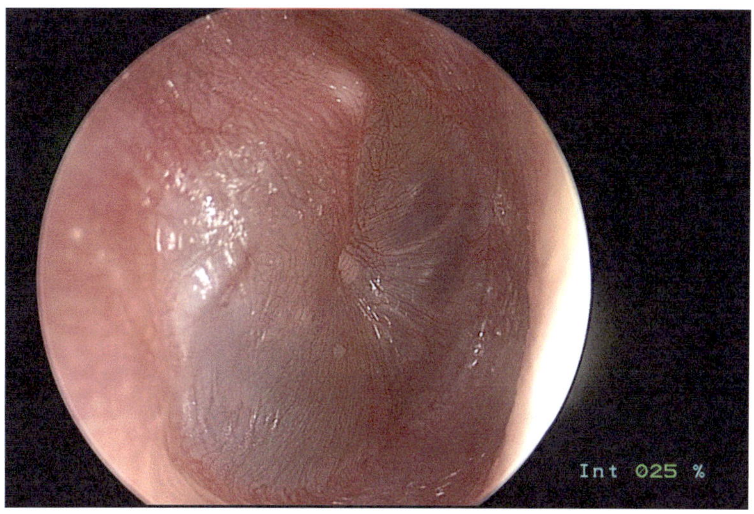

Fig. 3.3 Mucoid effusion with bubbles in right middle ear

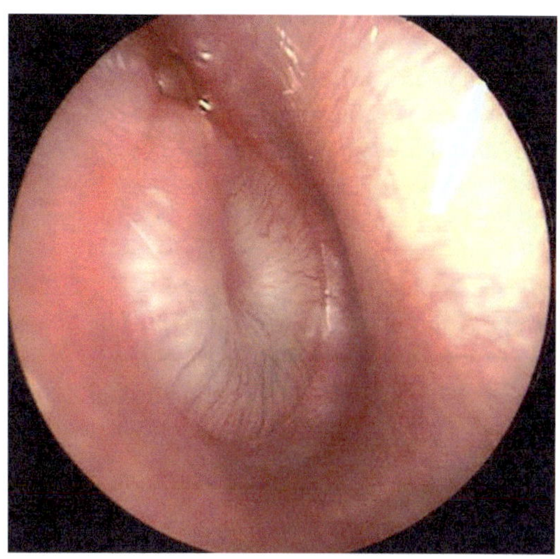

Fig. 3.4 AOM of right ear

Tympanocentesis was performed but no culture was obtained. Of the acute visits in the study, MEE was found in 84.9 and 81.8 % at the two sites. Of the exam findings, a cloudy, bulging TM with impaired mobility was the best predictor of AOM. Impaired mobility had the highest sensitivity (95 %) and specificity (85 %). Individually, cloudiness was 74 % sensitive and 93 % specific. Bulging TM was only 51 % sensitive, but 97 % specific. Several other studies support the value of the bulging TM on physical exam [40, 41] moderate to severe bulging of the TM is the most important characteristic in the diagnosis of AOM [10].

In looking at the presenting symptoms of AOM, ear pain had the highest combined positive likelihood ratio (3.0–7.3) in a 2003 review by Rothman et al. [42]. In three studies cited, Niemela et al reported 54 % sensitivity and 82 % specificity of ear pain [43]. Heikkinen reported 60 % sensitivity and 92 % [44] and Ingvarsson reported 100 % sensitivity, though did not report specificity [45].

Despite its usefulness as a symptom to be used in the diagnosis of AOM, ear pain is only present in 50–60 % of children with AOM [42]. Other signs, restless, ear rubbing, fever, non-specific respiratory complaints, diarrhea were not helpful in diagnosis AOM.

Takata et al reviewed the accuracy of eight methods of diagnosing OME [46]. Pneumatic otoscopy was found to have the best performance with a sensitivity of 94 % (95 % CI 92–96 %) and a specificity of 80 % (95 % CI 75–86 %). Pneumatic otoscopy was compared to acoustic reflectometer, portable tympanometry and several variations of professional tympanometry. All included studies used myringotomy as internal diagnostic comparison. Only one of the included studies on pneumatic otoscopy was performed by validated otoscopists [47]. Additionally, the author noted that audiometry, binocular microscopy and non-pneumatic otoscopy could not be included in the analysis because of inadequate evidence. In a small study, Rogers et al looked at 201 ears in 102 patients and found that binocular microscopy by a staff pediatric otolaryngologist was the most sensitive in diagnosing OME with 88.0 % sensitivity (95 % CI 81.4–94.7) and 89 % specific (95 % CI 83.1–94.9). Resident binocular microscopy was the next most sensitive, followed by staff pneumatic otoscopy and resident pneumatic otoscopy. Thus, as would be expected, there is improved performance garnered from additional years of training and experience. Of note, however, even the resident exam was more specific that the tympanometer 78.4 % (95 % CI 70.4–86.4) to 47.7 % (95 % CI 38.3–57.1).

Tympanometry

Tympanograms are widely used as an adjunct to the pneumatic otoscope in the clinical evaluation of children with otitis media. Most primary care clinics today use a low frequency probe tones (220–226 Hz) [48] and classify results as Jerger A, B or C [49]. Type A represents normal compliance of the tympanic membrane, Type B no compliance and Type C negative pressure in the middle ear space. Tympanometry with low frequency probe is reliable for infants greater than 4 months and has good inter-observer agreement of the curve patterns in routine clinical practice [50]. Despite the relatively low specificity for predicting MEE with a type B tympanogram, 47.7 % in the Rogers study and 74.5 % in the Takata study, tympanometry can guide the clinician in clinical decision making. If the definition of abnormal results on tympanogram are expanded to include both type B as well as type C2 (tympanic peak pressures between −200 and −400 daPa) the sensitivity and specificity, according to data from Takata, improve to 93.8 % (95 % CI 91.1–96.4) and 61.8 (95 % CI 41.5–82.1) respectively. Although not as precise as pneumatic otoscopy, this definition of abnormal result may be the most useful for ruling out OME [51].

Other modalities that have been used to assess the status of the middle ear and aid in diagnosis of otitis media are 1000 Hz tympanometry, multifrequency tympanometry and wideband acoustic transfer functions specifically wideband reflectance (WBR). Data suggest that these methods are useful in specific situations to determine the presence or absence of MEE, especially 1000 Hz tympanometry and WBR as applied to screening in infants. Continued research is needed to define their exact role as diagnostic tools [51]. Acoustic reflectometry (AR) is another tool that can be used in the diagnosis of MEE. Modern acoustic reflectometers analyze the frequency spectrum of reflected sound. They have been shown to be nearly equivalent to pneumatic otoscopy and tympanometry in terms of sensitivity and specificity [52]. AR offers a potential advantage over tympanometry and pneumatic otoscopy in that it does not require an airtight seal.

Hearing Testing

Audiometry may be used in the assessment of patients with otitis media. It is recommended when MEE has been present for 3 months or greater or when there is concern for speech delay, learning problems or when a significant hearing loss is suspected. Audiometric results with otitis can range from normal to moderate hearing loss (0–55 dB). The average hearing loss is 25 dB hearing level (HL) and approximately 20 % of ears exceed 35 dB HL [50]. The hearing loss is conductive in nature and secondary to the effusion in the middle ear space or the retraction of the TM. It causes an overall stiffening of the middle ear transduction mechanism (TM and ossicles) that generally affect lower frequencies before higher frequencies [7].

Conventional audiometry can be performed for children greater than 4 years of age. Screening conventional audiometry can be performed in the primary care setting. For younger children and for those for whom conventional audiometry is not appropriate, comprehensive audiologic assessment should be obtained. This includes air conduction and bone conduction thresholds for pure tones, speech detection and speech reception thresholds. For children aged 6–24 months visual reinforced audiometry may be used. Play audiometry is typically used for children 24–48 months [53]. Assessment of individual ear thresholds using either headphones or in canal inserts is typically possible with children older than 24 months. If this is not possible, then assessment is done under sound-field conditions and the responses can only comment on the better hearing ear.

Auditory brainstem response (ABR) testing and otoacoustic emission (OAE) testing are not tests of hearing but rather assessments of the integrity of the auditory pathway. They are objective measures used in situations when behavioral testing is not possible (e.g. newborn screening), but they should not be used as a substitute for behavioral audiometry [53].

Treatment

Medical

As it can be seen from the discussion above, the correct diagnosis of otitis media drives all further management of the patient. Risks of treatment need to be weighed against the natural history of otitis media. A recent Cochrane review reported that up to 82 % of children with acute otitis media will improve spontaneously [54]. In terms of treatment for otitis media, it can broadly be broken down into medical and surgical with the mainstays being antibiotics, both oral and oto-topical. The mainstay of surgical therapy is tympanostomy tubes.

The classic study by Howie on the bacterial etiology of otitis media using placebo therapy and serial tympanocenteses revealed that the spontaneous resolution rate of otitis media is, to a large extent, determined by the specific pathogen [55]. AOM caused by *S. pneumoniae* is less likely to resolve on its own than that caused by *H. influenzae*. By contrast, the vast majority of *M. catarrhalis* ear infections resolve with placebo and serial tympanocentesis. The fact that suppurative complications of otitis media such as mastoiditis are almost never caused by *M. catarrhalis* further underscores the low pathogenic potential of this organism in AOM.

Since 2004 the AAP and the American Academy of Family Practice have emphasized a selective approach to the treatment of otitis media with the publication of clinical practice guideline for the diagnosis and management of AOM [38]. In 2013, the AAP released a comprehensive peer-reviewed revision to this guideline that incorporated recent data on the effect of PCV on the microbiology of AOM, as well as address some of the controversial issues raised by the original guideline [10]. These guidelines provide specific and stringent criteria for the diagnosis of AOM, as well as an option for initial observation vs. therapy in selected patients. They also address appropriate choices on antibiotic agents, pain management and preventive measures.

The AAP guideline provides a number of clinical scenarios to determine whether antibiotics are indicated or observation is an option [10]. These are based on the clinical presentation, severity of symptoms and the age of the child, and include:

(a) Severe unilateral or bilateral AOM, characterized by moderate/severe otalgia, otalgia for at least 48 h or fever ≥39 C, should be immediately treated, irrespectively of the child's age.
(b) Similarly, treatment with antibiotic should be initiated immediately for AOM with otorrhea.
(c) Non-severe bilateral otitis media in young children (6–23 months) should also be treated with antibiotics.
(d) Non-severe unilateral AOM in young children (6–23 months) should be either treated with antibiotics or observation with close follow up can be an option based on a joint decision with the caregivers.
(e) Non-severe AOM (unilateral or bilateral) in children 24 months or older should be either treated with antibiotics or offered observation based on a joint decision with the caregivers.

The guideline also emphasizes that if observation is elected, antibiotic therapy should be started if the child worsens or fails to improve within 48–72 h [10].

Most experts agree that amoxicillin for a full course of 10 days continues to be an effective agent following the introduction of PCV and should remain as the first-line agent of choice. Advantages of amoxicillin include reasonable efficacy in AOM, a good safety profile, low rates of gastrointestinal upset, acceptable palatability, and inexpensive cost compared with other commonly used second-line antibiotics. High-dose amoxicillin (80–90 mg/kg/day) is preferred to avoid suboptimal concentrations of amoxicillin in middle ear effusion [56, 57]. Despite the fact that high-dose amoxicillin is unlikely to be effective against β-lactamase–producing *H. influenzae* (56–64 % β-lactamase–positive) and *M. catarrhalis* (virtually 100 % β-lactamase-positive), current data support its effectiveness in new-onset AOM, although its continued effectiveness will need to be monitored [22].

Of the available FDA-approved antibiotic therapies for AOM (Table 3.2), only a handful are endorsed by the current AAP guideline [10], as there is concern or lack of information about the effectiveness of the rest of them. Intramuscular ceftriaxone, although recommended by the AAP as second-or third-line treatment, is not commonly used by clinicians for uncomplicated refractory AOM.

The most commonly used second-line agent is amoxicillin-clavulanic acid. A formulation of this antibiotic that contains these agents in a 14:1 ratio allows for a high-dose regimen without excessive rates of diarrhea and has improved tolerability [58]. Amoxicillin-clavulanate is also preferred in a patient who has received amoxicillin in the past 30 days or has a history of recurrent AOM unresponsive to amoxicillin [10].

Several acceptable alternative initial therapies are available for penicillin-allergic patients. Cefpodoxime, cefuroxime, and cefdinir have been found to be reasonably effective in the treatment of AOM [10, 38]. Although in the past caution has been emphasized when prescribing cephalosporins to

Table 3.2 Currently available FDA-approved antibiotics for AOM

FDA-approved antibiotics for the treatments of AOM				
Frequency of use	Penicillins	Cephalosporins	Macrolides	Others
Common	Amoxicillin	Cefdinir		
	Amoxicillin-clavulanate	Cefprozil		
Uncommon		Cefaclor	Azithromycin	
		Cefixime	Clarithromycin	
		Cefpodoxime proxetil		
		Ceftibuten		
		Cefuroxime		
		Ceftriaxone		
Rare		Cephalexin	Erythromycin	Trimethoprim-sulfamethoxazole
			Ethylsuccinate/sulfisoxazole	

Source: Data from [22]

patients with true penicillin allergy, recent studies have shown that the true incidence of cross-sensitivity is almost negligible with the 2nd and 3rd generation cephalosporins endorsed by the APP guideline (cefpodoxime, cefuroxime and cefdinir) [59, 60].

Clindamycin has activity against most strains of the pneumococcus, but no activity against *H. influenzae* or *M. catarrhalis*, and its use should probably be reserved for cases in which *S. pneumoniae* has been cultured from middle ear fluid, or when this organism is strongly suspected. If clindamycin is used in an empirical fashion in a patient that has failed with a conventional regimen, it may be prudent to give it in combination with an agent that is β-lactamase stable, such as a second or third generation cephalosporin.

Studies have shown that one intramuscular injection of ceftriaxone (50 mg/kg) is as effective as a 10-day course of amoxicillin-clavulanate for the initial treatment of AOM [61]. For treatment of previously unresponsive cases, 3 consecutive days of therapy is superior to a single injection [62]. However, the use of ceftriaxone for treatment of otitis media should not be routine. A single dose of intramuscular ceftriaxone has been shown to increase penicillin resistance among the pneumococci colonizing the nasopharynx [63]. Although some refractory cases of AOM due to multiple resistant organisms will respond to a 3-consecutive-day schedule of intramuscular ceftriaxone [10], this approach to therapy is painful and often inconvenient.

Linezolid and levofloxacin are newer antibiotics that are not approved by the FDA for the treatment of AOM but may be indicated for the treatment of multidrug resistant strains, usually after bacteriologic confirmation has been established [10]. In fact, levofloxacin is a quinolone antibiotic that has not been approved for use in children, but has been successfully used for the treatment of pediatric otitis media [64], including cases due to multidrug-resistant *S. pneumoniae* serotype 19A [65].

Table 3.3 summarizes the recommended dosages for first- and subsequent-line antibiotics for the treatment of AOM. It includes those antibiotics endorsed by the AAP guideline [10], as well as levofloxacin as a 3rd or 4th option. Although this quinolone was not included in the AAP otitis media guideline, it was considered as an option in the contemporaneous AAP guideline for the treatment of acute bacterial sinusitis, a condition with similar microbiology to AOM, because of it potent activity against *H. influenzae. M. catarrhalis* and many multi-resistant strains of *S. pneumoniae* [66]. Linezolid, an oxazolidinone, has remarkable activity against resistant Gram-positive organisms, but its high cost, precludes it from being a viable choice, except in selected cases.

A child with no improvement after consecutive courses of two or three different antibiotics should probably undergo tympanocentesis. This has the benefit of draining the pus, which may be therapeutic, in addition to enabling a sample to be obtained for culture and sensitivity testing.

Tablet 3.3 Recommended antibiotic dosages for the treatment of AOM

Antibiotic	Dosage
First-line treatment	
Amoxicillin	80–90 mg/kg/day in 2 divided doses
Amoxicillin-clavulanate	90 mg/kg/day of amoxicillin component in 2 divided doses
Alternative treatment	
Cefdinir	14 mg/kg/day in 1 or 2 doses
Cefuroxime	30 mg/kg/day in 2 divided doses
Cefpodoxime	10 mg/kg/day in 2 divided doses
Ceftriaxone (IM or IV)	50 mg/kg/day for 1–3 days
Clindamycin (with or without 3rd-generation cephalosporin)	30 mg/kg/day in 3 divided doses
Levofloxacin	20 mg/kg/day in 2 divided doses

Source: Data from [10, 66]

Persistent Middle Ear Effusion

Effusion is still present in about 50 % of children 10 days after treatment [67], especially those younger than 24 months [68]. With time, the effusion resolves: 90 % are resolved within 3 months. After that time, few cases resolve [67]. Persistence of middle-ear fluid after acute otitis media occurs more commonly in white children under 2 years of age and can cause transiently impaired hearing, although long-term follow-up reveals normal hearing and normal speech and language development in most [69]. When an episode of AOM results in persistence of middle ear fluid for 3 months and the tympanic membrane remains immobile, consultation with an otolaryngologist is advisable.

Bullous Myringitis

As discussed previously, this condition should be considered a variant of AOM, and treated appropriately. If there are associated middle or lower respiratory findings, it may be reasonable to consider therapy with a macrolide, although data about the efficacy of this approach are lacking.

Neonatal Otitis Media

In the first 3 months of life, hospitalized infants, especially those in intensive care units, may have *S. aureus* or enteric gram-negative bacilli recovered on tympanocentesis [70], whereas infants this age seen as outpatients are likely to have the conventional pathogens [68].

Other Treatment

Oral decongestants and antihistamines were of no value for AOM or for chronic effusion in two controlled studies [33, 71]. In the third study, antihistamines for AOM were associated with a longer duration of middle ear effusion [72]. In many children, antihistamines produce sedation, masking the neurologic symptoms of rare complications such as meningitis or brain abscess. However, antihistamines may be helpful in recurrent OME in children with documented allergic problems. The use of nonsedating antihistamines in children with this condition has not been evaluated [24].

Allergies and upper respiratory infections appear to disrupt Eustachian tube function. Prevention of otitis media by symptomatic treatment of allergies has not been demonstrated. The incidence of AOM is decreased in children given influenza vaccination [73, 74] so its use, along with that of PCV-13, should be strongly encouraged [10].

Analgesics

In recent years, the importance of including an assessment of pain in the management of AOM has been emphasized [10, 38]. Acetaminophen or ibuprofen may be used for relief of ear pain. Topical application of anesthetic ear drops, may be of some value in pain relief and may soften earwax for easier removal. These preparations are especially useful in the first 2 or 3 days of therapy but their effect may be limited to 30 min or less after instillation [75].

Surgical

The surgical treatment of otitis media consists of myringotomy typically with the placement of tympanostomy tubes. This procedure is performed over 660,000 times in children under 15 in the United States [7]. It is a brief and safe, outpatient procedure that is typically performed under general anesthesia so as to reduce patient discomfort and movement although it can also be performed in the office without general anesthesia. There are a wide variety of tubes that are commercially available that vary in inner lumen diameter, shaft length, and flange length. They are placed in the tympanic membrane in an incision in the inferior aspect of the tympanic membrane (Fig. 3.5). They migrate out of the tympanic membrane, typically over the course of 1–2 years. While in place, the tubes serve to regulate pressure changes in the middle ear, decreasing the likelihood of infection, decreasing the discomfort associated with infection and allowing the use of oto-topical drops in the case of infection.

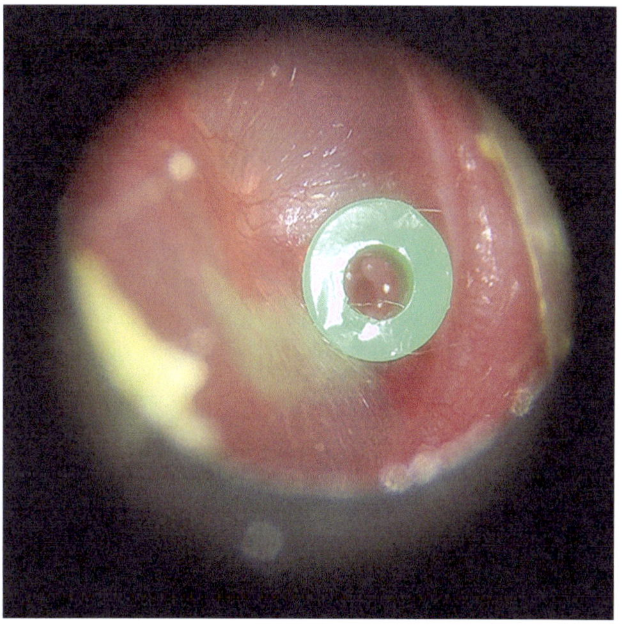

Fig. 3.5 Tympanostomy tube in right tympanic membrane

There is debate as to the indications for tympanostomy tubes. In an attempt to answer questions related to tympanostomy tubes and clarify indications for tubes the American Academy of Otolaryngology—Head & Neck Surgery (AAO-HNS) published a guideline for tympanostomy tubes [76]. This multidisciplinary guideline supports the insertion of tympanostomy tubes as a therapeutic option in children who have:

1. Recurrent infection, defined as 3 or more infections in 6 months or 4 or more in a year, with abnormal otoscopic findings on exam at time of evaluation by otolaryngologist.
2. Persistent MEE for greater than 3 months with associated difficulty with hearing.

Other recommendations include NOT offering tympanostomy tubes in cases of AOM/OME of short duration (less than 3 months) and when pre-operative otoscopic evaluation for tube candidacy by the surgeon is completely normal. These recommendations stem from the natural history of AOM/OME to improve spontaneously [77] and the acknowledged difficulty in accurate diagnosis of AOM, respectively.

Complications with tympanostomy tubes are infrequent and typically minor. Brief periods of tube otorrhea are reported by over 25 % of patients. This drainage is the hallmark of acute otitis media with functioning tympanostomy tubes and may be considered one of the benefits of the tubes. Persistent perforation after tube extrusion is seen in 1–4 % of patients. Myringosclerosis is also seen in up to 33 % of patients after PE tubes. Other complications include granulation tissue formation and atrophy of portions of tympanic membrane [78].

Conclusion

The diagnosis of otitis media can be difficult for even the most experienced of clinicians. It is a disease that primarily affects younger children who can be difficult to examine at best. Additionally, there is no gold-standard for diagnosis of otitis media. Recent studies and guidelines continue to refine the diagnostic criteria, with significant emphasis on physical exam findings, so as to help the clinician make an accurate diagnosis which informs all other decisions of therapy and management. Management and treatment are aimed at effectively curing the infection, quickly relieving symptoms, and preventing recurrence and rare complications. Recent advances in vaccination have resulted in significant changes in the treatment and management of otitis media. Continuing research is needed as the disease process continues to evolve and to determine the optimal prevention and treatment paradigms and the most appropriate candidates for surgical management.

References

1. Centers for Disease Control and Prevention. Table 2: top 5 diagnoses at visits to office-based physicians and hospital outpatient departments by patient age and sex. National Ambulatory Health Survey 2008. Atlanta: Centers for Disease Control and Prevention; 2008.
2. Grijalva CG, Nuorti JP, Griffin MR. Antibiotic prescription rates for acute respiratory tract infections in US ambulatory settings. JAMA. 2009;302(7):758–66.
3. McCaig LF, Besser RE, Hughes JM. Trends in antimicrobial prescribing rates for children and adolescents. JAMA. 2002;287(23):3096–102.
4. Casselbrant ML, Mandel EM. Epidemiology. In: Rosenfeld RM, Bluestone CD, editors. Evidence based otitis media. 2nd ed. Hamilton: Decker; 2003.
5. Rosenfeld RM, Bluestone CD, editors. Evidence-based otitis media. 2nd ed. Hamilton: B.C. Decker; 2003. p. 529.

6. Block SL, Harrison CJ, Hedrick J, Tyler R, Smith A, Hedrick R. Restricted use of antibiotic prophylaxis for recurrent acute otitis media in the era of penicillin non-susceptible Streptococcus pneumoniae. Int J Pediatr Otorhinolaryngol. 2001;61(1):47–60.
7. Stach BA. Audiologic evaluation of otologic/neurologic disease. In: Guyla AJ, Minor LB, Poe DS, editors. Glasscock Shambaugh, surgery of the ear. 6th ed. Connecticut: People's Medical Publishing House; 2010. p. 189–221.
8. Advisory Committee on Immunization Practices. Preventing pneumococcal disease among infants and young children. Recommendations of the Advisory Committee on Immunization Practices (ACIP). MMWR Recomm Rep. 2000;49(RR-9):1–35.
9. Brixner DI. Improving acute otitis media outcomes through proper antibiotic use and adherence. Am J Manag Care. 2005;11(6 Suppl):S202–10.
10. Lieberthal AS, Carroll AE, Chonmaitree T, Ganiats TG, Hoberman A, Jackson MA, et al. The diagnosis and management of acute otitis media. Pediatrics. 2013;131(3):e964–99.
11. Marom T, Tan A, Wilkinson GS, Pierson KS, Freeman JL, Chonmaitree T. Trends in otitis media-related health care use in the United States, 2001–2011. JAMA Pediatr. 2014;168(1):68–75. PMCID: 3947317.
12. Klein JO, Bluestone CD. Otitis media. In: Cherry JD, Harrison GJ, Kaplan SL, Hotez PJ, Steinbach WJ, editors. Feigin and Cherry's textbook of pediatric infectious diseases. 7th ed. Philadelphia: Saunders Elsevier; 2014. p. 209–40.
13. Casey JR, Pichichero ME. Changes in frequency and pathogens causing acute otitis media in 1995–2003. Pediatr Infect Dis J. 2004;23(9):824–8.
14. Block SL, Hedrick J, Harrison CJ, Tyler R, Smith A, Findlay R, et al. Community-wide vaccination with the heptavalent pneumococcal conjugate significantly alters the microbiology of acute otitis media. Pediatr Infect Dis J. 2004;23(9):829–33.
15. Jacobs MR, Anon J, Appelbaum PC. Mechanisms of resistance among respiratory tract pathogens. Clin Lab Med. 2004;24(2):419–53.
16. Centers for Disease Control and Prevention. Licensure of a 13-valent pneumococcal conjugate vaccine (PCV13) and recommendations for use among children—Advisory Committee on Immunization Practices (ACIP), 2010. MMWR Morb Mortal Wkly Rep. 2010;59(9):258–61.
17. Fireman B, Black SB, Shinefield HR, Lee J, Lewis E, Ray P. Impact of the pneumococcal conjugate vaccine on otitis media. Pediatr Infect Dis J. 2003;22(1):10–6.
18. Eskola J, Kilpi T, Palmu A, Jokinen J, Haapakoski J, Herva E, et al. Efficacy of a pneumococcal conjugate vaccine against acute otitis media. N Engl J Med. 2001;344(6):403–9.
19. Grijalva CG, Poehling KA, Nuorti JP, Zhu Y, Martin SW, Edwards KM, et al. National impact of universal childhood immunization with pneumococcal conjugate vaccine on outpatient medical care visits in the United States. Pediatrics. 2006;118(3):865–73.
20. Poehling KA, Szilagyi PG, Grijalva CG, Martin SW, LaFleur B, Mitchel E, et al. Reduction of frequent otitis media and pressure-equalizing tube insertions in children after introduction of pneumococcal conjugate vaccine. Pediatrics. 2007;119(4):707–15.
21. Garbutt J, Rosenbloom I, Wu J, Storch GA. Empiric first-line antibiotic treatment of acute otitis in the era of the heptavalent pneumococcal conjugate vaccine. Pediatrics. 2006;117(6):e1087–94.
22. Block SL, Correa AG. Update on the management of pediatric acute otitis media and acute bacterial sinusitis. Contemp Pediatr. 2006;23(12):1–10.
23. Ben-Shimol S, Givon-Lavi N, Leibovitz E, Raiz S, Greenberg D, Dagan R. Near-elimination of otitis media caused by 13-valent pneumococcal conjugate vaccine (PCV) serotypes in southern Israel shortly after sequential introduction of 7-valent/13-valent PCV. Clin Infect Dis. 2014;59(12):1724–32.
24. Fisher RG, Boyce TG. Moffet's pediatric infectious diseases. 4th ed. Philadelphia: Lippincott Williams & Wilkins; 2005.
25. Henderson FW, Collier AM, Sanyal MA, Watkins JM, Fairclough DL, Clyde Jr WA, et al. A longitudinal study of respiratory viruses and bacteria in the etiology of acute otitis media with effusion. N Engl J Med. 1982;306(23):1377–83.
26. Tetzlaff TR, Ashworth C, Nelson JD. Otitis media in children less than 12 weeks of age. Pediatrics. 1977;59(6):827–32.
27. Bonadio WA, Jeruc W, Anderson Y, Smith D. Systemic infection due to group B beta-hemolytic streptococcus in children. A review of 75 outpatient-evaluated cases during 13 years. Clin Pediatr. 1992;31(4):230–3.
28. Shaw CB, Obermyer N, Wetmore SJ, Spirou GA, Farr RW. Incidence of adenovirus and respiratory syncytial virus in chronic otitis media with effusion using the polymerase chain reaction. Otolaryngol Head Neck Surg. 1995;113(3):234–41.
29. Pitkaranta A, Jero J, Arruda E, Virolainen A, Hayden FG. Polymerase chain reaction-based detection of rhinovirus, respiratory syncytial virus, and coronavirus in otitis media with effusion. J Pediatr. 1998;133(3):390–4.
30. Chonmaitree T, Howie VM, Truant AL. Presence of respiratory viruses in middle ear fluids and nasal wash specimens from children with acute otitis media. Pediatrics. 1986;77(5):698–702.

31. Rezes S, Soderlund-Venermo M, Roivainen M, Kemppainen K, Szabo Z, Sziklai I, et al. Human bocavirus and rhino-enteroviruses in childhood otitis media with effusion. J Clin Virol. 2009;46(3):234–7.
32. Patel JA, Reisner B, Vizirinia N, Owen M, Chonmaitree T, Howie V. Bacteriologic failure of amoxicillin-clavulanate in treatment of acute otitis media caused by nontypeable Haemophilus influenzae. J Pediatr. 1995;126(5 Pt 1):799–806.
33. Heikkinen T, Thint M, Chonmaitree T. Prevalence of various respiratory viruses in the middle ear during acute otitis media. N Engl J Med. 1999;340(4):260–4.
34. Fisher RG, Gruber WC, Edwards KM, Reed GW, Tollefson SJ, Thompson JM, et al. Twenty years of outpatient respiratory syncytial virus infection: a framework for vaccine efficacy trials. Pediatrics. 1997;99(2), E7.
35. Rifkind D, Chanock R, Kravetz H, Johnson K, Knight V. Ear involvement (myringitis) and primary atypical pneumonia following inoculation of volunteers with Eaton agent. Am Rev Respir Dis. 1962;85:479–89.
36. Roberts DB. The etiology of bullous myringitis and the role of mycoplasmas in ear disease: a review. Pediatrics. 1980;65(4):761–6.
37. Isaacson G. Endoscopic anatomy of the pediatric middle ear. Otolaryngol Head Neck Surg. 2014;150(1):6–15.
38. American Academy of Pediatrics Subcommittee on Management of Acute Otitis Media. Diagnosis and management of acute otitis media. Pediatrics. 2004;113(5):1451–65.
39. Karma PH, Penttila MA, Sipila MM, Kataja MJ. Otoscopic diagnosis of middle ear effusion in acute and non-acute otitis media. I. The value of different otoscopic findings. Int J Pediatr Otorhinolaryngol. 1989;17(1):37–49.
40. McCormick DP, Lim-Melia E, Saeed K, Baldwin CD, Chonmaitree T. Otitis media: can clinical findings predict bacterial or viral etiology? Pediatr Infect Dis J. 2000;19(3):256–8. Epub 2000/04/05. eng.
41. Schwartz RH, Stool SE, Rodriguez WJ, Grundfast KM. Acute otitis media: toward a more precise definition. Clin Pediatr. 1981;20(9):549–54. Epub 1981/09/01. eng.
42. Rothman R, Owens T, Simel DL. Does this child have acute otitis media? JAMA. 2003;290(12):1633–40. Epub 2003/09/25. eng.
43. Niemela M, Uhari M, Jounio-Ervasti K, Luotonen J, Alho OP, Vierimaa E. Lack of specific symptomatology in children with acute otitis media. Pediatr Infect Dis J. 1994;13(9):765–8. Epub 1994/09/01. eng.
44. Heikkinen T, Ruuskanen O. Signs and symptoms predicting acute otitis media. Arch Pediatr Adolesc Med. 1995;149(1):26–9. Epub 1995/01/01. eng.
45. Ingvarsson L. Acute otalgia in children—findings and diagnosis. Acta Paediatr Scand. 1982;71(5):705–10. Epub 1982/09/01. eng.
46. Takata GS, Chan LS, Morphew T, Mangione-Smith R, Morton SC, Shekelle P. Evidence assessment of the accuracy of methods of diagnosing middle ear effusion in children with otitis media with effusion. Pediatrics. 2003;112(6 Pt 1):1379–87. Epub 2003/12/05. eng.
47. Paradise JL, Smith CG, Bluestone CD. Tympanometric detection of middle ear effusion in infants and young children. Pediatrics. 1976;58(2):198–210. Epub 1976/08/01. eng.
48. Johnson KC. Audiologic assessment of children with suspected hearing loss. Otolaryngol Clin North Am. 2002;35(4):711–32. Epub 2002/12/19. eng.
49. Jerger J. Clinical experience with impedance audiometry. Arch Otolaryngol. 1970;92(4):311–24. Epub 1970/10/01. eng.
50. Rosenfeld RM, Culpepper L, Doyle KJ, Grundfast KM, Hoberman A, Kenna MA, et al. Clinical practice guideline: otitis media with effusion. Otolaryngol Head Neck Surg. 2004;130(5 Suppl):S95–118. Epub 2004/05/13. eng.
51. Sanford CA, Schooling T, Frymark T. Determining the presence or absence of middle ear disorders: an evidence-based systematic review on the diagnostic accuracy of selected assessment instruments. Am J Audiol. 2012;21(2):251–68. Epub 2012/05/16. eng.
52. Teppo H, Revonta M. Comparison of old, professional and consumer model acoustic reflectometers in the detection of middle-ear fluid in children with recurrent acute otitis media or glue ear. Int J Pediatr Otorhinolaryngol. 2007;71(12):1865–72. Epub 2007/10/02. eng.
53. Cunningham M, Cox EO. Hearing assessment in infants and children: recommendations beyond neonatal screening. Pediatrics. 2003;111(2):436–40. Epub 2003/02/04. eng.
54. Venekamp RP, Sanders S, Glasziou PP, Del Mar CB, Rovers MM. Antibiotics for acute otitis media in children. Cochrane Database Syst Rev. 2013;1:Cd000219. Epub 2013/02/27. eng.
55. Howie VM. Natural history of otitis media. Ann Otol Rhinol Laryngol. 1975;84(2 PT2 SUPPL 19):67–72.
56. Seikel K, Shelton S, McCracken Jr GH. Middle ear fluid concentrations of amoxicillin after large dosages in children with acute otitis media. Pediatr Infect Dis J. 1997;16(7):710–1.
57. Harrison CJ, Welch DF. Middle ear effusion amoxicillin concentrations in acute otitis media. Pediatr Infect Dis J. 1998;17(7):657–8.
58. Hoberman A, Paradise JL, Burch DJ, Valinski WA, Hedrick JA, Aronovitz GH, et al. Equivalent efficacy and reduced occurrence of diarrhea from a new formulation of amoxicillin/clavulanate potassium (Augmentin) for treatment of acute otitis media in children. Pediatr Infect Dis J. 1997;16(5):463–70.
59. Pichichero ME. Use of selected cephalosporins in penicillin-allergic patients: a paradigm shift. Diagn Microbiol Infect Dis. 2007;57(3 Suppl):13S–8.

60. Pichichero ME, Casey JR. Safe use of selected cephalosporins in penicillin-allergic patients: a meta-analysis. Otolaryngol Head Neck Surg. 2007;136(3):340–7.
61. Varsano IB, Volovitz BM, Grossman JE. Effect of naproxen, a prostaglandin inhibitor, on acute otitis media and persistence of middle ear effusion in children. Ann Otol Rhinol Laryngol. 1989;98(5 Pt 1):389–92.
62. Leibovitz E, Piglansky L, Raiz S, Press J, Leiberman A, Dagan R. Bacteriologic and clinical efficacy of one day vs. three day intramuscular ceftriaxone for treatment of nonresponsive acute otitis media in children. Pediatr Infect Dis J. 2000;19(11):1040–5.
63. Heikkinen T, Saeed KA, McCormick DP, Baldwin C, Reisner BS, Chonmaitree T. A single intramuscular dose of ceftriaxone changes nasopharyngeal bacterial flora in children with acute otitis media. Acta Paediatr. 2000;89(11):1316–21.
64. Noel GJ, Blumer JL, Pichichero ME, Hedrick JA, Schwartz RH, Balis DA, et al. A randomized comparative study of levofloxacin versus amoxicillin/clavulanate for treatment of infants and young children with recurrent or persistent acute otitis media. Pediatr Infect Dis J. 2008;27(6):483–9.
65. Pichichero ME, Casey JR. Emergence of a multiresistant serotype 19A pneumococcal strain not included in the 7-valent conjugate vaccine as an otopathogen in children. JAMA. 2007;298(15):1772–8.
66. Wald ER, Applegate KE, Bordley C, Darrow DH, Glode MP, Marcy SM, et al. Clinical practice guideline for the diagnosis and management of acute bacterial sinusitis in children aged 1 to 18 years. Pediatrics. 2013;132(1): e262–80.
67. Schwartz RH, Rodriguez WJ, Grundfast KM. Duration of middle ear effusion after acute otitis media. Pediatr Infect Dis. 1984;3(3):204–7.
68. Shurin PA, Pelton SI, Donner A, Klein JO. Persistence of middle-ear effusion after acute otitis media in children. N Engl J Med. 1979;300(20):1121–3.
69. Roberts JE, Rosenfeld RM, Zeisel SA. Otitis media and speech and language: a meta-analysis of prospective studies. Pediatrics. 2004;113(3 Pt 1):e238–48.
70. Berman SA, Balkany TJ, Simmons MA. Otitis media in the neonatal intensive care unit. Pediatrics. 1978;62(2): 198–201.
71. Mandel EM, Rockette HE, Bluestone CD, Paradise JL, Nozza RJ. Efficacy of amoxicillin with and without decongestant-antihistamine for otitis media with effusion in children. Results of a double-blind, randomized trial. N Engl J Med. 1987;316(8):432–7.
72. Chonmaitree T, Saeed K, Uchida T, Heikkinen T, Baldwin CD, Freeman Jr DH, et al. A randomized, placebo-controlled trial of the effect of antihistamine or corticosteroid treatment in acute otitis media. J Pediatr. 2003;143(3):377–85.
73. Clements DA, Langdon L, Bland C, Walter E. Influenza A vaccine decreases the incidence of otitis media in 6- to 30-month-old children in day care. Arch Pediatr Adolesc Med. 1995;149(10):1113–7.
74. Heikkinen T, Block SL, Toback SL, Wu X, Ambrose CS. Effectiveness of intranasal live attenuated influenza vaccine against all-cause acute otitis media in children. Pediatr Infect Dis J. 2013;32(6):669–74.
75. Hoberman A, Paradise JL, Reynolds EA, Urkin J. Efficacy of Auralgan for treating ear pain in children with acute otitis media. Arch Pediatr Adolesc Med. 1997;151(7):675–8.
76. Rosenfeld RM, Schwartz SR, Pynnonen MA, Tunkel DE, Hussey HM, Fichera JS, et al. Clinical practice guideline: tympanostomy tubes in children. Otolaryngol Head Neck Surg. 2013;149(1 Suppl):S1–35.
77. Rosenfeld RM, Kay D. Natural history of untreated otitis media. Laryngoscope. 2003;113(10):1645–57. Epub 2003/10/02. eng.
78. Kay DJ, Nelson M, Rosenfeld RM. Meta-analysis of tympanostomy tube sequelae. Otolaryngol Head Neck Surg. 2001;124(4):374–80. Epub 2001/04/03. eng.

Chapter 4
Complications of Acute and Chronic Otitis Media

Nicholas J. Bennett, Scott R. Schoem, and Kyle Johnson

Introduction

Even though pediatric acute otitis media is very common, most children outgrow the underlying Eustachian tube dysfunction without any sequelae. However, a significant number will encounter mild or moderate degrees of complications with lingering effects into adulthood. These individuals will have permanent problems including hearing loss, speech articulation problems, eardrum perforation with occasional infections called otorrhea, and occasional pain and pressure issues due to lingering Eustachian tube dysfunction. A much smaller subpopulation will encounter serious or life-threatening intracranial complications.

In the preantibiotic era, complications of acute otitis media were very common with frequent hospital admissions due to intracranial complications such as meningitis, brain abscess and sigmoid sinus thrombosis. The incidence drastically decreased in the 1960s through the 1980s, only to re-emerge with the advent of antibiotic resistance and some degree of clinical complacency that antibiotics alone would cure acute mastoiditis. In nations with reduced access to adequate medical care, acute otitis media and mastoiditis leads to much higher complication rates and permanent disabilities.

This chapter discusses both common and uncommon complications of acute otitis media. The authors also introduce promising current and future research endeavors to alleviate Eustachian tube dysfunction.

N.J. Bennett, M.B.B.Chir., Ph.D.
Division of Infectious Diseases and Immunology, Connecticut Children's Medical Center, Hartford, CT, USA

S.R. Schoem, M.D.
Department of Otolaryngology, Connecticut Children's Medical Center, Hartford, CT, USA

K. Johnson, M.D. (✉)
Department of Otolaryngology, University of Connecticut School of Health Sciences, 263 Farmington Avenue, Farmington, CT 06030, USA
e-mail: Kjohnson@resident.uchc.edu

T.A. Valdez, J.G. Vallejo (eds.), *Infectious Diseases in Pediatric Otolaryngology*,
DOI 10.1007/978-3-319-21744-4_4

Normal Anatomy and Function

The middle ear is an air containing space in the temporal bone medial to the eardrum. The eardrum itself is approximately 1 cm square and is composed of 4 layers: squamous epithelium laterally, radial and circular fibrous layers, and mucosa medially. Attached to the medial surface of the eardrum is a chain of bony ossicles known as the malleus, incus, and stapes. The footplate of the stapes rests in the oval window of the cochlea [1]. Sound is conducted from the external world and the external auditory canal to the cochlea through mechanical vibration of the eardrum and ossicles. This mechanical energy is transduced into neural signals in the cochlea and conducted to the brain via the eighth cranial nerve [2]. This conduction of sound through the middle ear functions optimally when air in the middle ear space is at roughly the same pressure as air in the outside world. Unfortunately, the body tends to readily resorb air in any space in the body. Resorption of air in the middle ear leads to a negative pressure system, which then dampens vibrations in the eardrum and ossicles. The body overcomes this tendency to negative pressure in the middle ear with a valve connecting the middle ear space and the nasopharynx, known as the Eustachian tube. The Eustachian tube consists of a bony portion in the temporal bone that descends in a medial to lateral direction as it runs anteriorly from the temporal bone. The anteroinferior aspect of the Eustachian tube consists of a C-shaped cartilage connected to several muscles with a mucosal covering. The orifice of the Eustachian tube is closed in its resting position but opens during swallowing with contraction of the tensor veli palatini muscle, which is the primary dilator of the tube and attaches to the soft palate. Opening of the Eustachian tube orifice allows for air to enter and equalize the pressure of the middle ear space, allowing normal function of the auditory apparatus [3].

Importantly, the temporal bone is in close proximity to the skull base. The temporal bone is pyramidal in shape with its base located laterally and the apex located medially immediately adjacent to the cavernous sinus. The superior aspect of the temporal bone forms part of the floor of the middle cranial fossa, while the posterior wall of the temporal bone constitutes a large portion of the anterior floor of the posterior cranial fossa. Also along the posterior wall of the temporal bone is the sigmoid sinus. Anteriorly, the temporal bone connects to the sphenoid bone creating the roof of the infratemporal fossa. Also immediately anterior to the temporal bone lies the glenoid fossa where the temporomandibular joint articulates [1]. The parotid gland abuts the anterior aspect of the temporal bone at its lateral extent. In addition to the air containing middle ear space housed in the temporal bone, another space known as the mastoid resides posterior to the middle ear within the temporal bone. The mastoid is a usually aerated spaced with multiple air cells divided by bony septae. The mastoid connects with the attic or superior aspect of the middle ear space anteriorly through a space known as the aditus ad antrum. Thus aeration of the mastoid air cells is accomplished via appropriate function of the Eustachian tube as described above. The close proximity of these several structures to the temporal bone accounts for their involvement in complicated forms of otitis media as discussed below.

Pathophysiology

In some individuals, Eustachian tube function is insufficient to allow for consistent, sufficient aeration of the middle ear space. This is particularly true of young children, owing largely to the fact that their Eustachian tubes are shorter and oriented more horizontally than in adults, thus predisposing them to more frequent bouts of otitis media. The immature nature of young children also predisposes them to frequent viral upper respiratory infections [4]. Inflammation in the region of the nasopharynx from a URI leads to edema and swelling of the Eustachian tube orifice. This edema may temporarily worsen Eustachian tube function. When the Eustachian tube is unable to open for an extended period of time, the air in the middle ear is absorbed to the point that negative pressure develops within the middle ear space, retracting the eardrum medially [5]. As this negative pressure builds, it allows for accumulation of serous fluid excreted by the mucosal cells lining the middle ear. The fluid can then become secondarily infected as the negative pressure in the middle ear provides a pressure differential to draw bacteria-containing secretions from the nasopharynx, leading to acute otitis media (AOM) [6]. Infection of the fluid leads to influx of white blood cells to combat the infection and release of inflammatory mediators. The increased cell count in the fluid leads to increased osmolarity of the fluid, leading to further influx of fluid into the middle ear space. However, given that the space is primarily fixed due to its bony confines, increased pressure in the middle ear space leads to bulging of the eardrum laterally. Stretching of the eardrum and inflammation of the mucosa are the primary causes of the symptoms of AOM. If left unchecked, the infection can spread posteriorly via the aditus ad antrum to involve the mastoid air space, leading to mastoiditis. Progression of AOM to include intracranial complications is most commonly believed to be due to hematogenous dissemination or direct extension through preexisting pathways from the temporal bone to adjacent structures [7]. Fortunately the routine use of antibiotics has made complications of otitis media much less common than they were in the pre-antibiotic era.

Microbiology

The microbiology of otitis media (OM) is similar to that of other respiratory tract infections, and almost exclusively the causative agents are either viruses or bacteria. Fungal infections are rare and are more typically seen in the context of chronic infections or otitis externa. Mycobacterial infections are very rare.

Common viruses that can cause otitis media include respiratory syncitial virus (RSV), influenza, parainfluenza, and metapneumovirus. Prophylaxis for RSV in the form of monoclonal antibody injections for at-risk infants reduces the rate of OM, as does influenza vaccination. Viral infections are generally self-limited and do not require treatment or preventative antibiotics "just in case". Secondary bacterial infections can and do occur. Even in cases where a viral cause is identified, it is wise to watch for signs of worsening infection and act accordingly.

The routine identification of causative organisms in the setting of OM is no longer done. This requires tympanocentesis, which is unlikely to be performed in the outpatient setting. Historically, *Streptococcus pneumoniae*, *Haemophilus influenzae* and *Moraxella catarrhalis* were the predominant organisms responsible for OM. *S. pneumoniae* and some strains of *H. influenzae* are encapsulated organisms, with a polysaccharide coat that surrounds the bacterial cell and provides a degree of immune evasion. Younger children, in particular those under the age of two, are unable to mount a vigorous and lasting response to polysaccharide antigens. The ability to recognize and respond adequately to these bacteria improves with age, and above the age of 5 years the risk of serious infection is much lower. (See Chap. 3 for causes of Otitis Media in the era of PCV13.)

S. pneumoniae is a gram-positive coccus, often described as "lancet shaped" on gram stain, with a polysaccharide capsule. The capsule provides a degree of immune evasion as primary B cell responses against polysaccharides are blunted in the first few years of life. It is a predominant bacterial pathogen associated with respiratory tract diseases, such as OM, sinusitis, pneumonia, bronchitis, bacteremia and meningitis. There are over 90 capsular serotypes of *S. pneumoniae*, but the majority of invasive disease is caused by only a few strains.

H. influenzae is a gram-negative cocco-bacillus, which can appear pleomorphic on gram stain when grown in liquid media. It can also be encapsulated, with the more serious capsular type being *H. influenzae* type B. Non-typeable *H. influenzae* are less likely to cause invasive disease, but can still contribute to

OM and some lower respiratory tract infections, and in vaccinated children the non-typeable strains are likely to be the predominant type.

Moraxella catarrhalis is a gram-negative diplococcus, which often has a beta-lactamase enzyme present. Unlike the other two predominant pathogens, there is no evidence that it has a capsule to provide immune evasion. No vaccine exists for the organism, although it does appear that certain outer proteins are immunogenic. It is far less likely to cause serious invasive disease, such as bacteremia or meningitis. It is a cause of some cases of pneumonia and bronchitis.

Mycoplasma pneumoniae is an atypical bacterium that lacks a cell wall, and as such is intrinsically resistant to beta-lactam antibiotics. It is a cause of upper and lower respiratory tract disease, and in particular is known for causing a bullous myringitis. Mycoplasma infection is more common in those aged 5 and older, and may be due to it being commonly acquired in the school setting. There is no vaccine, but it is readily treated with macrolide antibiotics. Mycoplasma is not routinely cultured even if tympanocentesis is performed, due to the methods requiring prolonged incubation and microscopic examination, but PCR testing is available. Serology for mycoplasma IgM is sensitive but can be non-specific, and cold agglutinins may be a better test of acute disease [8, 9]. In general therapy for mycoplasma is empiric, as the time taken to obtain and confirm a diagnosis may be longer than the typical course of antibiotic therapy.

One aspect of the microbiology of OM is the formation of biofilms, which consist of mucus and bacterial flora, and which may provide protection from both the immune system and antibiotics. Non-pathogenic organisms that produce proteins that confer antibiotic-resistance may create a local environment in which antibiotic-susceptible organisms can flourish in the face of normally effective therapy. Biofilm formation has been shown to be common in those with chronic otitis media [10]. Staphylococcal species, including staphylococcus aureus and coagulase-negative staphylococcal species appear to be frequent isolates from biofilms although they are not a common cause of acute otitis media [11, 12].

The microbiology of OM favors the use of empiric narrow-spectrum therapy with beta-lactam antibiotics such as amoxicillin. Penicillin resistance in *S. pneumoniae* is mediated through a mutated penicillin-binding protein (PBP2x) and can be overcome with higher doses of antibiotic (80–90 mg/kg/day of amoxicillin, compared to 45 mg/kg/day in conventional dosing) [13]. Resistance in some strains of *H. influenzae* and Moraxella is through the production of a beta-lactamase enzyme that hydrolyzes the beta-lactam ring in penicillins, and can be overcome through the use of combination therapy with a penicillin and a beta-lactamase inhibitor such a clavulanic acid. Alternative agents may include oral cephalosporins with significant gram-negative activity such as second or third generation cephalosporins, although the oral bioavailability of these agents can be significantly less than that of amoxicillin. Macrolides such as azithromycin may have some activity, but resistance among pneumococcal isolates is relatively frequent and as such they would not be recommended as first-line agents. The fluoroquinolones, in particular levofloxacin, have excellent broad-spectrum activity against a wide range of respiratory pathogens, but should be used only as a drug of last resort in children due to concerns regarding side effects and the promotion of antibiotic resistance. The use of ciprofloxacin ear drops is a notable exception, as topical use may provide significant therapeutic effect while avoiding systemic side effects, particularly in cases of chronic OM with perforation.

Immune Deficiency

There are several immune deficiencies that predispose children to more frequent or severe OM, and frequent OM (more than eight in a year) may be the first sign of a problem with the immune system.

The most common problem is a defect in humoral immunity involving antibody responses. Naive B cells produce IgM, a pentameric molecule with high avidity but low affinity, as well as a surface IgD with identical antigen recognition to the secreted IgM. Antigen recognition, in particular in the context of concomitant T cell stimulation results first in a class-switch to one of the final immunoglobulin classes (IgG, IgA or IgE) and then a process of somatic hypermutation and affinity maturation to produce highly specific and effective antibodies.

The most serious antibody deficiencies involve a total loss of Immunoglobulin G (IgG). Bruton's Hypogammaglobulinemia is an X-linked disease where there is a total lack of B cells and as such no immune globulins are present. Children (almost exclusively boys) with Bruton's disease will present with frequent, recurrent infections including OM, but also more serious infections from pathogenic bacteria such as pneumococcal pneumonia or bacteremia. X-linked immunodeficiency with hyper IgM (XHIGM) is a class-switching failure and is due to a mutation in the T cell protein CD40-ligand. Children with mutations in the B cell protein CD40 may present with a similar phenotype but it is autosomal recessive. Children with hyper-IgM have absent IgG, IgA or IgE but develop very high levels of IgM as they age—IgM levels may be normal in infants and young children. They lack an ability to produce lasting immunity to infections, and in addition have a high risk of opportunistic infections from pneumocystis jirovecii and enterovirus. Without immune globulin replacement therapy these immune deficiencies are usually fatal in childhood.

IgG2 subclass deficiency is a specific isolated defect that predisposes the individual to infection from encapsulated organisms. IgG2 recognizes polysaccharide antigens as compared to the protein antigens recognized by IgG1 and IgG3, and because the predominant respiratory pathogens are pneumococcus and *H. influenzae*, infections from these organisms are then much more common. There will be no immunity to these organisms from either natural infection or from vaccination. IgG2 subclass deficiency can be treated with immune globulin replacement therapy to reduce the frequency and severity of infections.

IgA deficiency is a common finding (approximately 1 in 600 people) but in and of itself this may not actually pose a serious problem. IgA provides immunity at mucosal surfaces, being found in tears, saliva, breast milk and in the gastrointestinal tract. Those lacking IgA still have protection from serious encapsulated organisms through IgG subclass 2, so it may be prudent to test subclasses in those who are IgA-deficient. Isolated IgA deficiency is not amenable to immune globulin replacement therapy, and in fact those who are IgA-deficient often require low-IgA immune globulin products to avoid the risk of developing serious anaphylactic reactions through the development of anti-IgA IgE.

Children with Common Variable Immunodeficiency (CVID) present with recurrent or chronic respiratory infections, as well as chronic gastrointestinal complaints. They may have slightly low total IgG levels, or may even be within the normal range. They often have poor to absent responses to vaccinations, in particular the conjugated polysaccharide vaccines (pneumococcus and Hib). Some patients show an initial response to repeat vaccination, with a loss of immunity within 6–12 months. This is due to a defect in B cell memory, and in many instances may be a transient delay in the maturation of the immune system. Up to a third of children with recurrent OM may have a defect in polysaccharide immune memory [14], but how many of these go on to require long-term treatment for CVID is unclear.

Complement deficiencies are a collection of defects in the innate humoral immune system that can be broadly divided into early and late (terminal) complement deficiencies. Complement is particularly important in providing protection from encapsulated organisms, such as those that cause upper and lower respiratory tract infections. Children with terminal complement deficiencies are at a particular risk from invasive, recurrent infection with *Neisseria meningitidis*. Deficiency of the C3 or C4 components, which initiate the alternative complement pathway, is associated with recurrent upper and sometimes lower respiratory tract disease. Mannose binding protein (MBP) is another initiator of the complement cascade and very low levels of MBP are associated with recurrent upper respiratory tract infections, in particular sinusitis. Due to the extremely rapid degradation of the complement components in the blood, there is no replacement option for routine prophylaxis. Protection from infections usually is provided by prophylactic antibiotics.

An important immune deficiency syndrome associated with recurrent OM is that of 22q11.2 deletion syndrome (also known as DiGeorge Syndrome, Velocardiofacial Syndrome, and Shprintzen Syndrome). 22q11.2 deletion is frequently associated with immunologic abnormalities, the most well-known being thymic aplasia and T cell lymphopenia. This may result, rarely, in a severe immune deficiency requiring thymic transplant, but more commonly the child has low absolute T cell numbers, with preserved T cell function and a normal ratio of CD4+ helper and CD8+ cytotoxic T cells. Many children with 22q11.2del have significant problems with OM in the early years of childhood, and interestingly this has little bearing on their future likelihood of immune deficiency or dysfunction. It appears to be primarily an issue with the anatomy of the ear. Children with 22q11.2del may have small, cupped pinnae, and narrow, tortuous outer ear canals. Presumably similar changes are found internally that affect the normal fluid drainage and pressure equalization of the middle ear. In addition, people with 22q11.2del have a particular problem with healing of the tympanic membrane, and even when they no longer have problems with infections they may have persistent perforations of the ear drum that last well into adulthood. Caution should be exercised in the placement of pressure-equalizing tubes in these patients as the surgical defect may become permanent.

Some children with 22q11.2del go on to develop a CVID-like immune deficiency with low IgG or poor vaccine responses, and long-term followup and monitoring with a specialist is recommended.

Very severe immune deficiencies involving absence of T cells, HIV infection, or severe-combined immune deficiency (SCID) more typically present with more severe or unusual infections than isolated OM, and in the absence of more serious issues patients and families can generally be reassured that these conditions can be ruled out.

In general, if there is a suspicion of an immune deficiency contributing to the frequency of a particular child's ear infections, consultation with an infectious disease specialist or immunologist is recommended.

Immunization

Childhood vaccinations to the common bacterial pathogens of childhood have led to significant reductions in the risk of invasive infection from these organisms.

The two main organisms that have proven to be amenable to vaccination are *S. pneumoniae* and *H. influenzae*. Both have polysaccharide capsules that assist immune evasion, and which infants and younger children have difficulty mounting an effective immune response to. Plain polysaccharide vaccines have much lower effectiveness in children under the age of 2 years. The covalent modification of the antigen through conjugation with a protein toxoid (either tetanus or diphtheria toxoid) engages T cell help to the B cell responses, and promotes B cell memory. Conjugate vaccines can also be boosted through repeated dosing, something that in plain polysaccharide vaccines is generally not possible, and which may in fact induce B cell anergy to the target antigen.

The conjugated polysaccharide vaccine against pneumococcus has led to dramatic reductions in the rates of serious disease. A 7-valent vaccine introduced in 2000 lowered infections due to S. pneumoniae in young children by 80–90 %. In the decade following that, there was a small but significant rise in non-vaccine strains causing disease. Two in particular, 19A and 6A, were associated with more invasive disease, a higher rate of *S. pneumoniae*-related hemolytic uremic syndrome [15], and higher rates of antibiotic resistance. In 2010 a 13-valent vaccine was introduced that included these, and other serotypes, with the goal of addressing these issues. Early indications are that, at least in terms of invasive disease such as pneumonia, further gains have been realized.

The introduction of the conjugated Hib vaccine reduced infections by more than 99 %, with no sign of serotype replacement with other invasive strains. Much of the Haemophilus disease seen in the vaccine era is from non-typeable Haemophilus, and is far less serious.

Developmental Complications

Hearing Loss

Hearing loss is an important potential complication of otitis media, particularly in the chronic forms of the disease. Tympanic membrane perforations, chronic middle ear effusion, and erosion of the ossicles in the middle ear can all lead to conductive hearing loss. This occurs due to dampening of the vibrations as they travel through the eardrum and ossicles of the middle ear, in the case of chronic effusions, or frank disruption of the conductive system, in the case of ossicular erosion. Chronic suppurative otitis media (CSOM), in particular, is associated with permanent hearing loss in as many as half of patients affected with the disease, especially in developing nations where CSOM is more prevalent [16]. Formation of cholesteatoma (discussed below) can also lead to erosion through to the cochlea, leading to sensorineural hearing loss, although this is less common. In patients with less severe disease, the relationship between long term hearing loss and otitis media is less clear. Patients with middle ear effusions do suffer from a conductive hearing loss as long as the effusion is present [17]. However, studies have failed to definitively prove a long term hearing benefit to placement of PE tubes in children [18]. In fact, a Cochrane review in 2010 concluded that the hearing benefit obtained by the placement of PE tubes in children with documented hearing loss and otitis media with effusion was no better than the improvement in hearing that naturally occurs with age in children not treated surgically [19]. Therefore, according to the currently available body of literature, appropriately treated uncomplicated otitis media tends to have little lasting effect on a person's hearing. However, progression to chronic otitis media can have profound deleterious effects on hearing, particularly when diagnosis and treatment is delayed, such as in developing nations.

Speech Delay

Speech delay is an especially important concern in the pediatric population, as the first 2 years of life are a critical period for developing communicative abilities. During this time period, language development depends on exposure to language stimulus [20]. Hearing loss not corrected in the first several years of life is one major contributor to speech delay. However, the influence of recurrent acute otitis media (RAOM), particularly after the age of 2–3 years, on speech development is unclear. There is a theoretical possibility that any hearing loss during infancy or the toddler years, even if temporary, can have adverse effects on the development of speech and language. Multiple studies have attempted to evaluate the relationship between otitis media and speech development, with some finding a negative effect on speech development and others finding no effect. However, a recent meta analysis failed to find sufficient evidence from well-designed studies to establish a clear and indisputable adverse effect of otitis media on speech development [21]. That meta-analysis noted that otitis media with effusion potentially has a very small to no effect on speech development, but the authors felt this modest effect may have in fact been an overestimation due to pooled studies failing to control for known confounding factors such as low socioeconomic status. Fortunately, otherwise healthy children with uncomplicated otitis media, even when it is recurrent or persistent enough to warrant placement of tympanostomy tubes, do not appear to suffer from significant speech delay according to the currently available literature.

Intratemporal, Extracranial Complications

Eardrum Perforation

Typically, acute otitis media with rupture heals spontaneously without sequelae; however, repeated episodes of acute otitis media with rupture may result in persistent perforation. In addition, insertion of pressure equalizing ear tubes may lead to eardrum perforation with the rate of perforation depending on the size and construction of the tube (Fig. 4.1). The eardrum often has focal areas of myringosclerosis (scar plaques) or focal areas of retraction. Usually, these are visual findings on physician exam without any functional hearing deficit. Eardrum perforation should be distinguished from retraction. The advantage of eardrum perforation is protection against the slow, but steady negative pressure exerted against the undersurface of the eardrum leading to global retraction, permanent adhesive changes or development of cholesteatoma. Therefore, a perforation may be beneficial functioning as an ear tube without the appliance.

Several issues should be investigated before considering surgical closure of a long-standing eardrum perforation [22]. First, age plays a role. Closure at 5–6 years old, before the child may have outgrown Eustachian tube dysfunction, can lead to recollection of middle ear fluid and conductive hearing impairment, or retraction with potential ossicular erosion or cholesteatoma. Additionally, if the individual still has endogenous (not swimming related) ear infections with intermittent otorrhea, the perforation may well serve as an exit portal and be an asset rather than a liability.

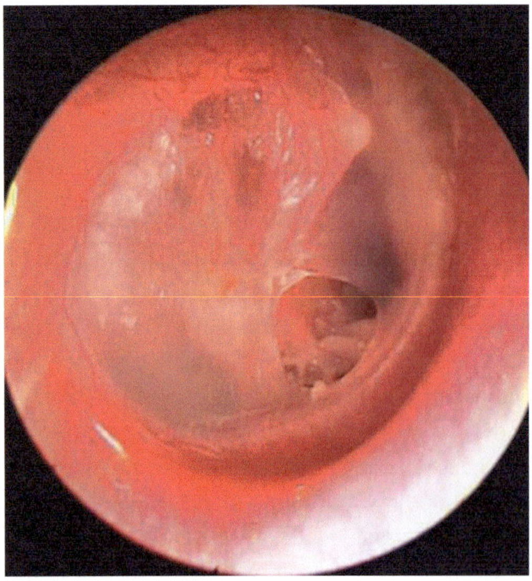

Fig. 4.1 Typical eardrum perforation following tympanostomy tube extrusion

The necessity of using a swim plug for eardrum perforation is controversial. Within the past two decades, recommendations have shifted from always using a plug to situational use depending on the type of water (pool, pond, lake, ocean) and depth of swimming [23]. Currently, most otolaryngologists recommend a plug for non-pool swimming and water exposure below 2–3 ft.

Surgical closure of persistent perforation is typically based on surgeon preference. However, a few guidelines are helpful. First, if the individual has a conductive hearing impairment greater than expected due to perforation alone, the ossicles should be examined as part of the procedure. This requires exploration of the middle ear (tympanoplasty) rather than attempt at closure of the perforation alone (myringoplasty). Second, even in the era of minimally invasive surgery, adequate exposure of the entire eardrum perforation and the size of the ear canal are important factors. If the ear canal accommodates only a 4or 4.5 mm speculum, enlargement of the ear canal or a postauricular approach may be necessary for success. Hearing results after tympanoplasty for perforation are not easily predictable [24]. Chronic middle ear disease may lead to acoustical changes that are not surgically correctable.

Adhesive Otitis Media

Consistent negative pressure due to ongoing Eustachian tube dysfunction acts as a vacuum on the undersurface of the eardrum leading to progressive eardrum retraction. When controlled early enough in the process via ventilation, the ear tube arrests the process. Without ventilation, ongoing severe negative pressure may lead to global retraction forming permanent adhesive scar bands from the undersurface of the eardrum to the ossicles and floor of the middle ear, collapse of the middle ear space and adhesive otitis media or "saran wrap" ear. Surprisingly, this may result in very minimal conductive hearing impairment if sound is conducted through the ossicles and oval window. However, in most cases, there is at least mild hearing impairment. The incus-stapes joint is often eroded and occasionally the stapes itself becomes eroded. Adhesive otitis media usually remains as a self-cleaning ear without formation of granulation tissue or cholesteatoma formation (Fig. 4.2).

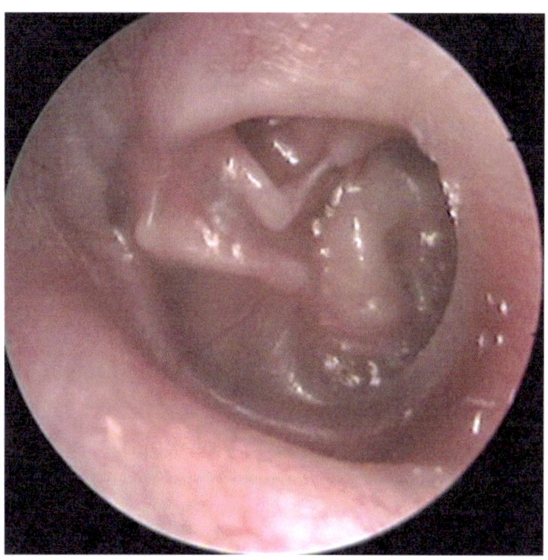

Fig. 4.2 Severe eardrum atelectasis after many years of Eustachian tube dysfunction

Treatment recommendations for this situation are controversial. Options include monitoring alone with periodic hearing assessment, placement of an ear tube through the eardrum for ventilation, placement of a subannular ear tube for ventilation [25, 26], and cartilage tympanoplasty [27, 28]. The use of transnasal balloon dilation of the Eustachian tube is currently experimental in adults.

Chronic Otorrhea

Whereas some eardrum perforations remain clean and dry, others may intermittently drain mucopurulent infection [29]. If the ear drains only a few times each year and resolves within 1–2 weeks using antibiotic ear drops, then there is little concern. However, if the drainage persists longer than 3 weeks or resumes drainage soon after cessation, then the ear may have chronic infection within the mastoid cavity or chronically infected mastoid cholesteatoma. Some individuals may have small eardrum perforations with occasional otorrhea during upper respiratory infections. If drainage persists longer than 3 weeks, a bacterial and fungal culture should be obtained to help guide therapy.

For unremitting drainage, CT scan with contrast of the mastoid may help determine if long-term antibiotics or mastoidectomy may be beneficial. MRI is oversensitive for detection of mastoid disease and does not detect bony defects, as does CT scan.

Ossicular Erosion

Long-term Eustachian tube dysfunction with negative pressure or chronic drainage may lead to erosion of the incus-stapes joint and further erosion of both the incus and stapes bones leading to conductive hearing impairment [30, 31]. Yet, there are no prospective studies addressing how long this process takes to occur and when is the proper time of intervention to arrest this process. Moreover, cholesteatoma formation may erode the ossicles leading to conductive hearing impairment.

Ossicular erosion may occur by direct pressure exerted by the retracted eardrum, ongoing infection with inflammation or enzymatic bony destruction due to cholesteatoma. Commonly, the lenticular process of the incus is involved with incus-stapes disarticulation. Continuation of the process leads to stapes erosion. Usually, the malleus is spared.

Despite advances in technology, ossicular replacement with prostheses remains only moderately successful. Presence of the stapes bone leads to a higher success rate of ossicular reconstruction than with absence of the stapes [32–34].

Facial Nerve Paralysis

At any time, acute otitis media may cause acute facial nerve paresis or paralysis [35–37]. This is a direct toxic effect of the bacteria rather than an erosive process of the bone surrounding the nerve sheath. Facial nerve weakness is more likely if there is a natural bone dehiscence within the middle ear with a direct toxic effect on the nerve sheath. Treatment is urgent myringotomy with ventilation tube placement and culture-directed antibiotic therapy. Prompt therapy leads to over 95 % return of facial nerve function. However, delayed therapy may impair resolution of facial nerve weakness with residual permanent injury.

Cholesteatoma (Keratoma)

The term cholesteatoma is a misnomer and has no meaning. The term was coined in the 1850s when the thought was that this represented a growth or "oma" of cholesterin. Even though the proper term is "keratoma": meaning "skin growth," The literature continues to perpetuate the word cholesteatoma and it seems difficult to purge this from our lexicon (Figs. 4.3 and 4.4).

Acquired cholesteatoma may occur in several ways. Classically taught, focal eardrum retraction of the posterior half of the eardrum may extend to and beyond the incus and stapes bones with erosion of the ossicles [38] along with trapping of skin debris and formation of granulation tissue. If instead, or in addition, the posterior, superior portion of the eardrum called the pars flaccida retracts from the attic region behind to the antrum of the mastoid, this is termed an attic retraction cholesteatoma. An attic retraction cholesteatoma does not usually lead to ossicular damage unless there is a concurrent

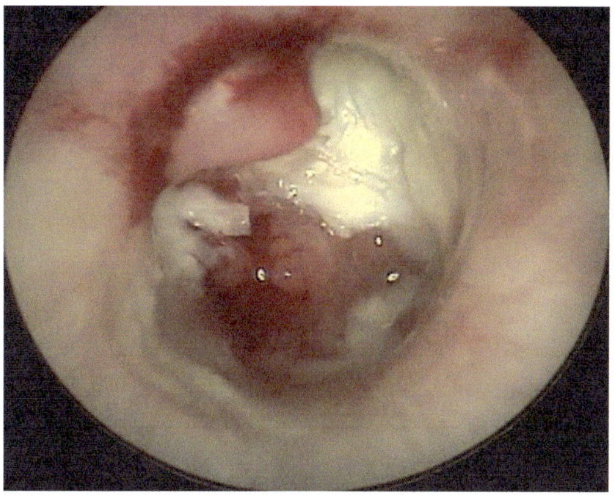

Fig. 4.3 Photo of middle ear cholesteatoma with granulation tissue

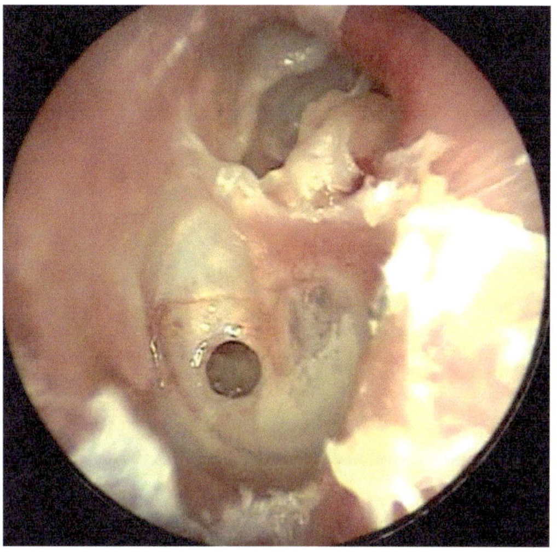

Fig. 4.4 Photo of attic retraction cholesteatoma and eardrum perforation

middle ear component tracking towards to incus and stapes. Other mechanisms of cholesteatoma formation include implantation of skin behind the eardrum after repeated eardrum rupture due to acute infection or occasionally due to a surgically created perforation as with ear ventilation tubes. Acquired cholesteatomas may remain clean and dry or may become chronically infected with mixed aerobic and anaerobic bacteria.

The cholesteatoma dissolves bone both by direct extension and by halisteresis (bone resorption through enzymatic destruction). This process may become very destructive with erosion of the bone separating the mastoid from the middle cranial fossa called the tegmen. The bone covering the floor of the mastoid may also erode with extension to the posterior fossa. Infection may then lead to intratemporal, intracranial complications. Treatment is surgical and may require several, staged surgeries for successful keratoma removal and ossicular reconstruction [39–42]. Pediatric ossicular reconstruction is less successful than in the adult population.

Acute Mastoiditis

An acute middle ear infection by definition leads to infection in the mastoid cavity via direct extension through the attic region of the middle ear, which is the portion of the middle ear cavity superior to the eardrum. Therefore, radiographically, the mastoid cavity will be expected to have infection just as the middle ear. However, an acute otitis media with radiographic fluid in the mastoid does not equate clinically with a diagnosis of acute mastoiditis. Rather, the diagnosis of acute mastoiditis depends on clinical findings. Early findings are fever, pain and erythema and edema behind the ear over the mastoid bone equating with the largest air cell of the mastoid called the antrum (Fig. 4.5). Next, as the mastoid diploic veins become engorged and develops venous congestion, the swelling increases pushing the conchal bowl of the ear outward and then downward (proptosis). Internally, the infection dissolves the trabecular network of bony partitions within the honey-combed mastoid cavity leading to coalescent mastoiditis. The cortex may then erode externally leading to a subperiosteal abscess and/ or internally leading to an epidural abscess or brain abscess. A Bezold abscess develops when the

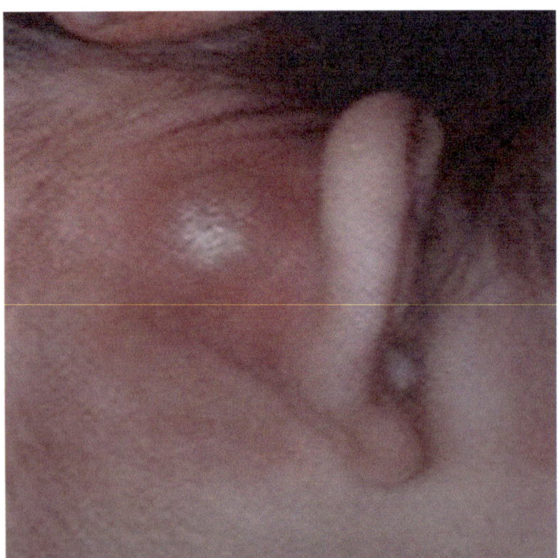

Fig. 4.5 Clinical photo of early mastoiditis

infection erodes through the mastoid tip into the neck. Gradenigo syndrome is the triad of deep unremitting ear pain, ear drainage and Cranial Nerve VI (abducens) paralysis.

The incidence of acute mastoiditis has declined since introduction of the heptavalent pneumococcal conjugate vaccine (PCV7) in 2000 [43, 44]. However, the clinician must guard against a false sense of security regarding the efficacy of intravenous antibiotic therapy alone, without prompt surgical intervention to arrest the infectious process, especially in the presence of intracranial complications [45, 46].

Intratemporal, Intracranial Complications

The overall incidence of intracranial complications has declined dramatically. However, masked symptoms and signs may lead to a false sense of security with delayed therapy or undertreatment. The clinician needs to be keenly aware of circumstances that warrant concern including deep unremitting ear pain, vertigo and only partial response to antibiotic therapy.

Advances in imaging technology have greatly enhanced the ability to make critical, life-saving decisions quickly. Magnetic resonance imaging with vascular flow studies help pinpoint the site and extent of disease.

Meningitis

The incidence of bacterial meningitis has greatly decreased in well-vaccinated populations. Vaccination with PCV 7 and PCV 13 has been instrumental in reduction of pneumococcal meningitis, with reductions in the order of 80–90 %, almost exclusively in vaccine serotypes [47].

Meningitis is a medical emergency, requiring immediate initiation of intravenous, broad-spectrum antibiotics (typically a third generation cephalosporin in combination with vancomycin to cover for resistant pneumococcus). It is a rare complication of otitis media and more typically occurs through hematogenous spread, subsequent to initial invasion of the retropharyngeal tissues by the pathogenic bacteria that are common oral flora. Meningitis can occur secondary to infection in adjacent structures, such as the frontal or mastoid air sinuses, and in that setting the onset may be sudden and catastrophic.

Although the diagnosis can be made clinically it usually requires a lumbar puncture be performed to obtain cerebrospinal fluid (CSF) for analysis, gram stain, and culture. Bacterial meningitis typically has high white cell counts in the CSF (1000's per microliter) with a neutrophil predominance, low glucose and high protein. Bacteria may or may not be visible on gram stain, but usually grow readily from fluid cultures. Antibiotic therapy should not be delayed for results, and in fact should ideally not be delayed by the attempts to perform the lumbar puncture. If the lumbar puncture cannot be performed quickly, empiric therapy followed by subsequent attempts to obtain CSF for analysis is the standard of care.

The duration of treatment varies by pathogen—from as short as a week for Neisseria meningitides to 3 weeks or more for enteric organisms. Consultation with an infectious disease specialist is recommended.

There is a risk of sensorineural hearing loss secondary to bacterial meningitis, and all patients who have meningitis should have a hearing test performed at the end of therapy.

Epidural Abscess

Acute mastoiditis may lead to an epidural abscess via direct extension of infection through natural dehiscences of bone to either the middle or posterior fossa. The most common site is extension through the tegmen bone separating the mastoid cavity from the middle cranial fossa (Figs. 4.6, 4.7 and 4.8). The presenting symptom is deep seated, throbbing pain from dural traction. Neurosurgical consultation should be obtained. When small, the abscess will usually resolve with mastoidectomy and culture directed intravenous antibiotics. When extensive, the intracranial abscess may require neurosurgical drainage [48].

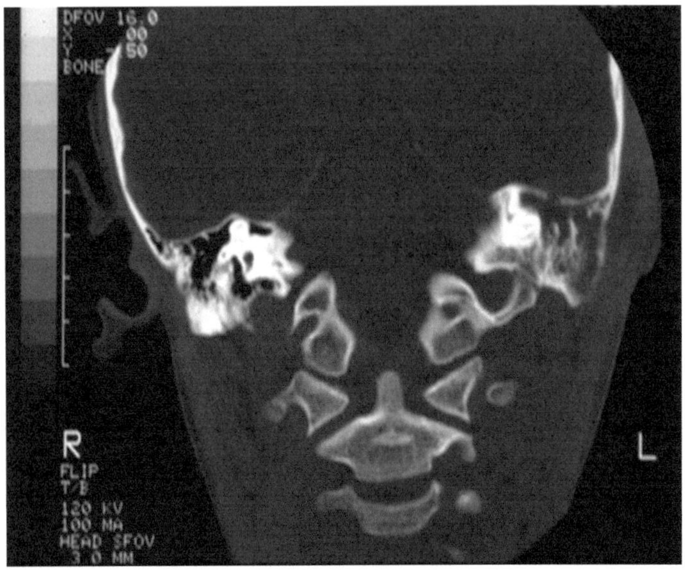

Fig. 4.6 CT scan of bony erosion of tegmen that separates mastoid from middle cranial fossa

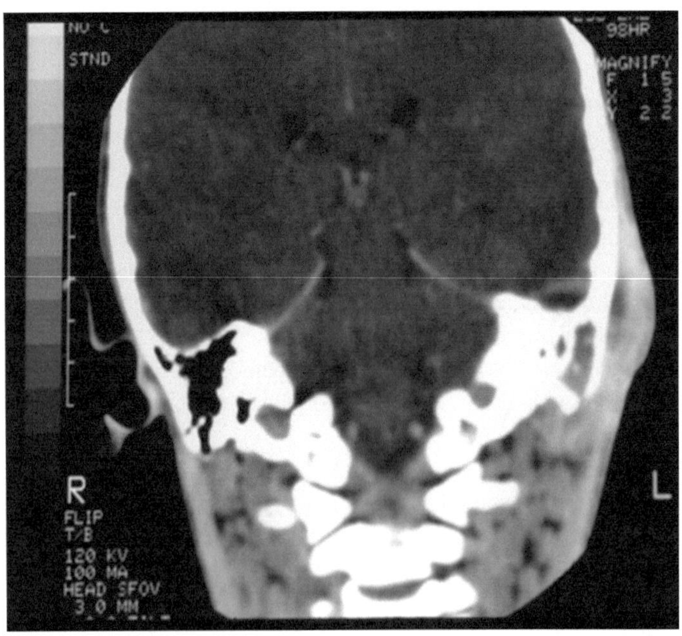

Fig. 4.7 CT scan from same patient of epidural abscess

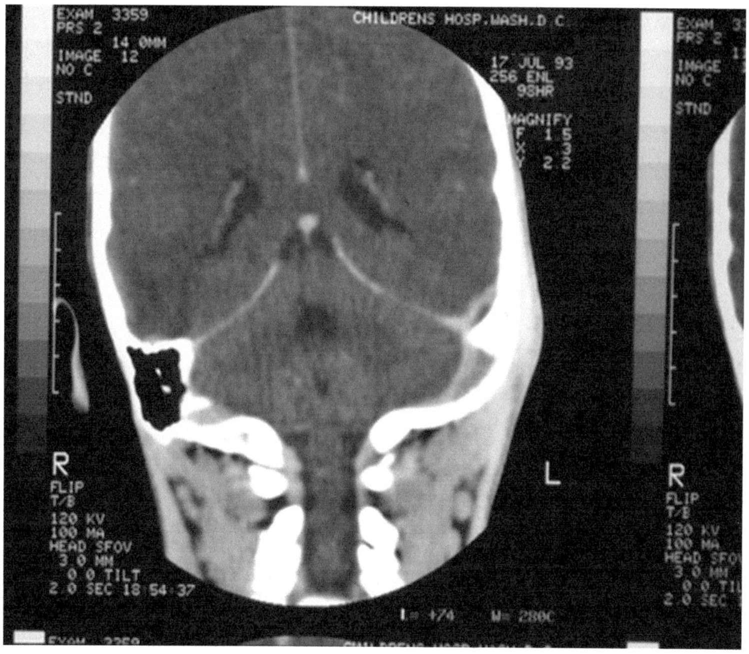

Fig. 4.8 CT scan from same patient of sigmoid sinus thrombosis

Sigmoid Sinus Thrombosis

In the preantibiotic era, sigmoid sinus thrombosis was a more frequent complication of acute mastoiditis. The classic sign of "picket fence" fever referred to the wide swings in temperature with high fever followed by resolution, and then resumption of high fever repeating the cycle. Although sinus thrombosis is still seen, the symptoms and signs are often muted by use of oral antibiotics and fever-reducing medications. Deep pain, fever, and high white blood cell count are cardinal features. When assessing for acute mastoiditis, CT scan with contrast may indicate suspicion for sinus thrombosis. A more conclusive follow up study is magnetic resonance imaging with venography.

Both medical and surgical therapy options are controversial. Surgically, some experts advocate only performing a mastoidectomy whereas others recommend uncapping the bone overlying the sinus, incising and evacuating clot from the sinus. Duration of intravenous antibiotic therapy also varies. In addition, opinions vary on whether anticoagulation therapy is required and for how long to treat based on risk of clot propagation and stroke [49].

Labyrinthitis

Labyrinthitis occurs when infection spreads through either the round window or oval window of the middle ear into the inner ear. This may lead to vertigo, sensorineural hearing loss or both [45, 48]. Myringotomy with culture may help guide antibiotic therapy and ventilation tube placement may speed up the recovery.

Brain Abscess

True brain abscess extends through the tegmen and dura into the temporal lobe, or via the sigmoid sinus into the posterior fossa [46, 48]. An infected cholesteatoma may also erode through the dura into the brain. Clinical presentation may include high fever, vertigo, seizures, severe headache, irritability and lethargy. More worrisome signs include visual field deficits, papilledema and hydrocephalus. Urgent and aggressive medical and surgical therapy is required.

References

1. Anson B, Donaldson J. Surgical anatomy of the temporal bone. 3rd ed. Philadelphia: Saunders; 1981.
2. Geisler CD. From sound to synapse. Oxford: Oxford University Press; 1998.
3. Cunsolo E, Marchioni D, Leo G, Incorvaia C, Presutti L. Functional anatomy of the Eustachian tube. Int J Immunopathol Pharmacol. 2010;23(1 Suppl):4–7.
4. Bluestone CD, Swarts JH. Human evolutionary history: consequences for the pathogenesis of otitis media. Otolaryngol Head Neck Surg. 2010;143(6):739–44.
5. Rettig E, Tunkel DE. Contemporary concepts in management of acute otitis media in children. Otolaryngol Clin North Am. 2014;47(5):651–72.
6. Rovers MM, Schilder AG, Zielhuis GA, et al. Otitis media. Lancet. 2004;363(9407):465–73.
7. Harker LA. Cranial and intracranial complications of acute and chronic otitis media. In: Snow JB, Ballenger JJ, editors. Ballenger's otorhinolaryngology head and neck surgery. 16th ed. Hamilton: Decker; 2003. p. 294–316.
8. Qu J, et al. Accuracy of IgM antibody testing, FQ-PCR and culture in laboratory diagnosis of acute infection by Mycoplasma pneumoniae in adults and adolescents with community-acquired pneumonia. BMC Infect Dis. 2013;13:172.
9. Shankar EM, et al. Serosurveillance of acute Mycoplasma pneumoniae infection among HIV infected patients with pulmonary complaints in Chennai, Southern India. J Infect. 2006;53(5):325–30.
10. Gu X, Keyoumu Y, Long L, Zhang H. Detection of bacterial biofilms in different types of chronic otitis media. Eur Arch Otorhinolaryngol. 2014;271(11):2877–83.
11. Zhao AS, et al. Impact of 13-valent pneumococcal conjugate vaccine on otitis media bacteriology. Int J Pediatr Otorhinolaryngol. 2014;78(3):499–503.
12. Casey JR, Adlowitz DG, Pichichero ME. New patterns in the otopathogens causing acute otitis media six to eight years after introduction of pneumococcal conjugate vaccine. Pediatr Infect Dis J. 2010;29(4):304–9.
13. Dagan R, et al. Bacteriologic and clinical efficacy of high dose amoxicillin/clavulanate in children with acute otitis media. Pediatr Infect Dis J. 2001;20(9):829–37.
14. Sharma SK, Casey JR, Pichichero ME. Reduced serum IgG responses to pneumococcal antigens in otitis-prone children may be due to poor memory B-cell generation. J Infect Dis. 2012;205(8):1225–9.
15. Bannerjee R, et al. Streptococcus pneumoniae-associated hemolytic uremic syndrome among children in North America. Pediatr Infect Dis J. 2011;30(9):736–9.
16. Jensen RG, Koch A, Homøe P. The risk of hearing loss in a population with a high prevalence of chronic suppurative otitis media. Int J Pediatr Otorhinolaryngol. 2013;77(9):1530–5.
17. Rovers MM, Stratman H, Ingels K, et al. The effect of short-term ventilation tubes versus watchful waiting on hearing in young children with persistent otitis media with effusion: a randomized trial. Ear Hear. 2001;22(3):191–9.
18. Khodaverdi M, Jørgensen G, Lange T, Stangerup SE, Drozdziewizc D, Tos M, Bonding P, Caye-Thomasen P. Hearing 25 years after surgical treatment of otitis media with effusion in early childhood. Int J Pediatr Otorhinolaryngol. 2013;77(2):241–7.
19. Browning GG, Rovers MM, Williamson I, Lous J, Burton MJ. Grommets (ventilation tubes) for hearing loss associated with otitis media with effusion in children. Cochrane Database Syst Rev. 2010;10, CD001801.
20. Tonn CR, Grundfast KM. What an otolaryngologist should know about evaluation of a child referred for delay in speech development. JAMA Otolaryngol Head Neck Surg. 2014;140(3):259–65.
21. Roberts JE, Rosenfeld RM, Zeisel SA. Otitis media and speech and language: a meta-analysis of prospective studies. Pediatrics. 2004;113(3 Pt 1):e238–48.
22. James AL, Papsin BC. Ten top considerations in pediatric tympanoplasty. Otolaryngol Head Neck Surg. 2012;147(6):992–8.
23. Derkay CS, Shroyer MN, Ashby J. Water precautions in children with tympanostomy tubes. Am J Otolaryngol. 1992;13(5):301–5.

24. Kent DT, Kitsko DJ, Wine T, Chi DH. Frequency-specific hearing outcomes in pediatric type 1 tympanoplasty. JAMA Otolaryngol Head Neck Surg. 2014;140(2):106–11.
25. Cloutier JF, Arcand P, Martinez J, Abela A, Quintal MC, Guerguerian AJ. Subannular ventilation tubes: retrospective study. J Otolaryngol. 2005;34(5):312–6.
26. Elluru RG, Dhanda R, Neely JG, Goebel JA. Anterior subannular T-tube for prolonged middle ear ventilation during tympanoplasty: evaluation of efficacy and complications. Otol Neurotol. 2001;22(6):761–5.
27. Friedman AB, Gluth MB, Moore PC, Dornhoffer JL. Outcomes of cartilage tympanoplasty in the pediatric population. Otolaryngol Head Neck Surg. 2013;148(2):297–301.
28. Velepic M, Starcevic R, Ticac R, Kunjundzic M. Cartilage palisade tympanoplasty in children and adults: long term results. Int J Pediatr Otorhinolaryngol. 2012;76(5):663–6.
29. Van Dongen TM, van der Heijden GJ, Freling HG, Venekamp RP, Schilder AG. Parent-reported otorrhea in children with tympanostomy tubes: incidence and predictors. PLoS One. 2013;8(7), e69062.
30. Guo Y, Liu Y, Lu QH, Zheng KH, Shi LJ, Wang QJ. CT two-dimensional reformation versus three-dimensional volume rendering with regard to surgical finding in the preoperative assessment of the ossicular chain in chronic suppurative otitis media. Eur J Radiol. 2013;82(9):1519–24.
31. Choi SA, Kang HM, Byun JY, Park MS, Yeo SG. Analysis of differences in facial nerve dehiscence and ossicular injury in chronic otitis media and cholesteatoma. Acta Otolaryngol. 2014;134(5):455–61.
32. Berenholz LP, Burkey LM, Lippy WH. Short- and long-term results of ossicular reconstruction using partial and total plastipore prostheses. Otol Neurotol. 2013;34(5):884–9.
33. Wolter NE, Holler T, Cushing SL, Chadha NK, Gordon KA, James AL, Papsin BC. Pediatric ossiculoplasty with titanium total ossicular replacement prosthesis. Laryngoscope. 2014;125(3):740–5. doi:10.1002/lary.24896.
34. Hess-Erga J, Moller P, Vassbotn FS. Long-term hearing result using Kurz titanium ossicular implants. Eur Arch Otorhinolaryngol. 2013;270(6):1817–21.
35. Pelligrini S, Gonzalez Macchi ME, Sommerfleck PA, Bernaldez PC. Intratemporal complications from acute otitis media in children: 17 cases in two years. Acta Otorrinolaringol Esp. 2012;63(1):21–5.
36. Elliott CA, Zalzal GH, Gottlieb WR. Acute otitis media and facial nerve paralysis in children. Ann Otol Rhinol Laryngol. 1996;105(1):58–62.
37. Evans AK, Licameli G, Brietzke S, Whittemore K, Kenna M. Pediatric facial paralysis: patients, management and outcomes. Int J Pediatr Otorhinolaryngol. 2005;69(11):1521–8.
38. Mohammadi G, Naderpour M, Mousaviagdas M. Ossicular erosion in patients requiring surgery for cholesteatoma. Iran J Otorhinolaryngol. 2012;24(68):125–8.
39. Diom ES, Cisse Z, Tall A, Ndiaye M, Pegbessou E, Ndiaye IC, Diallo BK, Diouf R, Diop EM. Management of acquired cholesteatoma in children: a 15 year review in ENT service of CHNU de FANN Dakar. Int J Pediatr Otorhinolaryngol. 2013;77(12):1998–2003.
40. Edfeldt L, Kinnefors A, Stromback K, Kobler S, Rask-Andersen H. Surgical treatment of paediatric cholesteatoma: long-term follow up in comparison with adults. Int J Pediatr Otorhinolaryngol. 2012;76(8):1091–7.
41. Shirazi MA, Muzaffar K, Leonetti JP, Marzo S. Surgical treatment of pediatric cholesteatomas. Laryngoscope. 2006;116(9):1603–7.
42. McRackan TR, Abdellatif WM, Wanna GB, Rivas A, Gupta N, Dietrich MS, Haynes DS. Evaluation of second look procedures for pediatric cholesteatomas. Otolaryngol Head Neck Surg. 2011;145(1):154–60.
43. Tamir SO, Roth Y, Dalal I, Goldfarb A, Marom T. Acute mastoiditis in the pneumococcal conjugate vaccine era. Clin Vaccine Immunol. 2014;21(8):1189–91.
44. Halgrimson WR, Chan KH, Abzug MJ, Perkins JN, Carosone-Link P, Simoes EA. Incidence of acute mastoiditis in Colorado children in the pneumococcal conjugate vaccine era. Pediatr Infect Dis J. 2014;33(5):453–7.
45. Maranhao AS, Andrade JS, Godofredo VR, Matos RC, Penido NO. Intratemporal complications of otitis media. Braz J Otorhinolaryngol. 2013;79(2):141–9.
46. Sun J, Sun J. Intratemporal complications of chronic otitis media. Eur Arch Otorhinolaryngol. 2014;271(11):2923–6.
47. Mvint TT, et al. The impact of 7-valent pneumococcal conjugate vaccine on invasive pneumococcal disease: a literature review. Adv Ther. 2013;30(2):127–51.
48. Isaacson B, Mirabal C, Kutz Jr JW, Lee KH, Roland PS. Pediatric otogenic intracranial abscesses. Otolaryngol Head Neck Surg. 2010;142(3):434–7.
49. Ulanovski D, Yacobovich J, Kornreich L, Shkalim V, Raveh E. Pediatric otogenic sigmoid sinus thrombosis: 12 year experience. Int J Pediatr Otorhinolaryngol. 2014;78(6):930–3.

Chapter 5
Inner Ear Infections

Corrie E. Roehm and Marisol Fernandez

Introduction

The inner ear can be affected by a variety of pathologies, including autoimmune processes, allergies, inflammatory processes [1] and infections. Depending on which portion of the inner ear is affected, clinical manifestations can include hearing loss, which can be unilateral or bilateral and vary from mild to severe loss or deafness, and difficulties with balance control. Several clinical entities are potentially associated with infections of the inner ear. These include acute labyrinthitis, labyrinthine neuritis, sudden sensorineural hearing loss (SSNHL) and Meniere's disease. This chapter will focus on common pediatric pathologies of congenital hearing loss, acute labyrinthitis, and labyrinthine neuritis.

Important to note in a chapter on infectious diseases of the inner ear is the practical difficulty of proving that a given infectious agent causes an infection in the human labyrinth. Non-invasive evaluations (physical examination, imaging, non-otologic laboratory testing from peripheral blood or tissue sampling) cannot definitively prove infectious causality [2]. In many studies, clinical association of an infection with symptoms of labyrinthine inflammation (vertigo, hearing loss) is confirmed with isolation of the agent at a non-otologic, peripheral site. Sampling from the inner ear directly poses significant risk to the inner ear structures, and is available only in intraoperative perilymph sampling, as during a cochlear implantation, or in postmortem temporal bone specimens. Polymerase chain reaction (PCR), tissue culture or electron microscopy detection of viral nucleic acid can prove presence of the infectious agent within inner ear structures, but is often remote to the acute infection, and can be difficult to demonstrate direct causality of pathophysiologic damage to the tissue. Animal models have also been utilized to demonstrate similar clinical symptoms and correlate this with inner ear pathologic specimens [3]. Temporal bone histologic studies do, however, provide useful information comparing differing tissue effects from various infectious agents, and will be included in this discussion where possible.

C.E. Roehm, M.D.
Department of Pediatric Otolaryngology, Dell Children's Hospital, Austin, TX, USA

M. Fernandez, M.D. (✉)
Department of Pediatric Infectious Diseases, Dell Children's Medical Center, Seton Healthcare Family, 1301 Barbara Jordan Blvd., Austin, TX 78723, USA
e-mail: mfernandez@sfcaustin.com

T.A. Valdez, J.G. Vallejo (eds.), *Infectious Diseases in Pediatric Otolaryngology*,
DOI 10.1007/978-3-319-21744-4_5

Anatomy

To better understand how infections affect the inner ear, it is important to understand temporal bone and inner ear anatomy. The inner ear is protected in the solid osseous otic capsule of the temporal bone and includes the cochlear (hearing) and the vestibular (balance) system (Fig. 5.1). Both systems are comprised of fluid-filled tubes of the membranous labyrinth encased by osseous channels within the temporal bone, known as the bony labyrinth, that includes the cochlea, the semicircular canals, and the vestibule. Suspended inside the bony labyrinth, the fluid-filled membranous labyrinth also contains three corresponding parts: the cochlear duct inside the cochlea, the semicircular ducts and cristae inside the semicircular canals, and the saccule and utricle inside the vestibule. In the spiral of the cochlea, the cochlear duct spans the width of the spiral, dividing it into three separate fluid-filled tubes, the scala vestibuli caudally (separated from the cochlear duct by the thin Reissner's membrane), the cochlear duct (or scala media) between, and the scala tympani dorsally (separated from the cochlear duct by the more architecturally complex basilar membrane and the spiral lamina). The basilar membrane houses the Organ of Corti, which, with its inner and outer hair cells, converts mechanical sound energy vibrating the basilar membrane into electrical impulses that transmit sound information to the cochlear nerve and into the auditory pathway. The tube of the membranous labyrinth is filled with endolymph, and is surrounded by perilymph that suspends it within the space of the bony labyrinth. In the cochlea, the scala vestibuli and scala tympani are filled with perilymph and connect at the helicotrema in the cochlear apex, while the scala media between them is filled with endolymph. The cochlear endolymph in the scala media

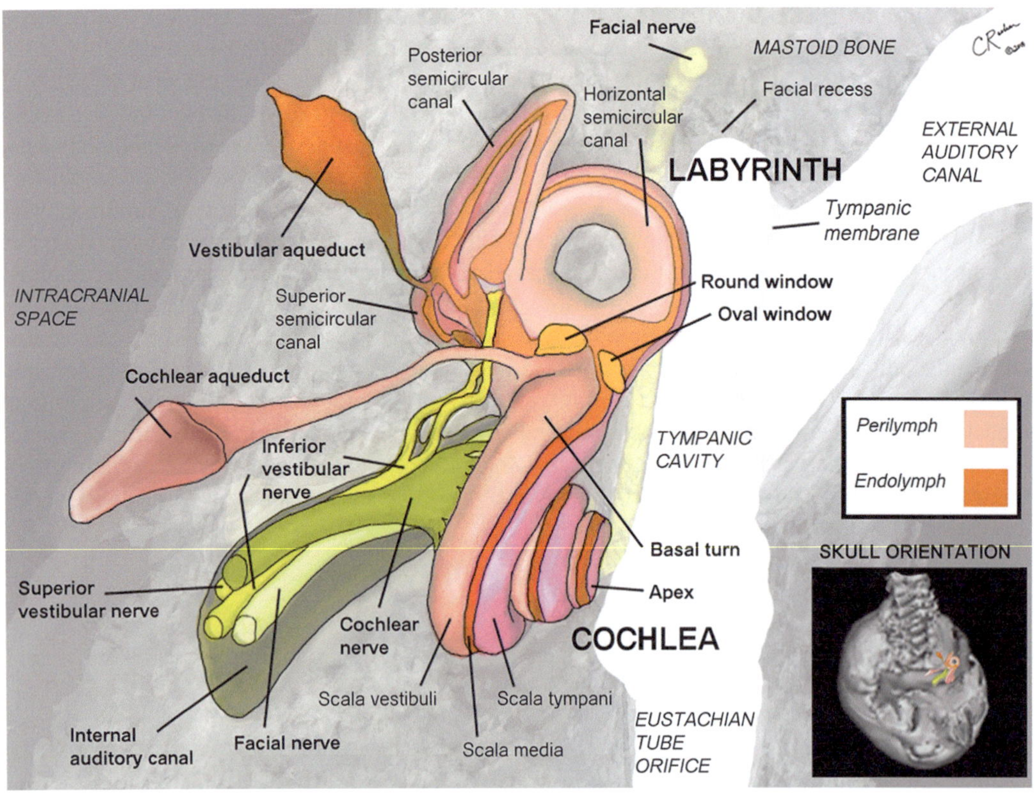

Fig. 5.1 Inner ear anatomy and surrounding structures. Endolymph (*orange*) fills the membranous labyrinth that is suspended within the bony labyrinth, cushioned by surrounding perilymph (*pink*). Right ear from an inferior oblique view (see skull orientation) to demonstrate the cochlear and vestibular aqueducts. © Corrie Roehm

continues into the vestibule through the ductus reuniens and the saccular duct. Small bony channels passing through the temporal bone connect the inner ear fluid spaces to the intracranial vault, including the vestibular aqueduct containing the endolymphatic sac, and the cochlear aqueduct. Endolymph extends out to the intracranial vault in the posterior fossa through the closed endolymphatic sac within the vestibular aqueduct. Perilymph is directly connected to the intracranial space and cerebrospinal fluid through the cochlear aqueduct. This hourglass-shaped open bony channel starts in the posterior fossa and ends in the scala tympani of the basal turn of the cochlea adjacent to the round window membrane. The cranial orifice of the cochlear aqueduct is covered with a dura-arachnoid sheath extending into the aqueduct for a variable length, and the bony walls of the cochlear aqueduct are lined with connective tissue that in one study occupied the entire duct volume in approximately 60 % of specimens, with a patent central cochlear duct lumen in 34 % [4]. The vestibular aqueduct and the internal auditory canal to the cochlear aperture are also potential connections to the CSF space if abnormally enlarged, as seen with enlarged vestibular aqueduct or dilated cochlear aperture. If the bony capsule of the inner ear is violated, perilymph will escape, driven by the hydrostatic pressure of CSF, and will be replaced by CSF moving into the cochlear aqueduct that is slowly transitioned into perilymph as it enters the inner ear. Persisting leaks of perilymph can occur in a perilymph fistula. The oval and round window membranes are thin separations between the inner ear and the middle ear or tympanic space, and also provide potential entrance to the inner ear.

Inner Ear Infections

Infections affecting the inner ear can be classified as primary (infections that intrinsically involve the inner ear), or secondary (infections that affect the inner ear by extension from contiguous anatomic structures) (Table 5.1). Pathogens can reach the inner ear by multiple routes, including hematogenously, via the meninges, through anatomic connections in the temporal bone between the cerebrospinal fluid and the inner ear (cochlear duct, vestibular aqueduct), from the middle ear through the oval or round window, or through abnormal congenital or acquired dehiscence of the otic capsule [5]. Vertical infections include maternal to fetal transmission of pathogens across the placental membranes, resulting in congenital infections. Pathogens can also enter the inner ear through colonization of intracochlear implants [6], particularly in now-discontinued implant models utilizing an intracochlear spacer or electrode positioner [7]. Cochlear implants are increasingly used in pediatrics for the treatment of severe to profound sensorineural hearing loss and can become secondarily infected,

Table 5.1 Organisms associated with inner ear infections

Conditions associated with primary inner ear infections	Conditions associated with secondary inner ear infections
Vestibular neuritis	Bacterial meningitis
Labyrinthitis	Cochlear implants
Labyrinthitis ossificans	Middle ear infections
Infectious agents associated with primary infections	**Infectious agents associated with secondary infections**
Cytomegalovirus	*Streptococcus pneumoniae*
Rubella	*Haemophilus influenza* type b
Measles	*Staphylococcus aureus*
Syphilis	Group A *streptococcus*
Toxoplasmosis	*Pseudomonas aeruginosa*
Herpes virus simplex/Varicella zoster	Fungus
Parvovirus B 19	*Mycobacterium tuberculosis*
Mycoplasma pneumoniae	Atypical mycobacterium

introducing infection into the inner ear along the intracochlear electrode through surgical openings into the cochlea including the round window membrane or a cochleostomy. A study conducted to describe the microbial flora associated with infected and non-infected cochlear implants, based on indication for removal, found all tested implants to have evidence of microbes [6]. The bacterial species involved was different depending on whether the indication for removal was infection or another cause. *Staphylococcus aureus* was more commonly isolated from infected cochlear implants. Biofilm formation has also been recognized as a cause of cochlear implant failures, even when infection was not the indication for implant removal [8].

Etiologies of Primary Inner Ear Infections

Cytomegalovirus (CMV)

CMV belongs to the family of the herpesvirus group and it can remain latent in tissues after initial infection. The route of acquisition of CMV infection includes horizontal transmission (person to person), via the respiratory tract, urinary, genital tract or contact with infected bodily fluids, or by transfusion of CMV infected blood products; and vertical transmission (mother to infant). Vertical transmission can result in congenital infection, which can be associated with hearing loss.

Vertical transmission can occur at any time during pregnancy or at the time of birth. Vertical transmission occurs in about 30 % of infected mothers, but not all fetuses are affected. Congenital CMV infection occurs in about 1 % of all live-born infants and the majority of infected neonates appear healthy at birth. Symptomatic congenital infection can be acquired at any time during pregnancy, but congenital infection with severe sequalae is most likely associated with primary maternal infection in the first half of pregnancy.

Horizontally acquired CMV infection, even in neonates, can be symptomatic affecting multiple organ systems, but it is not associated with hearing loss.

Congenital CMV infection is the leading cause of sensorineural hearing loss [9].

Hearing loss can be present at birth and diagnosed with universal newborn hearing screening, or it can develop months to years later. The hearing loss is typically progressive through childhood. The deficit can be unilateral or bilateral, with bilateral hearing loss developing in 37 % of congenitally infected symptomatic infants [9]. Congenital CMV hearing loss involves cochlear damage primarily in the scala media and the marginal cell layer of the stria vascularis, with associated generalized inflammation in the organ of Corti, the cochlear nerve and spiral ganglia [10]. In a study of human fetuses at 21 weeks gestation with known CMV infection, virus was isolated from the inner ear fluid in 45 % of the fetuses studied, and in more than half both inner ears were infected with multiple structures involved [11]. A recent study of 76 pediatric patient receiving cochlear implants, found that more than 14 % were due to CMV. Perilymph fluid obtained at the time of implant placement, was compared to CMV from dried blood spots, and in one case of congenital CMV infection, viral strains were found to be genotypically identical [12]. The onset of progressive hearing loss usually occurs during the preschool years. But this decline in hearing has also been observed in school age children with congenital CMV. This finding underlies the importance of early diagnosis of CMV infection and possibility of offering close audiologic evaluation for congenitally infected neonates. Evidence of disseminated infection at birth (petechial, thrombocytopenia, intrauterine growth retardation, hepatitis or hepatosplenomegaly) is predictive of hearing loss, with about a third to half of children with symptomatic CMV infection developing hearing loss [13].

Diagnosis of congenital CMV infection is by definition confirmed within the first 3 weeks of life. Viral culture of the urine evaluating for CMV is a non-invasive standard diagnostic approach, and should be considered in neonates that are found to have abnormal hearing tests [14]. CMV detection by PCR technology of blood or cerebrospinal fluid has become readily available in commercial laboratories and can also be used for diagnosis. An approach for diagnosis of asymptomatic congenitally infected neonates needs to be standardized. Neonates with hearing loss, should be evaluated by an otorhinolaryngologists and tested for CMV infection. If CMV testing is positive, referral to a pediatric infectious disease specialist is recommended for further evaluation and treatment.

Regarding therapeutic approaches for congenital CMV infection, ganciclovir has been used for the past several decades. A randomized controlled trial using ganciclovir intravenously for 6 weeks in neonates with symptomatic CMV infection, involving the central nervous system showed hearing improvement or maintenance of normal hearing in about 80 % of the infant treated at 6 month follow up [15]. Development of neutropenia is common during therapy as well as liver enzyme abnormalities, and these should be monitored.

A study evaluating the use of prolonged (6 months) oral valganciclovir in symptomatic infants with congenital CMV has shown that language and receptive communication scores were superior in the group of infants receiving 6 months of oral valganciclovir with normal hearing also more likely to occur at 6 month follow up (46 % vs. 56 %), 12 month follow up (50 % vs. 65 %) and 24 month follow up (60 % vs. 68 %) [16]. A similar study in Europe has shown promising results [17].

A therapeutic dilemma remains in otherwise well appearing neonates who are found to have hearing loss and test positive for CMV, but have no radiologic evidence of CNS involvement. There may be a role for oral valganciclovir in this population.

Rubella

Rubella virus is a positive-stranded RNA virus. It belongs to the Togaviridae family. Maternal infection can result in congenital rubella syndrome. Fetal involvement earlier in pregnancy results in a higher incidence of congenital defects. Infection occurring during the third trimester of pregnancy results more commonly in deafness and retinopathy. The association between congenital rubella and deafness was first recognized in the 1940s and the virus has been shown to infect the inner ear [18].

Hearing is affected in 68–93 % of infected infants. As seen with CMV infection, hearing loss can be unilateral or bilateral and progressive ([19, 20]).

The diagnosis should be suspected when there is maternal history of infection during pregnancy or if the infant presents with clinical manifestations compatible with congenital rubella syndrome, including cataracts, congenital heart disease, hearing impairment, pigmentary retinopathy, microcephaly and developmental delay. The risk of congenital infection and defects is highest during the first 12 weeks of pregnancy, and decreases after the 12th week, with rare defects after the 20th week of gestation [21]. Serology testing with rubella IgM can provide information, but with higher risk of false positive compared to culture results [22]. The virus can be isolated in culture, up to 1 year after infection in specimens from throat, urine, blood and CSF.

There is no antiviral therapy available for congenital rubella infection. The most important preventive measure is maternal vaccination against rubella. Routine rubella immunization as part of the MMR, is recommended at 12–15 months of age, with a second dose prior to school entry at 4–6 years. Rubella vaccine should not be given to pregnant women or to those women considering pregnancy within 3 months of vaccine, but women that are found to be rubella non-immune should be vaccinated at the time of delivery.

Mumps

Mumps virus is an enveloped negative-stranded RNA virus, and it belongs to the Paramyxoviridae family. Infection with this virus is acquired via contact with infected respiratory secretions. After local viral replication in the nasopharyngeal region, there is a phase of viremia that allows the mumps virus to infect the central nervous system, salivary glandular tissue and testis most commonly. Although involvement of the inner ear is not frequently reported, association of mumps infection with hearing loss is well recognized [23]. Hearing loss is usually unilateral and in most cases reversible.

The association of mumps inner ear infection as the cause of hearing loss was reported in a 26 year with prior history of otosclerosis who 2 years after successful stapedectomy, developed mumps and subsequent unilateral hearing loss. At the time of surgical exploration to rule out complications from the otosclerosis process or a perilymph fistula, culture of the perilymph was positive for mumps [24].

Mumps is suspected in patients with parotitis and it can be confirmed using serology (presence of positive IgM or rising IgG levels). Viral culture, in special media for mumps, from pharynx, CSF or urine can also be performed. PCR is also available from the Centers for Disease Control and Prevention or commercial laboratories of buccal or oral swabs.

There is no specific antiviral therapy against this infection. Vaccination remains the most important tool for prevention. Two doses of mumps vaccine, as part of the MMR, are recommended at 12–15 months and 4–6 years of age.

Measles

Measles (Rubeola) belongs to the Paramyxoviridae family and it is formed by a single-stranded negative-sense RNA genome. After the incubation period (8–12 days), infected patients develop fever, hacking cough, conjunctivitis (nonpurulent), and coryza. Within 48–72 h, Koplik spots develop, and a generalized rash usually appears at the peak of respiratory symptoms.

The most common complication in pediatric patients infected with measles is acute otitis media, but hearing loss is not a frequent event. Measles was reported to be the cause of hearing loss in 13 % of African children with hearing impairment of known etiology [25].

Pathologic changes of the temporal bone with associated severe necrotizing otitis media has been reported in four fatal cases of measles infection. Half of the patients had inner ear changes, similar to those seen in congenital rubella syndrome [26].

Severe hearing loss after measles vaccination has been reported and it is usually associated with encephalitis [27]. These cases are rare and should not have a negative impact on recommendations regarding vaccination.

Measles is diagnosed in patients with compatible clinical presentation. Serologic testing can help confirm the diagnosis. Increasing IgM levels, when comparing acute and convalescent serum, indicate recent infection. Culture of this virus is difficult, and serology is the recommended diagnostic tool.

No specific antiviral therapy exists. Vaccination is effective in preventing disease development.

Syphilis

Syphilis is caused by *Treponema pallidum*. Congenital infection is acquired by the infant from an infected mother, via the placenta. Transmission to the fetus can occur in any stage of syphilitic infection.

Clinical complications of congenital syphilis develop later in life, including sensorineural hearing loss (related to osteochondritis of otic capsule and cochlear architecture degeneration), keratitis and Hutchinson's teeth. Eighth nerve deafness often starts with high frequency hearing loss when the child is between 8 and 10 years of age [28]. Hearing loss is usually bilateral and it can fluctuate. Meniere's disease can also develop as a consequence of syphilis infection. Otosyphilis has been associated with development of endolymphatic hydrops. Temporal bone changes including microgummata, bone reabsorption, or new bone formation have been described in specimens belonging to patients with proven syphilis [29]. Literature from the 1960s describes a group of patients treated with steroids, showing improvement in more than 50 %. Patients were treated with penicillin at the time of diagnosis, if they had never received therapy [30]. A case report of bilateral deafness associated with acquired syphilis, non-primary, showed that medical therapy restored unilateral hearing [31]. Other studies have shown variable response to antibiotics and steroids [32].

Screening for syphilis during early pregnancy, and providing antibiotic treatment to infected mothers, is the best preventive measure against congenital syphilis. Women should be retested at the time of delivery.

In patients that present with sensorineural hearing loss of unknown etiology, luetic, or syphilitic, inner ear disease should be included in the differential diagnosis. If serologic tests as nontreponemal (RPR or VDRL) confirmed by treponemal tests (MHATP or AFT-ABS) are found to be positive, the patient should receive steroids and antibiotics [33]. Penicillin remains the drug of choice, and in cases of otosyphilis, the same regimen used for treatment of neurosyphilis is recommended: Intravenous Aqueous Crystalline Penicillin G for 14 days [34].

Toxoplasmosis

Toxoplasma gondii is an intracellular protozoan parasite and it the cause of toxoplasmosis. Infection occurs when bradyzoites are ingested, during laboratory accidents, via blood transfusion or organ transplantation with infected specimens of tissue or transplacentally. If a pregnant woman acquires the infection early in pregnancy, fetal tissue necrosis usually occurs and affects many tissues, including brain and eye. If the infection is acquired later in pregnancy, the fetus is less severely affected.

Delayed onset, or progressive, hearing loss is reported in up 26 % of in utero acquired toxoplasmosis cases, and those children should undergo audiologic follow up. The incidence of hearing loss correlates with incomplete treatment or lack of treatment for congenitally acquired toxoplasmosis [35]. None of the children that received complete therapy, consisting of 12 months of antiparasitic treatment with Pyrimethamine, Sulfadiazine and Leucovorin, and before they were 2½ years old, developed hearing loss [36]. Audiologic re-evaluation is recommended at 24–30 months of age. For those children with incomplete or no treatment, audiologic evaluation should be performed yearly, until they can reliably complete behavioral audiologic testing [36].

In a histopathology study of temporal bones of nine newborns who died from congenital toxoplasmosis, 37 % had free or encysted organisms in the temporal bone, and in two of those infants numerous encysted organisms were found inside the inner ear without evidence of tissue necrosis or an inflammatory response. Cystic forms are not associated with an inflammatory response. Hearing loss may be secondary to delayed reactivation of the cystic form to the active tachyzoite, which could be prevented by treatment [37]. Serologic and molecular diagnostic testing in suspected cases of congenital toxoplasmosis should be performed at reference laboratories, and includes testing of blood and CSF. Treatment of congenitally-acquired toxoplasmosis requires combination therapy of one year duration to have a positive impact on hearing outcomes [37–39].

Herpes Virus Simplex (HSV)

HSV type 1 and 2 has been implicated in cases of sudden, sensorineural hearing loss in children. As with many other herpes viruses, three mechanisms of involvement have been postulated. The first is direct invasion of the cochlea or cochlear nerve. Second, reactivation of the virus in the inner ear can cause cellular inflammatory changes. Lastly, an immune response in the inner ear can be precipitated by distant HSV infection. Direct inoculation of HSV into the inner ear of guinea pigs results in similar pathologic changes to those seen in the temporal bone of adults with sudden hearing loss [40]. However, sudden onset of hearing loss appears to be multifactorial, and not only attributable to viral infections like HSV [3].

The evaluation of sudden sensorineural hearing loss should include serum HSV 1 and 2 PCR as well as serologic evaluation for HSV1 and 2 (IgM and IgG) that could demonstrate seroconversion.

The drug of choice for the treatment of HSV infections is acyclovir. In older children, if there is no evidence of clinical encephalitis, oral therapy with valacyclovir can be considered.

Parvovirus B19

This small, non-enveloped DNA virus is the cause of erythema infectiosum or fifth disease. It is transmitted person to person and humans are its only host. Symptoms involving the inner ear are uncommon. Case reports have described adults presenting with dizziness and hearing difficulties, but the mechanism of involvement is unknown. It is possible that an autoimmune process is ultimately the cause [41].

Parvovirus B-19 infection can be diagnosed using serologic testing (IgM and IgG) or molecular testing including PCR of the blood.

There is no antiviral therapy effective against parvovirus, but if hearing loss is related to an autoimmune response, the use of immunotherapy (intravenous immunoglobulin) can be of benefit.

Mycoplasma pneumoniae

There have been a few reported cases of sensorineural hearing loss associated with *Mycoplasma pneumoniae* infection. In some cases hearing loss has been bilateral, and in all cases occurred early in the course of infection. About half of the patients recovered hearing capacity after receiving treatment with a macrolide. Some patients were also treated with steroids [42]. The diagnosis of these cases was made with the use of antibody testing against mycoplasma [42]. However, the diagnosis of mycoplasma infection can be challenging as serology and polymerase chain reaction do not differentiate infection from asymptomatic colonization. Testing of acute and convalescent paired serum, showing a fourfold increase in titer indicates infection.

Primary Inner Ear Infections

Vestibular Neuritis

Vestibular neuritis describes inflammation of the inner ear and specifically the vestibular nerve, causing an acute onset of vertigo with imbalance, and possible nausea or vomiting, but with no associated hearing loss. Other clinical synonyms include vestibular paralysis, acute labyrinthitis, vestibular neuropathy and vestibular ganglionitis. The acute phase of symptoms in vestibular neuritis lasts from several hours to several days, with abrupt onset of severe and continuous vertigo, and mild imbalance that can persist for several weeks after an episode. Specific clinical signs include continuous vertigo worsened with head movement, spontaneous nystagmus, reduced or absent responses on caloric testing, and autonomic symptoms like clammy skin, fatigue and pallor [43]. The timeline of vertigo lasting over several hours to days suggests vestibular neuritis instead of other causes of peripheral vertigo with shorter or longer vertiginous episodes.

The infectious causes of vestibular neuritis have not been clearly identified. However, the presence of a preceding viral upper respiratory infection suggests a viral etiology, with previous studies isolating HSV DNA [44, 45]. *Borrelia burgdorferi*, the cause of Lyme disease, has also been implicated [46]. The differential diagnosis of vestibular neuritis includes other peripheral vestibular disorders like Meniere's disease, vestibular atelectasia, complications of chronic middle ear disease like labyrinthine fistula or cerebellar abscess [44], and perilymph fistulas, as well as central issues including vertebrobasilar insufficiency or early anterior inferior cerebellar artery infarction, Wallenberg's syndrome, migraine-associated vertigo, presyncopal dizziness, paraneoplastic syndrome, drug-induced vertigo, immune-mediated inner ear disorder [47], multiple sclerosis, or skull base tumors.

The diagnosis of vestibular neuritis primarily rests on a thorough history, including the timeline of vertigo symptoms, and a physical exam evaluating the ear, cranial nerves, tuning fork testing, cerebellar and gait testing, a head thrust test, and a neurological examination. Differentiation between central and peripheral vertigo can be made clinically by evaluating the direction and type of nystagmus, a head-thrust test, and a full neurologic assessment for any associated abnormalities. Peripheral vestibular disorders will produce a mixed horizontal and rotational nystagmus that does not change direction with changes in gaze position, while central nystagmus is typically purely vertical, horizontal or rotational and changes fast-twitch direction with gaze shift [43]. Nystagmus in vestibular neuritis typically is horizontal, rotary and spontaneous, with fast phase away from the involved ear and is reduced with fixation. Head thrust testing can demonstrate vestibular function differences between the ears by stimulating the horizontal vestibuloocular reflex (VOR). Typically, vestibular neuritis is unilateral, and loss of one labyrinth's function causes a positive head thrust test, while central lesions causing vertigo would have a negative (normal) head thrust test. However, patients with lateral pontine and cerebellar strokes can rarely have a positive head thrust test, and any vascular risk factors or associated clinical features should be carefully considered before excluding central lesions [48]. Formal vestibular testing can be considered with caloric testing or video nystagmography, although this may be difficult to obtain in the acute setting. Vestibular evoked myogenic potential (VEMP) testing can isolate the affected vestibular nerve to the inferior vestibular nerve through the cervical VEMP (cVEMP) that assesses the sacculocollic reflex, or the superior vestibular nerve through ocular VEMP (oVEMP) that assesses the crossed vestibuloocular reflex [49]. Imaging is not often needed, but can be considered based on the history and examination, with contrast tomography (CT) of the temporal bone to evaluate trauma or chronic ear disease, or magnetic resonance imaging (MRI) being preferred to further evaluate any neurologic abnormalities on physical exam. Treatment of vestibular neuritis is primarily supportive, with antiemetics and intravenous hydration if needed, and vestibular suppressants during the acute phase. Steroid use has been studied, with relative benefit to placebo or antiviral treatment [50], primarily by accelerating the return of normal vestibular function, although this is controversial, and steroid use does not clearly improve long-term outcome [44]. Some studies recommended initiating steroids for patients presenting within 3 days of symptom onset without risk factors for steroid complications, and to use vestibular suppressants and antiemetics only briefly for the first several days to avoid impeding central vestibular compensation in the subacute phase and prolonging symptoms [51]. After the acute phase, vestibular rehabilitation is useful to improve central compensation as the vestibular function slowly returns. Temporal bone pathology in vestibular neuritis has not been frequently reported, in part because the clinical course of the disease is benign and short-lived. Limited available histological data from several studies [46] showed atrophy of the superior division of the vestibular nerve, with partial or total neuronal loss, and atrophy of the corresponding horizontal and superior ampullae and cristae hair cells. Temporal bone histologic evaluation of the anatomic differences between the inferior/singular and superior vestibular nerves [52] demonstrated that the bony canal of the superior vestibular nerve and its corresponding arteriole is longer and narrower than the singular nerve, increasing the risk of neural edema causing entrapment and potential ischemia.

Labyrinthitis

Labyrinthitis is a peripheral vestibulopathy clinically characterized by an acute onset of vertigo, often with nausea and vomiting as seen in vestibular neuritis, but in contrast to vestibular neuritis also involves an associated hearing loss. Labyrinthitis can be serous, or purulent, or a "toxic" labyrinthitis caused by inflammation from bacterial or fungal toxins or inflammatory cell mediators entering the inner ear without direct labyrinthine infection [53]. Hearing loss occurs in labyrinthitis with panlabyrinthine inflammation involving the cochlea. Clinical synonyms of labyrinthitis include acute labyrinthitis, acute vestibular neuropathy, viral neurolabyrinthitis, vestibular neuronitis, and vestibular neurolabyrinthitis. Labyrinthitis presents acutely with vertigo, nausea and possible vomiting, hearing loss and difficulty ambulating and vision changes or blurring due to persistent spontaneous nystagmus. These symptoms worsen over several hours, peaking within 1–2 days and resolving gradually over several weeks with a benign course, usually recovering normal vestibular function completely within 1–3 months, although persisting dysfunction is possible, particularly in older patients. Hearing loss can be minimal or not present, or can be severe, and has variable recovery depending on the severity and etiology of the labyrinthitis. A preceding mild upper respiratory or viral illness often occurs 1–2 weeks before the onset of labyrinthitis symptoms. On examination, a full otologic and neurologic examination will typically show normal otoscopic findings and neurologic functioning aside from the peripheral vestibular findings. Patients will often present with nausea or vomiting and nystagmus during the acute phase, and possibly a mild positional vertigo component worsening with head movement. Head thrust testing in acute labyrinthitis may be positive if asymmetric labyrinth involvement is present and causing an imbalance of vestibular function between the ears, as in vestibular neuritis. Further formal vestibular testing can be considered with caloric testing, along with tuning fork and audiometric testing if hearing loss is present. Imaging is typically not necessary, but may be useful for patients with clinical features consistent with other differential diagnoses, including intracranial infection or masses, stroke or temporal bone masses or trauma. The differential diagnosis in labyrinthitis includes ischemic acute labyrinthitis, labyrinthine fistula, cholesteatoma or other erosive temporal bone mass, temporal bone trauma, benign positional vertigo, Meniere's disease, drug-induced vertigo, acoustic neuroma, or vertebrobasilar stroke. Infectious etiologies suspected in labyrinthitis include viruses (HSV-1 [3], mumps, measles), bacteria (*Streptococcus pneumoniae*, *Haemophilus influenzae*, *Neisseria meningitides*, *Borrelia burgdorferi* and *Treponema pallidum* and other organisms including fungal species [54, 55]. Other potential causes include immune mediated inner ear disease [47] and microvascular ischemic labyrinthine damage.

Care for labyrinthitis is supportive, with initial bed rest for severe vertigo through the acute phase, and increasing activity as tolerated to promote more rapid central vestibular compensation. Antiemetics and vestibular suppressants are effective adjunctive therapies during the acute phase to address symptoms, and steroids and antivirals have been utilized with unclear efficacy [56, 57]. In the subacute phase, vestibular rehabilitation can be helpful to encourage central vestibular compensation, particularly in older patients.

Temporal bone pathology in suppurative labyrinthitis shows severe destruction of the membranous labyrinth [58] with purulent changes of the perilymph fluid, often with sparing of the endolymph, and potential delayed ectopic ossification of the intralabyrinthine space, known as labyrinthitis ossificans. Labyrinthine infections with viruses and fungi show varying degrees of labyrinthine damage, but ossification is less common [54].

Labyrinthitis Ossificans

Purulent labyrinthitis caused by *Streptococcus pneumoniae* or *Haemophilus influenza* is associated with significant intralabyrinthine damage caused by a neutrophil-driven acute inflammatory response. This results in severe vertigo and hearing loss in the acute phase of infection [59]. As the infection and acute inflammation resolves, macrophage and fibroblast invasion of the damaged tissue may trigger permanent scarring of the membranous labyrinth. Primitive multipotential mesenchymal cells can migrate into this fibrosis and transition to osteoblasts, forming ectopic bone that then obliterates the intralabyrinthine space [60, 61]. This ossification of the labyrinth is called labyrinthitis ossificans, and can make cochlear implantation difficult or impossible in severe cases. Imaging with CT or MRI can show early fibrotic intracochlear changes and direct timing of cochlear implantation [62].

Secondary Inner Ear Infections

Secondary inner ear infections usually are bacterial or fungal in origin, and result from contiguous spread of infection from adjacent anatomical sites including the intracranial space, the tympanic cavity and the mastoid or petrous bones. A normal otic capsule has several sites of entry into the inner ear (Fig. 5.2), from the tympanic space through the membrane-ringed oval window and thin membranous round window, through natural bony openings in the otic capsule like the internal auditory canal through perineural or perivascular spaces, the vestibular aqueduct, or the cochlear aqueduct that

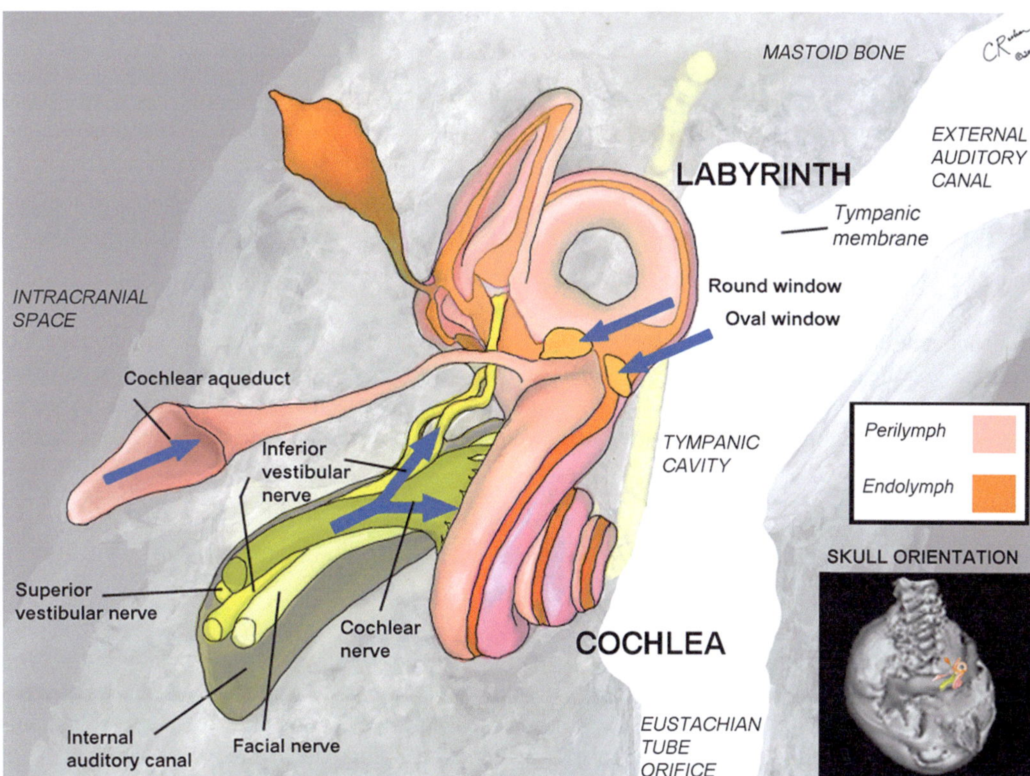

Fig. 5.2 Natural entry points into the inner ear. The oval and round windows are thin membranous barriers between the inner ear and the tympanic cavity. The cochlear aqueduct, and the perivascular and perineural spaces within the internal auditory canal, connect the intracranial space to the inner ear. © Corrie Roehm

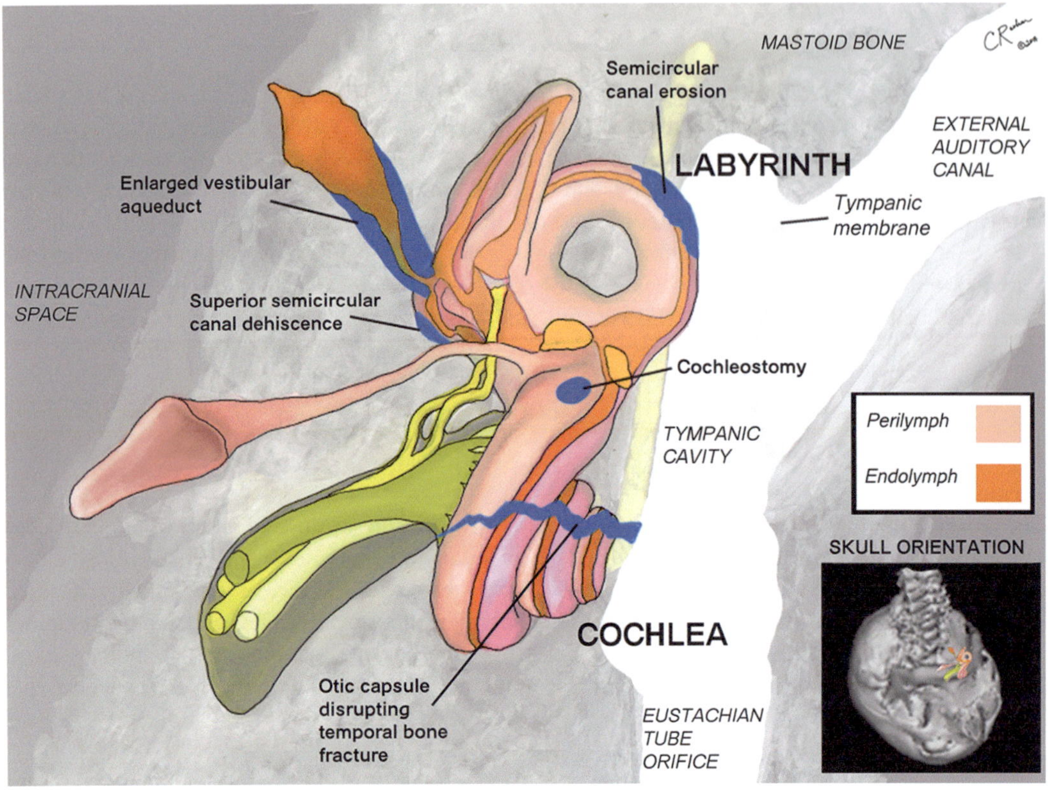

Fig. 5.3 Abnormal entry points into the inner ear. Anatomic abnormalities include enlarged vestibular aqueduct or superior semicircular canal dehiscence. Acquired bony openings include erosion into the bony labyrinth, temporal bone fractures disrupting the otic capsule or surgically created openings like a cochleostomy for cochlear implant insertion. © Corrie Roehm

connects the subarachnoid space to the scala tympani in the basal turn of the cochlea. Anatomic abnormalities in the otic capsule like Mondini or common cavity malformations, superior semicircular canal dehiscence, labyrinthine fistula, enlarged cochlear aperture or enlarged vestibular aqueduct can also provide access to the inner ear. Acquired bony openings into the inner ear can occur from erosive tumors, cholesteatomas, temporal bone trauma with otic capsule fracture or otologic surgeries like stapedectomy, translabyrinthine or labyrinthectomy procedures, or cochlear implantation (Fig. 5.3).

Meningitis

Viral and bacterial meningitis infections can extend into the inner ear, with resulting labyrinthitis and vertigo or hearing loss. Hearing loss is the most common identifiable complication of bacterial meningitis. The incidence of hearing loss has been reported between 10 and 40 % of pediatric patients recovering from bacterial meningitis [63, 64]. Hearing loss can fluctuate and recovery has been documented [65]. Several studies demonstrated permanent sensorineural hearing loss in 10 % of children with bacterial meningitis overall, affecting 20–31 % of *Streptococcus pneumoniae* infections, 0–10 %

of *Neisseria meningitidis* infections and 6–12 % of *Hemophilus influenzae* infections [66, 67]. Adult literature reports an incidence of about 20 % of hearing loss with pneumococcal meningitis [68]. The likelihood of hearing loss varies with the infecting bacteria, with the highest risk being from *Streptococcus pneumoniae* and *H. influenzae type b*, [69, 63] and is caused by direct inflammatory damage to the cochlea including the basilar membrane and Organ of Corti and to the spiral ganglia neurons [61]. Meningitis appears to affect the cochlea more frequently than the vestibular labyrinth [70], potentially due to a common pathway of infection from CSF through the cochlear aqueduct that inserts directly into the basal turn of the cochlea. Meningitic labyrinthitis typically presents with vertigo, nausea and vomiting with ataxia in most patients. Hearing loss occurs in a subset of 10–15 % of patients early in the course of meningitis, although delayed hearing loss onset is not uncommon. The hearing loss is usually permanent, involving all frequencies with severe or profound sensorineural hearing loss in ~10 % of meningitis patients. In approximately 15 % of meningitis patients hearing loss is transient [66], and resolution of the hearing loss is more likely if the initial hearing loss is mild or moderate [71]. Spinal fluid glucose of less than 20 mg/mL, elevated CSF protein and development of seizures have been found to be risk factors for development of hearing loss [72, 73].

In an animal model, severe sepsis was also associated with inner ear involvement and subsequent development of hearing loss. Histological evaluation of the inner ear of infected animals showed the presence of apoptosis in the supporting cells of the organ of Corti [74].

Diagnostic testing includes a full audiometric evaluation and neurologic and otologic examination, with adjunctive imaging with MRI with gadolinium showing contrast uptake in the labyrinth. Treatment includes aggressive antibiotic treatment of the meningitis process with culture-directed antibiotic therapy. The use of steroids, more specifically dexamethasone, was shown to be beneficial in reducing hearing loss complications in cases of *Haemophilus influenzae* type b meningitis [75]. This approach is yet unclear for other pathogens, including *Streptococcus pneumoniae* [3]. Given the risk of hearing loss, a comprehensive audiologic evaluation is recommended for all patients during the acute phase of meningitis and continuing after recovery, with hearing aid amplification or cochlear implantation if needed for hearing habilitation. Imaging evaluating for labyrinthitis ossificans is recommended if hearing loss is present, and some centers will monitor with repeat audiologic assessments before cochlear implantation given the small chance of hearing recovery, and implant once radiologic evidence of ossification is present, while other centers implant quickly after confirming radiologic evidence of ossification to improve the likelihood of a complete cochlear implant insertion.

Cochlear Implants

Inner ear infections resulting from the presence of cochlear implants can present as an infection affecting the device itself or related to increased complications resulting from otitis media during the first 2 months after implantation [76].

Children who develop acute otitis media after cochlear implants have increased risk for mastoiditis, meningitis and labyrinthitis, and require aggressive surgical and antimicrobial treatment to prevent further complications [77]. *Streptococcus pneumoniae* is not only one of the most common causes of meningitis among pediatric patients, but it is also implicated in central nervous system infections after cochlear implants.

It is important that children undergoing cochlear implant placement should have received all age appropriate dosages of vaccinations against *Haemophilus influenzae* type b and *Streptococcus pneumoniae* at least 2 weeks before surgery.

Other organisms including chronic *Pseudomonas aeruginosa* infections of cochlear implants have been reported, and they are difficult to treat, often requiring prolonged medical therapy with anti-pseudomonal antibiotics, with potential concomitant removal of the device [78].

Otitis Externa, Otitis Media and Mastoiditis

The middle ear and inner ear are separated only by the thin round and oval window membranes. This close anatomic proximity explains how infections of the middle ear can secondarily affect the inner ear [79]. The passage of toxins and inflammatory substances also play a role in secondary inner ear inflammation [80].

One potential complication of otitis media is the development of labyrinthitis, when infection spreads into the inner ear. This usually occurs suddenly, with associated development of vertigo and hearing loss. This complication is rare, due to the widespread use of antibiotics in the treatment of otitis media. However, it can account for up to 40 % of complications from otitis media [81].

Streptococcus pneumoniae is among the most common organisms causing acute otitis media. Other organisms have been reported to affect the inner ear by contiguous spread, including *group A streptococcus* and *Staphylococcus aureus* [82]. *Pseudomonas aeruginosa* is a well-known cause of otitis externa, including necrotizing changes in immunocompromised children. Malignant external otitis externa can also result in osteomyelitis of temporal bone and associated septic thrombosis of intracranial venous sinuses and extension into the inner ear structures [83]. Pseudomonas infection has also been reported as a cause of labyrinthitis after traumatic violation of the otic capsule [84].

Mycobacteria tuberculosis and non-tuberculous mycobacteria have been implicated in infections of the middle ear, but occur rarely [85]. Inner ear changes including inflammation of the facial nerve in the internal auditory canal with a serous labyrinthitis has been proven histologically. Patients can have abnormal tympanic membranes, typically edematous and thickened, but without obvious inflammation or perforation, and culture-negative labyrinthitis [86]. Infection with mycobacterium should be considered in patients with subacute otitis media, evidence of labyrinthitis and cranial nerve palsy [87]. Infections require prolonged antimicrobial therapy, usually in conjunction with surgical treatment. This infection should be considered in culture negative labyrinthitis.

Mycotic infections affecting the middle ear with subsequent involvement of the inner ear are rare, and they primarily affect pediatric patients that are immunocompromised or have had extensive otologic surgery. Infections can also spread to the inner ear as consequence of systemic fungal infection affecting the temporal bone. Medical treatment requires the use of systemic antifungals, combined with surgical debridement of affected tissue. Mortality is high and complications from surgical and medical treatment can be extensive.

References

1. Weinreich H, Agrawal Y. The link between allergy and Meniere's disease. Curr Opin Otolaryngol Head Neck Surg. 2014;22(3):227–30.
2. Davis L, Johnsson L. Viral infections of the inner ear: clinical, virologic, and pathologic studies in humans and animals. Am J Otolaryngol. 1983;4:347–62.
3. Beyea J, Agrawal S, Parnes L. Recent advances in viral inner ear disorders. Curr Opin Otolaryngol Head Neck Surg. 2012;20(5):404–8.
4. Gopen Q, Rosowski J, Merchant S. Anatomy of the normal human cochlear aqueduct with functional implications. Hear Res. 1997;107:9–22.

5. Yorgancilar E, Akkus Z, Gun R, Yildirim M, Bakir S, Kinis V. Temporal bone erosion in patients with chronic suppurative otitis media. B-ENT. 2013;9(1):17–22.
6. Antonelli P, Ojano-Dirain C. Microbial flora of cochlear implants by gene pyrosequencing. Otol Neurotol. 2013;34(7):e65–71.
7. Cunningham C, Slattery W, Luxford W. Postoperative infection in cochlear implant patients. Otolaryngol Head Neck Surg. 2004;131:109–14.
8. Ruellan K, Frijns J, Bloemberg G, Hautefort C, Van den Abbeele T, Lamers G. Detection of bacterial biofilm on cochlear implants removed because of device failure, without evidence of infection. Otol Neurotol. 2010;31(8):1320–4.
9. Pass R, Stagno S, Myers G, Alford C. Outcome of symptomatic congenital cytomegalovirus infection: results of long-term longitudinal follow-up. Pediatrics. 1980;66:758–62.
10. Teissier N, Delezoide A, Mas A. Inner ear lesions in congenital cytomegalovirus infection of human fetuses. Acta Neuropathol. 2011;122:763–74.
11. Gabrielli L, Bonasoni M, Santini D, Piccirilli G, Chiereghin A, Guerra B. Human fetal inner ear involvement in congenital cytomegalovirus infection. Acta Neuropathol Commun. 2013;1:63.
12. De Vries J, Vesseur A, Rotteveel L, Korver A, Rusman L. Cytomegalovirus DNA detection in dried blood spots and perilymphatic fluids from pediatric and adult cochlear implant recipients with prelingual deafness. J Clin Virol. 2013;56(2):113–7.
13. Rivera L, Boppana S, Fowler K, Britt W, Stagno S, Pass R. Predictors of hearing loss in children with symptomatic congenital cytomegalovirus infection. Pediatrics. 2002;110(4):762–7.
14. Park A, Duval M, McVicar S, Bale J, Hohler N, Carey JC. A diagnostic paradigm including cytomegalovirus testing for idiopathic pediatric sensorineural hearing loss. Laryngoscope. 2014;124(11):2624–9.
15. Kimberlin D, Lin C-Y, Sanchez P, Demmler G, Danker W, The SM, NIAID, Collaborative Antiviral Study Group. Effect of ganciclovir therapy on hearing in symptomatic congenital cytomegalovirus disease involving the central nervous system: a randomized, controlled trial. J Pediatr. 2003;143:17–26.
16. Kimberlin D. Six months versus six weeks of oral valganciclovir for infants with symptomatic congenital cytomegalovirus (CMV) disease with and without central nervous system (CNS) involvement: Results of a Phase III, randomized, double-blind, placebo-controlled, multinational study. Proceeding of the Infectious Diseases Society of America 2013. Oral abstract session. 5 Oct 2013.
17. Amir J, Wolf D, Levy I. Treatment of symptomatic congenital cytomegalovirus infection with intravenous ganciclovir followed by long term oral valganciclovir. Eur J Pediatr. 2010;169(9):1061–7.
18. Gussen R. Middle and inner ear changes in congenital rubella. Am J Otolaryngol. 1981;2(4):314–20.
19. Roizen N. Etiology of hearing loss in children. Nongenetic causes. Pediatr Clin North Am. 1999;46:49–64.
20. Ward P, Honrubia V, Moore B. Inner ear pathology in deafness due to maternal rubella. Arch Otolaryngol. 1968;87(1):22–8.
21. Miller E, Cradock-Watson J, Pollock T. Consequences of confirmed maternal rubella at successive stages of pregnancy. Lancet. 1982;2(8302):781–4.
22. Dimech W, Panagiotopoulos L, Marler J, Laven N, Leeson S, Dax E. Evaluation of three immunoassays used for detection of anti-rubella virus immunoglobulin M antibodies. Clin Diagn Lab Immunol. 2005;12(9):1104.
23. Everberg G. Deafness following mumps. Acta Otolaryngol. 1957;48:397–403.
24. Westmore G, Pickard B, Stern H. Isolation of mumps virus from the inner ear after sudden deafness. Br Med J. 1979;6(1):14–5.
25. Dunmade A, Segun-Busari S, Olajide TG, Ologe FE. Profound bilateral sensorineural hearing loss in Nigerian children: any shift in etiology? J Deaf Stud Deaf Educ. 2007;12(1):112–8.
26. Bordley J, Kapur Y. Histopathologic changes in the temporal bone resulting from measles infection. Arch Otolaryngol. 1977;103(3):162–8.
27. Hulbert T, Larsen R, Davis C, Holtom P. Bilateral hearing loss after measles and rubella vaccination in an adult. N Engl J Med. 1991;325(2):134.
28. Woods C. Syphilis in children: congenital and acquired. Semin Pediatr Infect Dis. 2005;16(4):245–57.
29. Miller M, Makary C, Lopez I, Ishiyama A. Endolymphatic hydrops in otologic syphilis: a temporal bone study. Otol Neurotol. 2010;31(4):681–6.
30. Morrison A. Management of severe deafness in adults. The otologist's contribution. Proc R Soc Med. 1969;62: 959–65.
31. Nadol J. Hearing loss of acquired syphilis: diagnosis confirmed by incudectomy. Laryngoscope. 1975; 85(11):1888–97.
32. Zoller M, Wilson W, Nadol J. Treatment of syphilitic hearing loss. Combined penicillin and steroid therapy in 29 patients. Ann Otol Rhinol Laryngol. 1979;88(2):160–5.
33. Hughes G, Rutherford I. Predictive value of serologic tests for syphilis in otology. Ann Otol Rhinol Laryngol. 1986;95(3):250–9.

34. Workowski K, Berman S, Centers for Disease Control and Prevention. Sexually transmitted diseases treatment guidelines, 2006. MMWR Recomm Rep. 2006;55(RR-11):1–94.
35. Brown E, Chau J, Atashband S, Westerberg B, Kozak F. A systematic review of neonatal toxoplasmosis exposure and sensorineural hearing loss. Int J Pediatr Otorhinolaryngol. 2009;73(5):707–11.
36. McLeod R, Boyer K, Karrison T, Kasza K, Swisher C, Roizen N, Toxoplasmosis study group. Outcome of treatment for congenital toxoplasmosis, 1981–2004: the national collaborative Chicago-based, congenital toxoplasmosis study. Clin Infect Dis. 2006;42(10):1383–94.
37. Salviz M, Montoya J, Nadol J, Santos F. Otopathology in congenital toxoplasmosis. Otol Neurotol. 2013; 34(6):1165–9.
38. Eichenwald H. A study of congenital toxoplasmosis, with particular emphasis on clinical manifestations, sequelae, and therapy. In: Siim JC, editor. Human toxoplasmosis. Copenhagen: Munksgaard; 1960. p. 41–9.
39. Wilson C, Remington J, Stagno S, Reynolds D. Development of adverse sequelae in children born with subclinical congenital Toxoplasma infection. Pediatrics. 1980;66(5):767–74.
40. Nomura Y, Kurata T, Saito Y. Cochlear changes after herpes simplex virus infection. Acta Otolaryngol. 1985;99(3-4):419–27.
41. Nara M, Shirata Y, Kikuchi T, Hongo M. Adult human parvovirus-B19 infection presenting with hearing difficulty and dizziness. Tohoku J Exp Med. 2011;224(1):57–9.
42. Okada T, Kato I, Miho I, Minami S, Kinoshita H, Akao I. Acute sensorineural hearing loss caused by Mycoplasma pneumoniae. Acta Otolaryngol Suppl. 1996;522:22–5.
43. Baloh R. Vestibular neuritis. N Engl J Med. 2003;348:1027–32.
44. Goddard J, Fayad J. Vestibular neuritis. Otolaryngol Clin North Am. 2011;44:361–5.
45. Furata Y, Takasu T, Sato K. Latent herpes simplex virus type 1 in human geniculate ganglia. Acta Neuropathol. 1992;84:39–44.
46. Baloh R, Ishiyama A, Wackym P. Vestibular neuritis: clinical–pathological correlation. Otolaryngol Head Neck Surg. 1996;114:586–92.
47. Stone J, Francis H. Immune-mediated inner ear disease. Curr Opin Rheumatol. 2000;12:32–40.
48. Newman-Toker D, Kattah J, Alvernia J, Wang D. Normal head impulse test differentiates acute cerebellar strokes from vestibular neuritis. Neurology. 2008;70:2378–85.
49. Lin C, Young Y. Identifying the affected branches of vestibular nerve in vestibular neuritis. Acta Otolaryngol. 2011;131:921–8.
50. Strupp M, Zingler V, Arbusow V. Methylprednisolone, valacyclovir or the combination for vestibular neuritis. N Engl J Med. 2004;351:354–61.
51. Walker M. Treatment of vestibular neuritis. Curr Treat Options Neurol. 2009;11:41–5.
52. Goebel J, O'Mara W, Gianoli G. Anatomic considerations in vestibular neuritis. Otol Neurotol. 2001;22:512–8.
53. Juhn S, Juhn T, Lin J, Rhee C. Effects of inflammatory mediators on middle ear pathology and on inner ear function. Ann N Y Acad Sci. 1997;830:130–42.
54. Gussen R, Canalis R. Mucormycosis of the temporal bone. Ann Otol Rhinol Laryngol. 1982;91:27.
55. Rothenberg R. Syphilitic hearing loss. South Med J. 1979;72:118.
56. Fishman J, Burgess C, Waddell A. Corticosteroids for the treatment of idiopathic acute vestibular dysfunction (vestibular neuritis). Cochrane Database Syst Rev. 2011; CD008607.
57. Amber K, Castano J, Angeli S. Prophylactic valacyclovir in a patient with recurrent vestibular disturbances secondary to vestibular neuritis. Am J Otolaryngol. 2012;33(4):487–8.
58. Igarashi M, Saito R, Alford B. Temporal bone findings in pneumococcal meningitis. Arch Otolaryngol Head Neck Surg. 1974;99:79.
59. Lin H, Fan Y, Wu K, Shu M, Yang C, Lin H. The incidence of tympanogenic labyrinthitis ossificans. J Laryngol Otol. 2014;128(7):618–20.
60. Xu H, Joglekar S, Paparella M. Labyrinthitis ossificans. Otol Neurotol. 2009;30:579–80.
61. Paparella M, Sugiura S. The pathology of suppurative labyrinthitis. Ann Otol Rhinol Laryngol. 1967;76:554.
62. Isaacson B, Booth T, Kutz J. Labyrinthitis ossificans: how accurate is MRI in predicting cochlear obstruction? Otolaryngol Head Neck Surg. 2009;140:692–6.
63. Baraff L, Lee S, Schriger D. Outcomes of bacterial meningitis in children: a meta-analysis. Pediatr Infect Dis J. 1993;12:389–94.
64. Karanja L, Oburra H, Masinde P, Wamalwa D. Prevalence of hearing loss in children following bacterial meningitis in a tertiary referral hospital. BMC Res Notes. 2014;11(7):138.
65. Roine I, Pelkonen T, Cruzeiro M, Kataja M, Aarnisalo A, Peltola H. Fluctuation in hearing thresholds during recovery from childhood bacterial meningitis. Pediatr Infect Dis J. 2014;33(3):253–7.
66. Dodge P, Davis H, Feigin R. Prospective evaluation of hearing impairment as sequela of acute bacterial meningitis. N Engl J Med. 1984;311:869.
67. McIntyre P, Berkey C, King SM, Schaad UB, Kilpi T, Kanra GY, Perez CM. Dexamethasone as adjunctive therapy in bacterial meningitis: a meta-analysis of randomized clinical trials since 1988. JAMA. 1997;278(11):925–31.

68. De Gans J, van de Beek D. Dexamethasone in adults with bacterial meningitis. N Engl J Med. 2002;347:1549.
69. Wellman M, Sommer D, McKenna J. Sensorineural hearing loss in postmeningitic children. Otol Neurotol. 2003;24:907.
70. Merchand S, Gopen Q. A human temporal bone study of acute bacterial meningogenic labyrinthitis. Am J Otol. 1996;17:375.
71. Nadol H. Hearing loss as a sequela of meningitis. Laryngoscope. 1978;38:739.
72. Karanja B, Oburra H, Masinde P, Wamalwa D. Risk factors for hearing loss in children following bacterial meningitis in a tertiary referral hospital. Int J Otolaryngol. 2013;2013:354725.
73. Kutz J, Simon L, Chennupati S, Giannoni C, Manolidis S. Clinical predictors for hearing loss in children with bacterial meningitis. Arch Otolaryngol Head Neck Surg. 2006;132(9):941–5.
74. Schmutzhard J, Glueckert R, Pritz C, Blumer M, Bitsche M, Lackner P. Sepsis otopathy: experimental sepsis leads to significant hearing impairment due to apoptosis and glutamate excitotoxicity in murine cochlea. Dis Model Mech. 2013;6(3):745–54.
75. Lebel M, Freij B, Syrogiannopoulos G, Charne D, Igarashi M, Stewart S. Dexamethasone therapy for bacterial meningitis. Results of two double-blind, placebo-controlled trials. N Engl J Med. 1988;319(15):964–71.
76. Rubin L, Papsin B. Cochlear implants in children: surgical site infections and prevention and treatment of acute otitis media and meningitis. Pediatrics. 2010;126(2):381–91.
77. Osborn H, Cushing S, Gordon K, James A, Papsin B. The management of acute mastoiditis in children with cochlear implants: saving the device. Cochlear Implants Int. 2013;14(5):252–6.
78. Germiller J, El-Kashlan H, Shah U. Chronic pseudomonas infections of cochlear implants. Otol Neurotol. 2005;26(2):196–201.
79. Hellstrom S, Eriksson P, Yoon Y, Johansson U. Interactions between the middle ear and the inner ear: bacterial products. Ann N Y Acad Sci. 1997;830:110–9.
80. Cureoglu S, Schachern P, Rinaldo A, Tsuprun V, Ferlito A, Paparella M. Round window membrane and labyrinthine pathological changes: an overview. Acta Otolaryngol. 2005;125(1):9–15.
81. Pellegrini S, Gonzalez M, Sommerfleck P, Bernáldez P. Intratemporal complications from acute otitis media in children: 17 cases in two years. Acta Otorrinolaringol Esp. 2012;63(1):21–5.
82. Hyden D, Akerlind B, Peebo M. Inner ear and facial nerve complications of acute otitis media with focus on bacteriology and virology. Acta Otolaryngol. 2006;126(50):460–6.
83. Sando I, Harada T, Okano Y, Saito R, Caparosa R. Temporal bone histopathology of necrotizing external otitis. A case report. Ann Otol Rhinol Laryngol. 1981;90(2 Pt 1):109–15.
84. Tanaka K, Matsuura S, Fukuda S, Terayama Y. Pseudomonas labyrinthitis. Arch Otorhinolaryngol. 1985;242(3):273–7.
85. Hwang G, Jung J, Yum G, Choi J. Tuberculous otitis media with facial paralysis combined with labyrinthitis. Korean J Audiol. 2013;17(1):27–9.
86. Nicolau Y, Northrop C, Eavey R. Tuberculous otitis in infants: temporal bone histopathology and clinical extrapolation. Otol Neurotol. 2006;27(5):667–71.
87. Dumas G, Schmerber S, Atallah I, Brion J, Righini C. Subacute tuberculous otitis media complicated by petrositis and meningitis. Rev Laryngol Otol Rhinol (Bord). 2012;133(4–5):221–4.

Part II
Nasal Cavity and Sinuses

Chapter 6
Nasal Soft Tissue Infections

Ronald J. Vilela

Introduction

Nasal soft tissue infections have been described under a variety of names, including nasal vestibulitis, nasal furunculosis, nasal vestibular furunculosis, nasal cellulitis, and nasal folliculitis. In this chapter, we will review relevant anatomy and the history of treatment of nasal soft tissue infections. There have not been any published articles that have looked at the incidence or prevalence of nasal vestibulitis. We will discuss how nasal soft tissue infections present. We will go over relevant microbiology and nasal carriage of bacteria, especially as it relates to *Staphylococcus aureus*. We will discuss diagnosis of nasal soft tissue infections and concluded the chapter with relevant treatment options. Special attention will be directed towards bacterial colonization of the nose as it pertains to both community acquired and nosocomial infections.

Relevant Anatomy

The nose is made up of various components including, but not limited to, skin, nasal mucosa, bone and cartilage. What gives the nose its structure and integrity are the nasal bones superiorly, the upper and lower lateral cartilages inferiorly, and the cartilaginous nasal septum. The nasal vestibule is made up of hair-bearing skin anteriorly and transitions to nasal mucosa posteriorly. The epithelial wall of the nostril interiorly is fully keratinized and includes sebaceous gland, apocrine sweat glands, and hair follicles [1]. The angular and nasolabial veins draining the nasal vestibule are valveless. Therefore, infections in this area have the potential to spread to structures such as the cavernous sinus via these facial veins if treatment is inadequate. This area has been called the "danger triangle" for this reason [2].

R.J. Vilela, M.D. (✉)
Department of Pediatric Otolaryngology—Head and Neck Surgery, Baylor College of Medicine, Houston, TX, USA

Texas Children's Hospital, Houston, TX, USA
e-mail: Ronald.Vilela@bcm.edu

T.A. Valdez, J.G. Vallejo (eds.), *Infectious Diseases in Pediatric Otolaryngology*,
DOI 10.1007/978-3-319-21744-4_6

Microbiology

The most common bacterial flora found in the nose includes coagulase-negative staphylococci (12–81 %) which includes *Staphylococcus epidermidis*, *Staphylococcus hominis* and *Staphylococcus haemolyticus*, aerobic diphtheroids (6–68 %), and *S. aureus* (6–34 %). Other aerobic species like *Streptococcus viridians*, pneumococci, meningococci, enteric bacteria and Moraxella species are also commonly found [3, 4].

S. aureus, one of the most common bacteria that cause nasal vestibulitis, produces penicillinase, a beta-lactamase that inactivates penicillin and extended-spectrum penicillins. Beta-lactamase inhibitors, such as potassium clavulanate help to overcome this resistance, unless methicillin-resistant *S. aureus* (MRSA) is present. MRSA accounts for 25–60 % of all strains of *S. aureus* in hospitals in the United States [4].

Immunosuppressed patients may be prone to infection with different pathogens such as *Pseudomonas aeruginosa*, mycobacteria, or invasive fungi like mucormycosis or aspergillus [5]. Herpes simplex virus, herpes zoster and other viruses can affect the nasal vestibule as well as the oral cavity and lips.

There have been a few case reports of rare organisms causing nasal vestibulitis in adult patients, but none in pediatric patients. *Nocardiopsis dassonvillei* was found in a 55-year-old diabetic patient in Mandya, Karnataka, India that recurred after a 10 day course of cefuroxime [6]. He fully recovered 4 weeks after receiving a week of clarithromycin and levofloxacin. *Burkholderia pseudomallei* was found to cause sinonasal Melioidosis and sepsis in 51-year-old diabetic man with hepatitis B who suffered from alcohol abuse in Melbourne, Australia who needed incision and drainage, debridement and endoscopic sinus surgery for infection of the nasal vestibule with a septal abscess [7]. He travelled from Vietnam, an endemic area for these particular bacteria. He was treated with IV meropenem, then IV ceftazidime for 8 weeks, followed by 3 months of Bactrim DS and doxycycline. Because of inadequately sterilized surgical equipment at a hospital in Mexico City, 22 (27.5 %) of 81 patients who underwent rhinoplasty from December 1987 to April 1988 developed nasal cellulitis due to *Mycobacterium chelonae* [8].

Diagnosis

Symptoms of typical nasal vestibulitis include localized pain and swelling of the nasal vestibule, usually of sudden onset [5]. Nose picking or excessive blowing can precipitate the disease process and can result in crusting or bleeding near the nasal hair follicles. Nasal steroid use does not usually precipitate nasal vestibulitis, but intranasal drug use can lead to chronic nasal sores with ulceration. Nasal obstruction is not usually present. On physical examination, the nose can be swollen, tender to palpation, crusting, erythematous and warm. Sometimes a pimple-like lesion is present. A chronic nasal sore that does not heal after appropriate time and treatment may need to be biopsied to rule out other, more unusual causes such as systemic disease like Wegener's granulomatosis with polyangitis (GPA) or sarcoidosis, or more rarely, lethal midline granuloma or sinonasal lymphoma. A neoplastic process such as basal cell or squamous cell carcinoma should also be ruled out. Eczema can also be on the differential diagnosis as well [2]. Dahle and Sontheimer have mentioned in the past a term they coined the "Rudolf sign," as in *Rudolf the Red Nosed Reindeer*, in their case report of typical nasal vestibulitis that resolved with mupirocin ointment. The authors describe the "Rudolf sign" as unilateral, or sometimes bilateral, tender erythema of the nasal tip [9]. Involvement of both sides of the nose is rare, as is frank abscess. Systemic symptoms such as fever and chills are very uncommon. Spontaneous resolution, though, is very common. Symptoms can be more common in winter months.

Nasal Colonization

There are many bacteria that can colonize the nose. Even if there is not a clear cut correlation between colonization and active nasal vestibulitis, nasal colonization has significant importance, especially with regard to invasive disease in other parts of the body. *Staphylococcus aureus* is by far the most studied, with the anterior nasal cavity being the most frequent carriage site [1]. Carrier status can be classified as persistent (20 %), intermittent (30 %) or non-carriage (50 %), with persistent carriers having a higher bacterial load and a higher risk of acquiring an infection than intermittent carriers [1]. Adults have lower persistent carriage rates than children with a transition from persistent to intermittent to non-carrier states during the adolescent years [1]. Carrier rates tend to be higher in white people, in men, in patients with diabetes mellitus, those undergoing hemodialysis, patients with end stage liver disease, patients with HIV, obese patients, patients with a history of stroke and patients skin diseases (psoriasis or eczema) that can pre-dispose them to skin infections [1]. Transmission of bacteria is usually via direct contact, but rarely can be transmitted via airborne dispersal. Family members tend to have the same carrier state. Being hospitalized is also an important risk factor for nasal carrier state. The second most common cause of hospital-acquired bloodstream infections is *S. aureus* with approximately 20 % of surgical patients acquiring at least one nosocomial infection [1]. This rate varies by institution. For community-acquired methicillin-resistant *Staphylococcus aureus* (MRSA), carrier rates are still low, but seem to be rapidly escalating in certain parts of the world.

A prospective observational study conducted at Brooke Army Medical Center in Ft. Sam Houston, Texas [10], determined the prevalence of nasal colonization with MRSA in patients hospitalized at five different units at the hospital. Colonization status was determined at admission and longitudinally over a 3 month period. Of the 26 patients who were initially colonized with MRSA, 5 (19 %) developed an infection involving MRSA. This was about 10 times the incidence in patients colonized with methicillin-susceptible *S. aureus* (MSSA), with a significant difference in relative risk (RR, 13; 95 % CI, 2.7–64; p<.01) for patients colonized with MRSA initially. Twelve (2.0 %) of the 595 patients who were initially not colonized with *S. aureus* developed MRSA infection, thus determining a higher relative risk (RR, 9.5; 95 % CI, 3.6–25; p<.01). Statistical analysis in this study showed MRSA infection to be more prevalent in older patients (mean age, 69 year) and in patients who were more prolonged admissions (mean length of stay, 16 days). Davis, et al., also mentioned that 12 (3.0 %) patients acquired MRSA colonization during their hospital admission. Nine of the 12 had no *S. aureus* colonization at admission while 3 were colonized with MSSA. There was a higher relative risk of MRSA infection (RR, 12; 95 % CI, 4.0–38; P<.01) for patients who acquire MRSA colonization during their hospitalization. This study is consistent with previous reports in the literature about the natural history of MRSA colonization in the nose.

Fritz, et al. studied the natural history of *S. aureus* nasal colonization in 1300 community children from October 2005 to June 2006 finding 34 % persistently carried S. aureus on three consecutive samplings, 50 % intermittently colonized and 16 % persistently non-colonized [11]. They found the following are factors that were independently associated with longitudinal MRSA colonization in multivariate analysis: 1. Prior MRSA colonization (adjusted OR [aOR] 12.5, 95 % CI, 2.1–75.7, p=.007), 2. Medicaid or no health insurance (aOR 10.2, 95 % CI, 1.7–61.3, p=.01), 3. Healthcare worker in the household (aOR 5.9, 95 % CI, 1.3–27.6, p=.02), and 4. Interval skin or soft tissue infection (SSTI) in a household member (aOR 6.5, 95 % CI 1.0–42.8, p=.05). Prior MSSA colonization (aOR 16.2, 95 % CI 5.9–44.4, p<.001), school attendance (aOR 3.8, 95 % CI 1.4–10.8, p=.01), and fingernail biting (aOR 3.1, 95 % CI 1.0–9.5, p=.05) were significant risk factors for longitudinal MSSA colonization. They found that contemporary MRSA colonization can resolve spontaneously. If multiple cultures were positive, then those individuals were more likely to stay colonized, thereby possibly allowing for better identification of those more at risk for developing recurrent SSTI.

A case–control study in 2005 out of Grady Memorial Hospital in Atlanta, Georgia, looked at the prevalence of MRSA colonization and risk factors associated to colonization [12]. The study also looked at the prevalence of nasal carriage of community-associated MRSA. Molecular typing and gene analysis of MRSA was also performed which showed that a significant proportion (2.2 %) of patients admitted were colonized with a particular clone of MRSA that is identified with community-association. MRSA was found in 53 (7.3 %) of the 726 nasal cultures performed with MSSA was found in 119 (16.3 %) and no *S. aureus* found in 554 (76.3 %). Of the 53 patients colonized with MRSA, only 7 (13 %) developed or were admitted with a diagnosed MRSA infection. Hospitalization within the past 12 months was an independent risk factor of MRSA colonization on multivariate analysis. Other risk factors included having a skin or soft tissue infection at the time of admission, use of any antimicrobial agents within the 3 months prior to admission, and HIV-seropositive status. There was increased risk of MRSA colonization in patients who were HIV-positive and had not received antibiotics within 3 months of admission, but not for HIV-positive patients who had received antibiotics within 3 months of admission. On the contrary, when compared to HIV-negative patients who had not received antibiotics 3 months prior to being admitted, there was also an increased risk of MRSA colonization for HIV-negative patients who had received antimicrobial within 3 months prior to admission. The authors suspect that prophylactic trimethoprim-sulfamethoxazole could possibly reduce colonization of MRSA in HIV-positive patients. The authors also found that there was an increased likelihood of MRSA colonization with increase numbers of risk factors present. They suggest that, if a certain number of risk factors exist, screening for MRSA colonization could be more cost effective than screening for all patients admitted.

A more recent study in 2009 sought to reclassify nasal carriage status from the above mentioned categories, to a simpler classification: persistent carriers versus others [13]. Belkin, et al. looked at 51 healthy volunteers for a duration of 6 months, monitoring their nasal cultures, antistaphylococcal antibodies, C-reactive protein levels and leukocyte counts before and after nasal mupirocin ointment twice daily for 5 days. After treatment, the volunteers were inoculated artificially with a mixture of *S. aureus* strains and nasal cultures were followed for up to 22 weeks. Screening showed 29 % to be non-carriers, 47 % intermittent carriers and 24 % persistent carriers. Four intermittent carriers and 4 persistent carriers still carried *S. aureus* after mupirocin treatment. In follow-up, median survival of *S. aureus* was significantly lower for non-carriers and intermittent carriers (4 days, 14 days, respectively) versus persistent carriers (>154 days) with significantly higher bacterial counts in persistent carriers. There was no apparent difference quantitatively in antistaphylococcal antibodies between the three types of carriers. The authors suggest that the differences in the non-carrier and intermittent carrier groups were not as significant as that of the persistent carrier type, perhaps meaning that non-carriage is incidental and likely to be intermittent carriers or that intermittent carriers might actually be non-carriers who harbor *S. aureus* only under environmental stress. They found that 11 of the 19 persistent carriers selected for their own resident strain after inoculation, suggesting that host-*S. aureus* interactions are highly specific.

A prospective, observational study performed by Zafar et al. analyzed the prevalence of *S. aureus* nasal colonization in patients and their household members who presented to two different hospitals with infections caused by community-associated MRSA (CA-MRSA) from September 2004 to February 2006 [14]. They found the relative risk for MRSA infection in 51 patients who had S. aureus recovered from nasal swabs was 2.30 (95 % CI, 1.06–5.00, p = .01). The relative risk in household members was 0.48 (95 % CI, .025–.083, p = .01) with the parents of the patient having the highest risk for colonization, followed by spouses and children or siblings.

A randomized, double-blind, placebo-controlled, multicenter trial by Bode, et al. in 2010 assessed whether treatment of the nostrils of rapidly identified nasal carriers of *S. aureus* with mupirocin and treatment of the skin with chlorhexidine gluconate soap could prevent nosocomial *S. aureus* infections. [15] Patients with planned admission to the hospital for a minimum of 14 days were screened at or prior to admission for nasal carriage of *S. aureus*. The *S. aureus* was rapidly identified with real-time PCR. Patients were then randomized into a treatment group where the patients were treated with mupirocin in the nose and chlorhexidine gluconate soap for the skin and a placebo group where patients were given both placebo ointment and placebo soap. Treatment was for 5 days and patients were monitored for hospital acquired *S. aureus* infections. A total of 1251 (18.8 %) of 6771 screened patients tested positive for *S. aureus* on PCR. A total of 918 patients were randomized into one of the two groups. They found that the cumulative incidence of health care-associated *S. aureus* infection was significantly lower in the treatment group versus the placebo group. In the treatment group, 17 (3.4 %) of the 504 patients developed nosocomial *S. aureus* infections as opposed to 37 (7.7 %) of the 413 patients in the placebo group. There was no statistically significant difference between surgical and nonsurgical patients for cumulative incidence of hospital associated *S. aureus* infections. Kaplan-Meier curves of their data showed significantly shorter time to infection in the placebo group than in the treatment group. The mean duration of hospital admission was significantly longer in the placebo group versus the treatment group by perhaps a day. All cause hospital mortality was not significantly different between the two groups. What was surprising about this study was that all strains of *S. aureus* were methicillin-sensitive and also susceptible to mupirocin. All of their data showed the risk of hospital-associated infections associated with *S. aureus* was reduced by 60 %.

A 2012 study from Turkey looked at nasal bacterial flora and colonization by MRSA in patients with a known diagnosis of allergic rhinitis [3]. The authors separated patients into one of two groups, a study group, which consisted of patient with allergic rhinitis, and a control group, consisting of patient without a history of allergic disease. Cultures were performed from nasal swabs of both groups. Methicillin-resistant coagulase-negative *S. aureus* was the most commonly colonized resistant bacteria in the study group. When looking at MRSA and methicillin-resistant coagulase-negative *S. aureus*, 15 (27.8 %) of 54 patients with allergic rhinitis were culture positive, whereas only 2 (4.0 %) of 50 patients in the control group were culture positive. Small sample sizes in this study make drawing conclusions difficult and more research is necessary, but their findings bring to light the importance of disorders related to allergic rhinitis.

A placebo-controlled, double-blind study from Columbia University in 1992 was performed to establish the efficacy and safety of mupirocin application to the anterior part of the nose for 5 days to try to eradicate nasal carriage of *S. aureus* [16]. Mupirocin is a topical antibiotic that binds to and inhibits bacterial isobenzyl-transfer RNS synthetase. This blocks bacterial protein synthesis. The authors cultured volunteer medical staff to screen for *S. aureus*. Patients were then separated into two groups. One group was given mupirocin topically inside each nostril twice daily for 5 days, with the other group given placebo. The placebo group showed persistence of *S. aureus* while the treatment group showed that 25 (74 %) of 34 patients were free of *S. aureus* at early follow-up. Follow-up occurred at 1, 2 and 4 week intervals with re-colonization occurring in 11 patients. Mupirocin is 95 % efficacious at eliminating the original strain of *S. aureus* at early follow-up with 79 % efficacy at 4 week follow-up. Only 41 % of patients showed persistent eradication of all *S. aureus* at 4 weeks. A finding that was very interesting was that six (18 %) of 34 patients treated had resistance to mupirocin. Chambers, et al. in 2004 hypothesized that using mupirocin in the nose will reduce nasal-to-hand transmission of colonizing bacteria to other cutaneous sites, but nasal colonization with the same strain will eventually occur because of the presence of that strain on other parts of the body [17].

Treatment

One of the earliest reported cases in the literature was in August of 1949 when a 25 day old African-American infant that developed a nasal septal abscess with associated orbital cellulitis that did not respond to a 10-day course of penicillin. Only after sulfadiazine and dihydrostreptomycin administration did the patient improve [18]. Topical aluminum chloride was once described along with antiseptics [9]. Another treatment described very early on for simple nasal vestibulitis by DeWeese in 1962 was the use of 5 % ammoniated mercury ointment, which he thought was much more effective than the commonly used Borofax ointment or sulfathiazole ointment that was common at that time [19]. Standard treatment of uncomplicated nasal vestibulitis included warm compresses and mupirocin, with cephalexin or culture-directed oral antibiotics if the infection appears to be widespread [5]. Community-acquired MRSA may be treated with antibiotics such as trimethoprim/sulfamethoxazole or clindamycin [4]. Saline irrigations and avoiding digital manipulation are advisable as an adjunct to treatment. Abscess formation, as one would expect, would require incision and drainage via an intranasal approach to avoid external scarring of the face with consideration for intravenous antibiotics.

Conclusion

Since there has not been a lot of literature published on nasal vestibulitis, most diagnosis and treatment options are based more on anecdotal evidence and case reports. Nasal carriage has been researched more in depth in order to mainly try to decrease the incidence of both community acquired and nosocomial soft tissue infections that may have their bacterial origins in the nasal cavity. More research is necessary to further elucidate colonization of the nose. Because of the simplicity of typical nasal vestibulitis, more thorough research, although desirable, may not be all that forthcoming in the future.

References

1. Wertheim HF, Melles DC, Vos MC, van Leeuwen W, van Belkum A, Verbrugh HA, Nouwen JL. The Role of nasal carriage in *Staphylococcus aureus* infections. Lancet Infect Dis. 2005;5(12):751–62.
2. Önerci TM. Nasal vestibulitis and nasal furunculosis and mucormycosis. In: Önerci TM, editor. Diagnosis in otorhinolaryngology. Berlin: Springer; 2010. p. 69–71.
3. Çevik C, Yula E, Yengil E, Gülmez Mİ, Akbay E. Identification of nasal bacterial flora profile and carriage rates of methicillin-resistant Staphylococcus aureus in patients with allergic rhinitis. Eur Arch Otorhinolaryngol. 2014;271(1):103–7.
4. Fairbanks DN. Pocket guide to antimicrobial therapy in otolaryngology—head and neck surgery. 13th ed. Alexandria: The American Academy of Otolaryngology—Head and Neck Surgery Foundation; 2007.
5. Wang MB. Etiologies of nasal symptoms: an overview. In: Feldweg AM, Corren J editors. UpToDate. UpToDate: Waltham. Accessed 16 Oct 2014.
6. Rudramurthy M, Sumangala B, Honnavar P, Madhav YB, Munegowda KC, Ravi D, Chakrabarti A. Nasal vestibulitis due to Nocardiopsis dassonvillei in a diabetic patient. J Med Microbiol. 2012;61(Pt 8):1168–73.
7. Lim RS, Flatman S, Dahm MC. Sinonasal melioidosis in a returned traveler presenting with nasal cellulitis and sinusitis. Case Rep Otolaryngol. 2013;2013:920352.
8. Soto LE, Bobadilla M, Villalobos Y, Sifuentes J, Avelar J, Arrieta M, Ponce de Leon S. Post-surgical nasal cellulitis outbreak due to Mycobacterium chelonae. J Hosp Infect. 1991;19(2):99–106.
9. Dahle KW, Sontheimer RD. The Rudolph sign of nasal vestibular furunculosis: questions raised by this common but under-recognized nasal mucocutaneous disorder. Dermatol Online J. 2012;18(3):6.
10. Davis KA, Stewart JJ, Crouch HK, Florez CE, Hospenthal DR. Methicillin-resistant Staphylococcus aureus (MRSA) nares colonization at hospital admission and its effect on subsequent MRSA infection. Clin Infect Dis. 2004;39(6):776–82.
11. Fritz SA, Krauss MJ, Epplin EK, Burnham CA, Garbutt J, Dunne WM, Hunstad DA, Storch GA. The natural history of contemporary *Staphylococcus aureus* nasal colonization in community children. Pediatr Infect Dis J. 2011;30(4):349–51.
12. Hidron AI, Kourbatova EV, Halvosa JS, Terrell BJ, McDougal LK, Tenover FC, Blumberg HM, King MD. Risk factors for colonization with methicillin-resistant Staphylococcus aureus (MRSA) in patients admitted to an urban hospital: emergence of community-associated MRSA nasal carriage. Clin Infect Dis. 2005;41(2):159–66.
13. van Belkum A, Verkaik NJ, de Vogel CP, Boelens HA, Verveer J, Nouwen JL, Verbrugh HA, Wertheim HF. Reclassification of Staphylococcus aureus nasal carriage types. J Infect Dis. 2009;199(12):1820–6.

14. Zafar U, Johnson LB, Hanna M, Riederer K, Sharma M, Fakih MG, Thirumoorthi MC, Farjo R, Khatib R. Prevalence of nasal colonization among patients with community-associated methicillin-resistant *Staphylococcus aureus* infection and their household contacts. Infect Control Hosp Epidemiol. 2007;28(8):966–9.
15. Bode LG, Kluytmans JA, Wertheim HF, Bogaers D, Vandenbroucke-Grauls CM, Roosendaal R, Troelstra A, Box AT, Voss A, van der Tweel I, van Belkum A, Verbrugh HA, Vos MC. Preventing surgical-site infections in nasal carriers of Staphylococcus aureus. N Engl J Med. 2010;362(1):9–17.
16. Scully BE, Briones F, Gu JW, Neu HC. Mupirocin treatment of nasal staphylococcal colonization. Arch Intern Med. 1992;152(2):353–6.
17. Chambers 3rd HF, Winston LG. Mupirocin prophylaxis misses by a nose. Ann Intern Med. 2004;140(6):484–5.
18. Hayden GD, Pastore PN, Kundert K. Abscess of the nasal septum and orbital cellulitis in an infant. AMA Arch Otolaryngol. 1950;52(5):773–5.
19. DeWeese DD. "Letters to the editor". Treatment for nasal vestibulitis. Arch Otolaryngol. 1962;76(2):99.

Chapter 7
Sinusitis

J. Chase McNeil and Yamilet Tirado

Introduction

Sinusitis is defined as an inflammation of the paranasal sinuses caused by a viral or bacterial infection, allergies and/or autoimmune diseases. Sinusitis is one of the most prevalent diseases in the United States, with more than 30 million cases of chronic sinusitis including all ages reported annually by the Centers for Disease Control and Prevention [1]. Children affected with sinusitis experience a negative change in their quality of life, as it is known to exacerbate other airway pathologies including reactive airway disease, chronic bronchitis and asthma, creating a substantial health care burden with a socio-economic impact of more than $5.8 billion per year in treatment costs [1].

The diagnosis of sinus infection is made by clinical history and supported by findings on physical exam. Signs and symptoms of sinusitis include headache, facial pain or pressure, thick nasal discharge of yellow/green color, fever, fatigue, bad breath, dental pain and ear pressure, among others (see Table 7.1). Approximately 6–8 upper respiratory tract infections (URTIs) occur in children per year, which usually present with similar symptoms but only 8–10 % progress to sinusitis [2]. Self-limiting URTIs may be difficult to distinguish from an acute sinus infection but the lack of improvement or worsening symptoms at 7–10 days is highly suggestive of acute sinusitis.

The American Academy of Pediatrics divides sinusitis into 5 different categories based on the duration and frequency of symptoms (see Fig. 7.1) [3]. Acute sinusitis is defined as symptoms of less than 4 weeks duration and strongly suggested by the presence of 2 major symptoms or 1 major and 2 minor symptoms (see Table 7.1). Subacute sinusitis is regarded as when symptoms last anywhere from 4 to 8 weeks. Chronic sinusitis is characterized by symptoms lasting longer than 90 days. Recurrent acute sinusitis, which is, defined as recurrent episodes each completely resolving in less than 2 weeks, separated by asymptomatic periods of at least 10 days. Acute exacerbation of chronic sinusitis is when patients with chronic sinusitis develop new acute respiratory symptoms.

J.C. McNeil, M.D.
Department of Pediatrics, Section of Infectious Diseases, Baylor College of Medicine, 1102 Bates St. Suite 1150, Houston, TX, USA
e-mail: jm140109@bcm.tmc.edu

Y. Tirado, M.D. (✉)
Department of Otolaryngology, Miami Children's Hospital, Miami, FL, USA
e-mail: yamilet.tirado@mch.com

T.A. Valdez, J.G. Vallejo (eds.), *Infectious Diseases in Pediatric Otolaryngology*,
DOI 10.1007/978-3-319-21744-4_7

Table 7.1 Signs and symptoms of sinusitis

Major symptoms	Minor symptoms
Facial pain/pressure	Dental pain
Nasal obstruction/congestion	Ear fullness/pain
Nasal discharge	Headache
Hyposmia/anosmia	Halitosis
Cough	Fever
	Fatigue

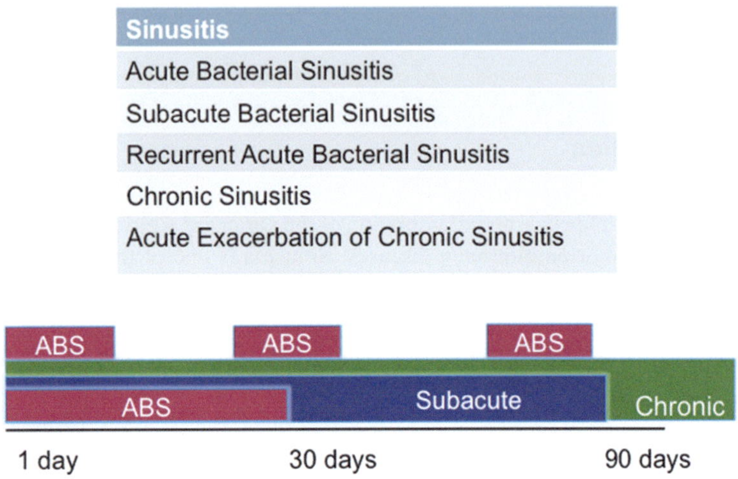

Fig. 7.1 Categories of sinusitis. ABS (acute bacterial sinusitis); chronic (chronic sinusitis)

Anatomy

The paranasal sinuses consist of air-filled paired cavities in the skull named after the bone in which it is located. The maxillary sinuses are located deep to the cheeks and under the eyes. The frontal sinuses are located above the eyes, the ethmoid sinuses between the eyes and the sphenoid sinuses located at the center of the skull behind the eyes. These cavities are involved in the humidification of air, voice resonance, and skull weight. Each of these sinuses drains through an ostium of approximately 1–3 mm in size into the nasal cavity.

The maxillary and the ethmoid sinuses are present at birth and slowly enlarge to adult size by puberty [4]. The maxillary sinuses have an inverted pyramidal shape and are the largest of the sinuses. The natural opening of the maxillary sinus is positioned superiorly on the medial maxillary wall and opens to the ostiomeatal complex, a confluence of sinus drainage from the frontal, anterior ethmoids and maxillary sinuses located between the middle and inferior turbinates. The ethmoid sinuses consist of a honeycomb of air cells that lie medial to the orbits and are separated from the orbits by the lamina papyracea. The ethmoid sinuses are divided into anterior and posterior cells. Infection of the ethmoids can easily spread to the orbit directly through bony dehiscences or by traversing the neurovascular foramina. The frontal sinuses arise from the anterior ethmoid air cells and start developing between the ages of 5–6 years and continue to develop until late adolescence [5]. The frontal sinuses are funnel-shaped structures with the posterior wall separating the sinus from the anterior cranial fossa. The diploic veins connect the vasculature of the sinus mucosa with the intracranial sinuses and veins, providing a potential route of infectious spread. The sphenoid sinus begins to develop between 3 and 5 years of age and continues to grow until late teenage years. The sphenoid sinus ostium is located on the anterosuperior surface of the sphenoid face, and drains with the posterior ethmoid cells into the superior meatus located between the middle and superior turbinates. The optic nerve and the carotid artery are located on the lateral wall of the sphenoid sinus and the pituitary fossa is located in the posterior aspect.

The sinus cavities are lined with pseudostratified ciliated epithelium, which contain globlet cells, and submucosal glands that produce two different layers of secretions. The deep layer consist of serous secretions permitting normal cilia motility and the superficial layer consist of mucinous/viscous secretions which increase viscosity to capture particles and pathogens. The cilia move mucus and debris from the sinus cavities into the nasopharynx.

Pathophysiology

For the paranasal sinuses to have normal function three main factors need to be present: a normal mucociliary function, patency of the sinus ostia, and thin/clear consistency of nasal secretions. The most common causes to disrupt the normal function of the sinuses in children are viral URTIs and allergic rhinitis. Mucosal edema and inflammation can be caused by viral infections, allergic rhinitis, immune disorders, gastroesophageal reflux disease (GERD), nasal obstruction, and/or anatomical abnormalities and systemic disorders. Prolonged sinus obstruction, variation in the character of nasal secretions and alterations in intranasal pressure can lead to bacterial growth, colonization and subsequently infection of the sinus cavities. Although inflammation in any of the sinuses can lead to obstruction of the sinus ostia, the most commonly involved sinuses in a sinus infection are the maxillary and the anterior ethmoid sinuses [6].

In an URTI, the nasal mucosa responds to the virus by producing mucus and recruiting white blood cells to the lining of the nose, inducing an inflammatory response leading to congestion and swelling of the nasal passages [7]. The resultant ostial obstruction creates sinus cavity hypoxia and mucus retention causing the cilia to function less efficiently, creating an environment for bacterial growth.

Allergy is involved in sinusitis due to an inflammatory obstruction of the sinonasal mucosa and ostia caused by the release of histamine and major basic protein by mast cells and eosinophils, respectively. These substances cause vasodilation, mucous secretion, nerve stimulation and smooth muscle contraction causing damage to the surrounding tissue resulting in rhinorrhea, itching, sneezing and postnasal drip [8]. Non-allergic environmental irritants such as cigarette smoke and household chemicals can directly affect the mucosa of the sinuses. In addition to allergy, immunologic compromise may be an important etiologic factor in patients with chronic, refractory sinusitis. Children with immune deficiencies will likely have a history of recurrent and refractory sinus infections associated with otitis media, bronchitis, and lower respiratory infections.

There is a higher prevalence of GERD in patients with refractory sinusitis, suggesting that reflux may be a contributing factor to the pathogenesis of chronic sinus infection. Acid from the stomach can directly injure the nasal mucosa leading to sinonasal edema and impaired mucociliary clearance. Nasopharyngeal reflux has been documented in children with symptoms of chronic sinusitis that present with coughing paroxysms [9]. Despite the low quality of evidence supporting this relationship, GERD treatment should be considered in patients with chronic sinusitis and reflux symptoms, particularly in those patients not responding to conventional sinusitis treatment [10].

Anatomical variations most commonly associated with nasal obstruction and sinus pathology are nasal septal deviation and concha bullosa, (see Fig. 7.2). Intranasal growths such as nasal polyps, benign or malignant tumors, and adenoid hypertrophy are contributing factors to sinus infections. Both anatomical abnormalities and intranasal growths can cause mechanical obstruction of the sinus ostia predisposing patients to sinusitis [11, 12]. However, studies in children have not found a relationship between sinus disease and anatomical variations, suggesting that other factors play a more essential role in the development of pediatric sinusitis. In addition, the adenoid pad can act as a nidus of bacteria contributing to recurrent or chronic bacterial sinusitis.

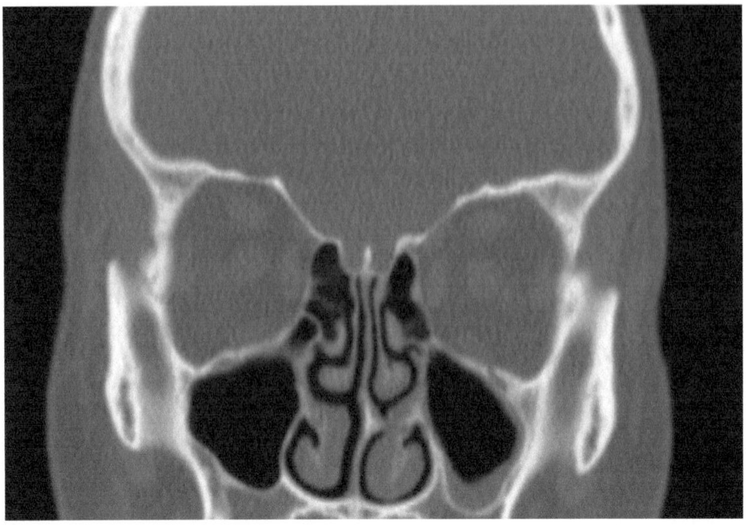

Fig. 7.2 Non-contrast CT sinus showing an area of nasal obstruction. Left septal spur impinging an enlarged inferior turbinate with mild mucosal thickening of the left maxillary sinus

Systemic diseases such as cystic fibrosis and primary ciliary dyskinesia can also alter the normal mucociliary function and cause sinus infections. Cystic fibrosis causes significant alteration in the quality of mucous secreted in the nasal cavities interrupting normal physiology [13]. Primary ciliary dyskinesia affects the cilia morphology and number therefore causing reduced mucous clearance from the respiratory tract and altering the defense mechanisms against environmental particles, bacterial and viral pathogens.

Microbiology

The specific data regarding the contemporary microbiology of sinus disease is limited and much of what is known in children is extrapolated from studies of either nasal colonization or otitis media. Studies of pediatric outpatients with acute otitis media who had middle ear fluid (MEF) and nasopharyngeal (NP) cultures obtained simultaneously have revealed that the middle ear pathogen was also co-isolated in NP culture in 100 % of cases. By contrast however, other pathogens were identified in the NP culture that were not present in the MEF in 47 % of cases [14]. Thus, while NP cultures may provide some information regarding potential otitis and sinus pathogens, the results are hardly definitive. While *Streptococcus pneumoniae* remains the predominant bacterial respiratory pathogen in children, the microbiology of pediatric respiratory disease has evolved tremendously over the past 14 years. This change is mainly the result of the introduction of the 7-valent followed by the 13-valent pneumococcal conjugate vaccines (PCV7 and PCV13). Following introduction of the PCV7 vaccine, a decline in sinus disease and otitis media due to serotypes of *S. pneumoniae* included in the vaccine was observed. Studies of children who underwent endoscopic sinus surgery (ESS) following introduction of PCV7, however, revealed an increase in the relative proportion of cases of sinusitis due to *S. pneumoniae* serotypes not included in the vaccine. Notably the antibiotic-resistant pneumococcal serotype 19A was most common among these non-vaccine serotypes [15]. The prevalence of serotype 19A *S. pneumoniae* as a sinus pathogen has since declined after widespread use of PCV13 (which includes serotype 19A) [16]. Furthermore, the proportion of cases of orbital abscesses due to *S. pneumoniae* has declined following introduction of the PCVs [17]. In addition, among isolates causing invasive disease, the percent of pneumococci non-susceptible to penicillin decreased in the post PCV-13 era [18]. Risk factors for infection with pneumococci resistant to penicillin and other antibiotics include age <2 years or >65 years, daycare attendance, medical comorbidities and recent antibiotic use [19, 20]. Studies of invasive pneumococcal disease have shown that among patients with previous antibiotic exposure, proximity to last antibiotic course predicted resistance to that particular antibiotic; such may be the case for pneumococcal sinusitis as well [21].

While the proportion of cases due to *S. pneumoniae* has declined, other pathogens have increased in frequency. Recent studies of young children with otitis media from Rochester, New York have demonstrated a decline in *S. pneumoniae* isolation from MEF culture and a relative increase in the prevalence of nontypeable-Haemophilus *influenzae* (NTHI). Work from New Zealand has demonstrated that *H. influenzae* can be identified from MEF through a combination of culture and PCR techniques in up to 60 % of children with otitis in the post-PCV era [22]. Studies in the United States have shown that NTHI may contribute to up to 41 % of cases in children, an increase from 25 % in the pre-PCV era [23]. *H. influenzae* can present therapeutic challenges in that many strains possess plasmid-encoded β-lactamases. Heilman et al. noted that 26 % of *H. influenzae* respiratory isolates were β-lactamase-positive [24], however there is tremendous variability around the globe. There has also been noted in recent years outside of the US the emergence of NTHI strains that are resistant to β-lactams through alternative mechanisms other than β-lactamases [25, 26]. The other predominant bacterial pathogen in acute sinusitis to consider in children is *Moraxella catarrhalis* [27]. *M. catarrhalis* accounts for up to 20 % of sinusitis pathogens in children [28]. While notably over 90 % of *M. catarrhalis* produce β-lactamases, susceptibility to other agents remains high [29, 30].

With the rise of community-acquired methicillin-resistant *Staphylococcus aureus* (MRSA), much interest has developed in the role that *S. aureus* may play in respiratory disease. *S. aureus* has been variably reported as a cause of acute bacterial sinusitis with reports ranging from 0 to >30 % of cases [31]. Many investigators have reported an increased in frequency of MRSA recovered from patients with sinus disease [32]. The exact prevalence of *S. aureus* in sinus disease is unclear as nasal colonization with *S. aureus*, in particular MRSA, has increased over time in healthy pediatric and adult controls. Thus, the prevalence of *S. aureus* as a pathogen of acute sinusitis has likely been over estimated by studies that have relied on NP culture for diagnosis alone. Notably, however, Huang et al. in Taiwan performed cultures of middle meatus drainage in adults and children with maxillary sinusitis and found MRSA in 2.7 % [33]. In contrast to its relatively small role in acute sinusitis, *S. aureus* can be a prominent cause of chronic sinusitis. In a 3 year review of cases of chronic sinusitis managed with ESS, Whitby et al. identified 56 cases of *S. aureus* sinusitis of which 21 % were MRSA [34]. Notably, in this study copathogens were isolated in 77 % of cases underscoring that chronic sinusitis is frequently a polymicrobial disease. Among patients with chronic sinusitis, other etiologies to consider include anaerobes, gram-negative bacilli and fungi. *Actinomyces* has rarely been reported as a cause of sinusitis in adults and children [35], often in the absence of dental caries that are typical for cervicofacial actinomycosis (Fig. 7.3). Allergic *Aspergillus* sinusitis is occasionally a cause of chronic sinusitis in children with negative cultures who have been refractory to antibiotics; patients typically have a history of atopy, recurrent sinusitis, nasal polyps and the identification of fungi on cultures/smears [36]. Such patients can be managed with thorough debridement and corticosteroids. Among patients with chronic, recurrent or refractory sinusitis consideration should also be given to an immunocompromising condition.

Atypical bacterial pathogens are very uncommon causes of sinusitis. *Chlamydia* (also referred to as *Chlamydophila*) *pneumoniae* can rarely be identified as causes of chronic sinusitis in adults or children [37, 38]. Among adults with sinusitis one group of investigators noted that 3.5 % had elevation of complement fixing anti-*Mycoplasma* antibodies [39]. Given that *Mycoplasma* antibodies cross react with other pathogens and have a long half-life, relying on this as a diagnostic tool is problematic. Lee et al. performed PCR for *Mycoplasma*, *C. pneumoniae* and *Legionella* from ethmoid sinus samples of 11 adults undergoing endoscopic sinus surgery for chronic sinusitis; none of these patients had molecular evidence of infection due to these pathogens [40]. Conversely, studies of military servicemen with *Mycoplasma pneumoniae* pneumonia found that nearly two-thirds had radiologic evidence

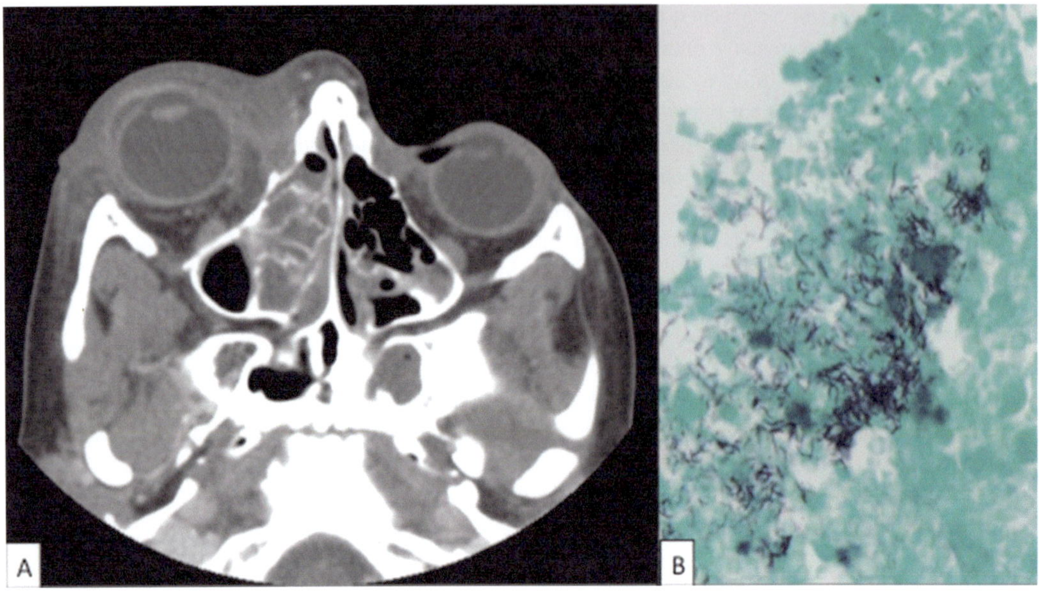

Fig. 7.3 Contrast enhanced CT scan of orbits with maxillary/ethmoid sinusitis due to Actinomyces israelii. (**a**) Contrast enhanced CT image of an 11-year old previously healthy boy with right-sided ethmoid sinus opacification and abscess in the medial, superior and inferior wall of the right orbit. He was taken to the operating room and histologic examination revealed sulfur granules and anaerobic cultures grew Actinomyces israelii. (**b**) ×40 magnification of specimen with filamentous branching bacterial organisms identified by MSN staining. Pathologic slide courtesy of Karen Eldin, MD, Dept of Pathology Baylor College of Medicine

of sinusitis [41]. Thus, for adults or older children with concomitant atypical pneumonia and sinusitis, *Mycoplasma* could be a potential etiology of disease. While it is believed that viral URTI may create inflammation at sinus ostia, impairing sinus drainage and predisposing to acute sinusitis, the direct role of viruses in infection is unclear. Rises in antibody titers to a number of viruses including influenza, adenovirus and parainfluenza virus have been documented to occur in the setting of acute sinusitis [39]. Other investigators have been able to demonstrate the presence of rhinovirus RNA in maxillary sinus epithelial cells of volunteers with clinically diagnosed sinusitis [42]. Given that viruses can continue to be shed for a period after resolution of an acute respiratory illness, the significance for etiology of the detection of these viruses in patients with sinusitis is unclear.

The diagnosis of sinusitis in a severely immunocompromised child is both a medical and surgical emergency because of the risk of invasive fungal infection. The primary fungi of concern include the Zygomycetes (also referred to as *Mucor*), *Aspergillus* spp. and as well as number of less common dematiaceous fungi (such as *Curvularia*, *Bipolaris*, *Fusarium* etc). Such patients are at risk for fungal extension into critical vessels as well as the CNS and aggressive surgical debridement is often necessary (Fig. 7.4). Rarely, acute infection in an otherwise healthy host can extend from the paranasal sinuses into the orbit (Fig. 7.5) or cranial vault. This complication occurs more often in boys (approximately 2:1 gender ratio) and intracranial extension typically occurs in older children (mean age of 11–13 years) [43, 44]. While typical acute sinusitis pathogens can be involved, particularly for intraorbital disease, other organisms predominant in intracranial infection. Common organisms associated with intracranial extension of sinusitis include *Streptococcus milleri* group, *Propionibacterium acnes* and *S. aureus* as well as anaerobes such as *Peptostreptococcus* spp., *Fusobacterium* spp. and *Prevotella* [43, 44]. Notably, both intracranial and intraorbital extension of sinus disease is frequently a polymicrobial infection [43, 45]. An additional rare complication of frontal sinusitis is the development of osteomyelitis of the frontal bone which if a subperiosteal abscess develops may manifest as the so-called Pott's puffy tumor.

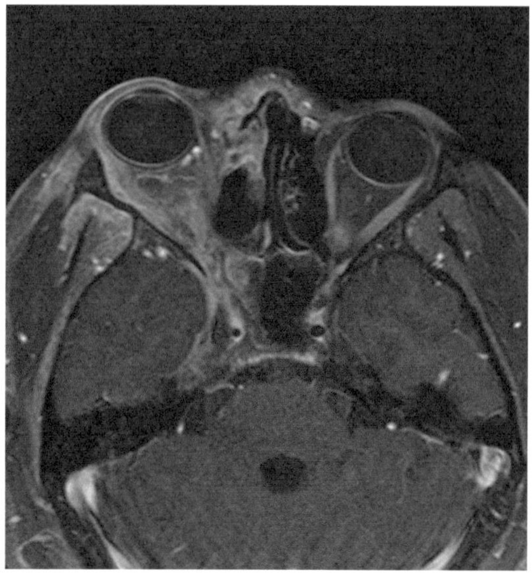

Fig. 7.4 Invasive fungal sinusitis with extension into the right orbit and intracranially. invasive fungal sinusitis in an adolescent with poorly controlled type 2 diabetes. T1-weighted MRI. Right maxillary sinus with extensive disease with extension into the right orbit. This patient presented with severe headaches and facial pain. He underwent debridement and was initiated promptly on voriconazole and amphotericin. Cultures grew Rhizopus. The child and his family denied radical surgical debridement. Despite maximal medical management the child's disease progressed and he subsequently expired

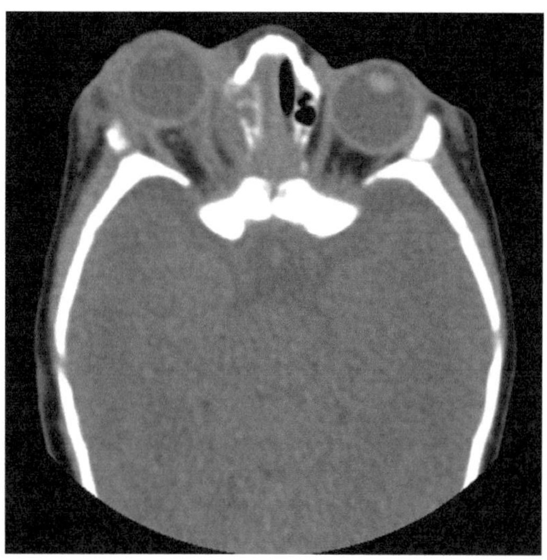

Fig. 7.5 Maxillary and ethmoid sinusitis with extension into right orbit. Nonenhanced CT of acute sinusitis with extension into the right orbit of a 6 year-old boy. Cultures grew S. pneumoniae

Epidemiology

Understanding the precise clinical epidemiology of sinusitis in children is difficult, in part due to the somewhat subjective nature of clinical diagnosis. Interestingly, sinusitis is not a problem limited to the modern era; there is archaeological evidence of chronic sinusitis in unearthed remains of both adults and children living in medieval Europe [46]. Estimates of the number of cases of sinusitis in adults and children in the United States based on diagnostic codes reach as high as 20 million per year [2]. Some investigators have estimated that acute bacterial sinusitis complicates as many as 8–10 % of viral URTIs in children [2, 47]. Furthermore, sinusitis accounts for 5–10 % of outpatient pediatric visits for which antibiotics are prescribed [48].

Sinusitis is more commonly diagnosed in boys than girls with at least a 1.8:1 gender ratio [49, 50]. The predominant age ranges for pediatric sinusitis vary in the literature from 3 to 12 years of age [49, 50]. In a study specifically examining children less than 3 years of age, Revai et al. noted that the proportion of URTIs complicated by sinusitis peaked in the second year of life [51]. In general, however, sinusitis can occur at any age with the notable caveat that it is an extremely rare diagnosis in infants.

Clinical Manifestations and Diagnosis

Symptoms of an acute pediatric sinus infection are similar to symptoms of a viral URTI, and are strongly suggested by the presence of nasal discharge, nasal obstruction, decreased sense of smell, cough, and/or facial pain/pressure. For patients in whom viral URTI symptoms have not resolved after 7–10 days, acute sinusitis should be suspected. The diagnosis of pediatric sinusitis is mostly clinical and supported by history and findings on physical exam.

Acute bacterial sinusitis is strongly suspected if two major symptoms or one major symptom and two minor symptoms are present (see Table 7.1). Physical examination may be challenging in a pediatric patient but presence of turbinate inflammation and erythema, mucopurulent secretions in the nasal floor, and pooling of secretions from the nasopharynx in the posterior pharynx are highly suggestive of bacterial sinusitis. Endoscopic evaluation can also visualize other abnormalities on exam such as adenoid hypertrophy, nasal polyps as well as to exclude foreign bodies or other causes of nasal obstruction [52]. The presence of nasal polyps on exam should prompt an evaluation for cystic fibrosis.

CBC, ESR, and blood cultures are rarely helpful in cases of uncomplicated acute sinus infection. In cases of recurrent or chronic sinus infections, allergy testing, laboratory evaluation of the immune system to rule out immunodeficiency, mucosal biopsy to rule out primary ciliary dyskinesia and genetic testing for cystic fibrosis should be considered.

A thorough history identifying symptoms for more than 10 days has been shown to significantly correlate with abnormal radiographs and positive cultures, therefore obviating the need for imaging in acute cases. Plain radiographs, including Water and Caldwell-Luc's views, are often ordered by clinicians to assist in the diagnosis of sinusitis but their roles is limited due to high false-positive rates and are not typically recommended in routine practice [53]. The gold standard for diagnosing bacterial sinusitis is maxillary sinus puncture with aspiration and cultures [54]. However, this procedure is usually done under anesthesia and thus is not practical except in children not responding to broad-spectrum antibiotics, patients who are toxic appearing or in immune deficient patients to target appropriate systemic antimicrobial therapy.

Children have thinner sinus walls and septa, higher bony porosity, open suture lines and larger vascular foramina in their cranial vault making them more susceptible to orbital and intracranial sinus complications than adults. Orbital complications are the most common and severity ranges from eyelid edema to subperiosteal and orbital abscesses (see Fig. 7.5) [55]. Decreased visual acuity, gaze restriction, proptosis, and diminished pupillary reflex are manifestation seen in children with orbital complications. Intracranial complications include meningitis, epidural and subdural abscess, cavernous and sagittal sinus thromboses, and intraparenchymal brain abscesses. Manifestations in pediatric patients with intracranial complications include fever, headaches, lethargy, seizures and neurologic deficits [56]. Otolaryngology and ophthalmology consultations are indicated in a patient with sinusitis and ophthalmologic findings, while otolaryngology and neurosurgery consultations are needed in a patient with sinusitis and neurological findings. Sinus complications are associated with increased morbidity and mortality therefore directed treatment and early management is strongly recommended [57].

CT scan is usually reserved for patients with suspected complications of sinusitis, those who are unresponsive to medical treatment, and patients under consideration for surgical intervention. CT is the gold standard in imaging of the sinuses as it gives better visualization providing higher resolution of bony structures. Axial and coronal views with limited cuts and *without* contrast usually suffice. Contrast is reserved for suspected suppuration and nasal masses. Mucosal changes, intrasinus collections or growths, and adjacent bone changes can also be visualized. MRI of the sinuses, orbits and brain is usually obtained in the presence of extensive disease and/or when multiple complications are suspected as it better characterize extension of local disease beyond the paranasal sinuses. MRI with contrast gadolinium allows better soft tissue differentiation and high spatial resolution images depicting fine details. A combination of CT and MRI is useful in cases of diagnostic difficulties [53].

Medical Management

While, in general infectious disease problems should be managed with a goal toward culture directed specific antimicrobial therapy, culture data is not typically available for acute sinusitis and therapy must be used empirically. Published guidelines for the management of acute bacterial sinusitis are available from both the Infectious Diseases Society of America (IDSA [58]) and the American Academy of Pediatrics (AAP [59]).

One challenge in the management of upper respiratory disease with or without fever in young children is distinguishing a viral rhinitis/rhinosinusitis from bacterial infection. Initiation of antimicrobial therapy is recommended when patients exhibit (a) persistent symptoms concerning for sinusitis lasting ≥10 days without clear clinical improvement, (b) onset with severe symptoms of high fever, purulent nasal discharge and/or facial pain lasting for at least 3–4 days or (c) worsening of symptoms after a period of initial improvement (so called “double sickening”). Patients with a toxic appearance or neurologic symptoms should undergo a thorough evaluation and receive broad-spectrum empiric therapy, as well as consideration of alternative diagnoses.

For initial empiric therapy in uncomplicated bacterial sinusitis in children the IDSA and AAP recommend initiation of amoxicillin-clavulanate. This recommendation is based on data, largely from studies of otitis media, which observed both a decline in the proportion of cases due to *S. pneumoniae* and a relative increase in the proportion of cases due to β-lactamase producing organisms, principally *H. influenzae* and *M. catarrhalis*. Use of a high dose of amoxicillin-clavulanate (90 mg/kg/day of the amoxicillin component divided twice daily) is recommended in regions with a prevalence of penicillin-resistant *S. pneumoniae* greater than 10 % or when risk factors for penicillin resistance exist (see Microbiology above). Potential problems with the high dose amoxicillin-clavulanate are the higher cost and greater gastrointestinal side effects.

For children with a history of type-I hypersensitivity to penicillins, the IDSA endorses the use of levofloxacin (10–20 mg/kg/day po every 12–24 h). While fluoroquinolones are not FDA approved for use in children and these agents have been typically avoided by pediatricians, a recent publication showed no increased incidence of musculoskeletal adverse events in children 5 years after receipt of levofloxacin compared to those who received a comparator agent [60]. By contrast, the AAP supports the use of cefdinir, cefuroxime or cefpodoxime for the treatment in β-lactam allergic patients due to low rates of cross-reactivity between these specific cephalosporins and penicillin [61, 62]. The IDSA, however, no longer recommends oral cephalosporins as monotherapy for acute bacterial sinusitis.

The oral cephalosporins with greatest in vitro activity against *S. pneumoniae* include cefdinir, cefixime, cefpodoxime and cefuroxime however there is tremendous variability by region. Among penicillin-intermediate *S. pneumoniae*, only 38 % were susceptible to cefuroxime or cefpodoxime and penicillin-resistant isolates were resistant to all oral cephalosporin examined in one study from Spain [63]. The parenteral third generation cephalosporins usually retain activity against penicillin-nonsusceptible pneumococci, however [64]. For this reason, both the IDSA and AAP support use of cefixime or cefpodoxime in combination with clindamycin for the management of acute sinusitis in children with a non-serious penicillin allergy, particularly in regions with high rates of penicillin-nonsusceptible *S. pneumoniae*. Doxycycline could be considered for penicillin allergic patients over the age of 8 years old. Linezolid, although not endorsed by national guidelines, is an additional option for treatment of sinusitis due to pneumococcus or *S. aureus*. Prolonged or frequent linezolid use is associated with significant adverse events including neutropenia, thrombocytopenia, peripheral neuropathy, optic neuritis and hypertensive crises. These adverse events, along with its high cost and lack of activity against *H. influenzae* or *M. catarrhalis* restrict the use of linezolid to patients with drug-resistant gram-positive organisms or with refractory disease. Similar to recommendations in children, for treatment of sinusitis in adults the IDSA recommends use of amoxicillin-clavulanate (500 mg/125 mg by mouth three times a day or 875 mg/125 mg by mouth twice daily) as first line therapy. High dose amoxicillin-clavulanate (2000 mg/ 125 mg twice daily) is recommended for adult patients failing first-line therapy or those at risk for drug-resistant organisms. Doxycycline (100 mg twice daily) or a respiratory fluoroquinolone (levofloxacin 500 mg daily or moxifloxacin 400 mg daily) can be considered in adults for second line therapy or in those with β-lactam allergies.

Macrolides are no longer recommended as monotherapy for acute sinusitis given rates of resistance among pneumococci of >30 % [65]. In particular the risk of macrolide resistant pneumococci is highest in children under 2-years-old. Trimethoprim-sulfamethoxazole is also no longer recommended as monotherapy due to increasing resistance. A survey of respiratory isolates from 2005 to 2007 revealed that 50 % of *S. pneumoniae* and 27 % of *H. influenzae* were resistant to trimethoprim-sulfamethoxazole [66]. For patients who fail to improve on standard therapy or particularly those who have chronic symptoms, strong consideration should be given to obtaining a sinus culture to specifically identify the offending pathogen.

For uncomplicated acute bacterial sinusitis in adults, most experts consider a course of therapy of 5–7 days sufficient for most patients. While differences in study designs exist, short course of therapy (3–5 days) has been shown to be as effective as longer course (>7 days) in adults [67]. In children, the IDSA recommends duration of 10–14 days based on the lack of data regarding shorter courses of therapy. The AAP recommends treating for 7 days beyond symptoms resolution, which for most patients is within 72 h of initiating antimicrobials.

Other non-antimicrobial therapies may be of benefit in select cases. Much of the data regarding adjunctive therapies is plagued by methodology problems and differences in definitions of disease and clinical outcomes making comparisons challenging. Among these adjunctive therapies include nasal saline irrigation, which has been used to clean debris from the nasal passages and to decrease the viscosity of secretions. A trial of patients receiving antimicrobials along with decongestants showed a benefit to children randomized to receive nasal saline washes in addition to the above agents compared to those who received antibiotics and decongestants alone [68]. Both antihistamines and decongestants have not been shown to affect duration of symptoms in children with acute bacterial sinusitis receiving antimicrobials.

Intranasal corticosteroids have the theoretical advantage of improving symptoms of congestion and facilitating sinus drainage by decreasing inflammation and swelling at sinus ostia. A number of studies in adults as well as adolescents have shown a benefit in symptoms to the use of intranasal steroids [69]. Barlan et al. performed a randomized trial of children with acute sinusitis treated with either amoxicillin-clavulanate plus intranasal budesonide compared to amoxicillin-clavulanate plus placebo for 3 weeks. The children who received budesonide had greater improvements in symptom scores at week two compared to the placebo group [70].

For severe presentations of sinusitis, including those associated with intracranial extension the IDSA recommends hospitalization and initiation of broad spectrum antimicrobial therapy with ampicillin-sulbactam (200–400 mg/kg/day every 6 h for children or 1.5–3 g every 6 h for adults), a third generation cephalosporin or a fluoroquinolone. Many experts in the field recommend a combination of vancomycin (15 mg/kg/dose IV q 6 h), cefotaxime (75 mg/kg/dose IV q 6 h) and metronidazole (7.5 mg/kg/dose IV q 6 h) for management of intracranial infection. Timely surgical evaluation is also critical in evaluation of these cases. Co-operative consultation with an infectious diseases specialist as well as otolaryngology and critical care medicine is recommended in the management of invasive fungal sinusitis in immunocompromised children.

Surgical Management

Surgical management is considered as a last resource in the pediatric population and is usually indicated in cases when medical management has failed or in the presence of acute complications. Studies have shown that adenoidectomy alone improves the symptoms of recurrent and chronic sinusitis in 50–60 % of children and therefore is usually first line surgical management [71]. Cultures of the maxillary sinus or middle meatus can also be performed at the time of adenoidectomy and assist in systemic antibiotic coverage. Pediatric patients presenting with orbital and/or intracranial complications from an acute sinus infection require urgent surgical consultation with intervention to prevent increased morbidity and mortality.

An atraumatic conservative surgical technique with functional endoscopic sinus surgery (FESS) and mucosal preservation is preferred in the pediatric population. Pediatric FESS is usually performed in patients that have failed medical therapy along with adenoidectomy or culture directed antibiotic treatment; patients with anatomical variations and/or intranasal growths such as tumors or nasal polyps (e.g., cystic fibrosis) patients with allergic fungal sinusitis; and patients with intraorbital or intracranial complications. FESS is mostly performed under intraoperative radiographic guidance and should only be considered after weighing the pros and cons of the procedure [72]. An uncinectomy, anterior ethmoidectomy and maxillary antrostomy are the most common forms of surgery with an overall success rate of approximately 80 %. Surgical intervention will aid in accessibility of the sinus cavities and drainage. Despite surgical therapy, patients continue to require postoperative nasal rinses and medical therapy.

Prior to FESS, balloon sinuplasty should be considered in those patients with significant symptoms who have failed medical treatment but have minimal anatomic findings on imaging [73]. The procedure consists of dilation of the sinus ostia with balloons under intraoperative radiographic guidance. As it is considered a newer technique, long-term data on the patency of the sinus ostia after balloon dilatation in children is not available yet. A comparative outcome analysis of FESS alone versus balloon sinuplasty in pediatric chronic sinusitis patients revealed that both are suitable treatments with similar outcomes, but patients after balloon sinuplasty required significantly less antibiotics in the post-operative period [74]. Although its use in the pediatric population is becoming popular, more controlled trials to determine its efficacy over conventional surgical treatment modalities are needed [75].

Prevention

Sinusitis can often be prevented with practicing good hand hygiene, avoiding close contact with people who have upper respiratory infections, removing children from crowded day cares, keeping up with the recommended immunizations and avoiding second hand smoking. Early data from Scandinavia have shown a decrease in pediatric hospitalizations related to sinusitis following introduction of PCV [76]. This would suggest that pneumococcal vaccination may serve as a preventative measure against, at least, severe cases of sinusitis. Other measures to minimize inflammation of the nasal mucosa which predisposes to sinusitis likely has a positive impact on decreasing frequency with which sinusitis occurs, though this is lacking in hard data. Such measures include treatment of allergic rhinitis with antihistamines and intranasal steroids as well as avoidance of environmental irritants such as cigarette smoke [77]. Cigarette smoke has been epidemiologically linked with increased risk of otitis media in children and laboratory research has demonstrated that smoke impairs ciliary function as well as promotes bacterial biofilm formation on nasal and sinus mucosa [78, 79].

While most acute episodes can be easily treated, certain patients are at risk for recurrence of disease. Recurrent and/or chronic sinusitis is best prevented by properly treating acute sinusitis and to assess and cure any associated underlying conditions. Patients with uncontrolled allergic rhinitis have a higher risk of recurrence as do those children with continued exposure to irritant such as chlorinated water or second-hand cigarette smoke. Thus all possible risk factors should as much as be mitigated in order to minimize the risk of reinfection.

Prognosis

The prognosis for acute bacterial sinusitis in children is excellent. In clinical trials of adults with sinusitis a substantial portion resolve their symptoms without specific antimicrobial therapy [80], up to 77 % at 2 weeks in one study [81]. Much of the literature regarding spontaneous resolution of symptoms is also hampered by methodological concerns such that many of the included patients may actually have viral URTIs and such data must be interpreted cautiously. This is supported by studies in pediatrics that have shown much lower rates of spontaneous resolution of sinusitis in children [82]. Nevertheless, antimicrobial therapy is indicated for adults and children once the diagnosis of acute bacterial sinusitis is made to minimize morbidity. The vast majority of patients resolve their symptoms within 48–72 h of initiating appropriate antimicrobial therapy. In a pediatric randomized placebo controlled trial 83 % of children with sinusitis had cure or significant symptom improvement within 3 days [83].

References

1. Centers for Disease Control and Prevention. Vital and health statistics: current estimates from the National Health Interview Survey, 1995. U.S. Dept of Health and Human Services, Centers for Disease Control and Prevention/ National Center for Health Statistics.
2. Ray NF, Baraniuk JN, Thamer M, et al. Healthcare expenditures for sinusitis in 1996: contributions of asthma, rhinitis, and other airway disorders. J Allergy Clin Immunol. 1999;103:408–14.
3. Wald ER, Guerra N, Byers C. Upper respiratory tract infections in young children: duration of and frequency of complications. Pediatrics. 1991;87:129–33.
4. Slavin RG. The diagnosis and management of sinusitis: a practice parameter update. J Allergy Clin Immunol. 2005;116(6 Suppl):13–47.
5. Wolf G, Anderhuber W, Kuhn F. Development of the paranasal sinuses in children: implications for paranasal sinus surgery. Ann Otol Rhinol Laryngol. 1993;102(9):705–11.
6. Wormald P-J. Surgery of the frontal recess and frontal sinus. Rhinology. 2005;43:82–5.
7. Hamilos DL. Chronic sinusitis. J Allergy Clin Immunol. 2000;106:213–27.
8. Osguthorpe JD, Hadley JA. Rhinosinusitis: current concepts in evaluation and management. Med Clin North Am. 1999;83(1):27–41.
9. Holgate ST. Asthma and allergy—disorders of civilization? QJM. 1998;91(3):171–84.
10. Phipps CD, Wood WE, Gibson WS, Cochran WJ. Gastroesophageal reflux contributing to chronic sinus disease in children: a prospective analysis. Arch Otolaryngol Head Neck Surg. 2000;126(7):831–6.

11. Dibase JK, Sharma VK. Does gastroesophageal reflux contribute to the development of chronic sinusitis? A review of the evidence. Dis Esophagus. 2006;19(6):419–24.
12. Sivasli E, Sirikçi A, Bayazýt YA, Gümüsburun E, Erbagci H, Bayram M, Kanlýkama M. Anatomic variations of the paranasal sinus area in pediatric patients with chronic sinusitis. Surg Radiol Anat. 2003;24(6):400–5.
13. Rosenstein BJ, Cutting GR. The diagnosis of cystic fibrosis: a consensus statement. Cystic Fibrosis Foundation Consensus Panel. J Pediatr. 1998;132(4):589–95.
14. Casey JR, Kaur R, Friedel VC, Pichichero ME. Acute otitis media otopathogens during 2008 to 2010 in Rochester, New York. Pediatr Infect Dis J. 2013;32:805–9.
15. McNeil JC, Hulten KG, Mason Jr EO, Kaplan SL. Serotype 19A is the most common Streptococcus pneumoniae isolate in children with chronic sinusitis. Pediatr Infect Dis J. 2009;28:766–8.
16. Olarte L, Hulten KG, Lamberth L, Mason Jr EO, Kaplan SL. Impact of the 13-valent pneumococcal conjugate vaccine on chronic sinusitis associated with Streptococcus pneumoniae in children. Pediatr Infect Dis J. 2014;33(10):1033–6.
17. Pena MT, Preciado D, Orestes M, Choi S. Orbital complications of acute sinusitis: changes in the post-pneumococcal vaccine era. JAMA Otolaryngol Head Neck Surg. 2013;139:223–7.
18. Kaplan SL, Barson WJ, Lin PL, Romero JR, Bradley JS, Tan TQ, Hoffman JA, Givner LB, Mason Jr EO. Early trends for invasive pneumococcal infections in children after the introduction of the 13-valent pneumococcal conjugate vaccine. Pediatr Infect Dis J. 2013;32:203–7.
19. Jacobs MR. Antimicrobial-resistant Streptococcus pneumoniae: trends and management. Expert Rev Anti Infect Ther. 2008;6:619–35.
20. Lynch 3rd JP, Zhanel GG. Streptococcus pneumoniae: epidemiology, risk factors, and strategies for prevention. Semin Respir Crit Care Med. 2009;30:189–209.
21. Kuster SP, Rudnick W, Shigayeva A, Green K, Baqi M, Gold WL, Lovinsky R, Muller MP, Powis JE, Rau N, Simor AE, Walmsley SL, Low DE, McGeer A, Toronto Invasive Bacterial Diseases Network. Previous antibiotic exposure and antimicrobial resistance in invasive pneumococcal disease: results from prospective surveillance. Clin Infect Dis. 2014;59:944–52.
22. Mills N, Best EJ, Murdoch D, Souter M, Neeff M, Anderson T, Salkeld L, Ahmad Z, Mahadevan M, Barber C, Brown C, Walker C, Walls T. What is behind the ear drum? The microbiology of otitis media and the nasopharyngeal flora in children in the era of pneumococcal vaccination. J Paediatr Child Health. 2015;21(3):300–6.
23. Brook I. Current issues in the management of acute bacterial sinusitis in children. Int J Pediatr Otorhinolaryngol. 2007;71:1653–61.
24. Heilmann KP, Rice CL, Miller AL, Miller NJ, Beekmann SE, Pfaller MA, Richter SS, Doern GV. Decreasing prevalence of beta-lactamase production among respiratory tract isolates of Haemophilus influenzae in the United States. Antimicrob Agents Chemother. 2005;49:2561–4.
25. Hotomi M, Fujihara K, Billal DS, Suzuki K, Nishimura T, Baba S, Yamanaka N. Genetic characteristics and clonal dissemination of beta-lactamase-negative ampicillin-resistant Haemophilus influenzae strains isolated from the upper respiratory tract of patients in Japan. Antimicrob Agents Chemother. 2007;51:3969–76.
26. Garcia-Cobos S, Campos J, Lazaro E, Roman F, Cercenado E, Garcia-Rey C, Perez-Vazquez M, Oteo J, de Abajo F. Ampicillin-resistant non-beta-lactamase-producing Haemophilus influenzae in Spain: recent emergence of clonal isolates with increased resistance to cefotaxime and cefixime. Antimicrob Agents Chemother. 2007; 51:2564–73.
27. Murphy TF, Parameswaran GI. Moraxella catarrhalis, a human respiratory tract pathogen. Clin Infect Dis. 2009;49:124–31.
28. Wald ER. Microbiology of acute and chronic sinusitis in children and adults. Am J Med Sci. 1998;316:13–20.
29. Sahm DF, Brown NP, Thornsberry C, Jones ME. Antimicrobial susceptibility profiles among common respiratory tract pathogens: a Global perspective. Postgrad Med. 2008;120:16–24.
30. Deshpande LM, Sader HS, Fritsche TR, Jones RN. Contemporary prevalence of BRO beta-lactamases in Moraxella catarrhalis: report from the SENTRY antimicrobial surveillance program (North America, 1997 to 2004). J Clin Microbiol. 2006;44:3775–7.
31. Payne SC, Benninger MS. Staphylococcus aureus is a major pathogen in acute bacterial rhinosinusitis: a meta-analysis. Clin Infect Dis. 2007;45:e121–7.
32. Brook I, Foote PA, Hausfeld JN. Increase in the frequency of recovery of meticillin-resistant Staphylococcus aureus in acute and chronic maxillary sinusitis. J Med Microbiol. 2008;57:1015–7.
33. Huang WH, Hung PK. Methicillin-resistant Staphylococcus aureus infections in acute rhinosinusitis. Laryngoscope. 2006;116:288–91.
34. Whitby CR, Kaplan SL, Mason Jr EO, Carrillo-Marquez M, Lamberth LB, Hammerman WA, Hulten KG. Staphylococcus aureus sinus infections in children. Int J Pediatr Otorhinolaryngol. 2011;75:118–21.
35. Woo HJ, Bae CH, Song SY, Choi YS, Kim YD. Actinomycosis of the paranasal sinus. Otolaryngol Head Neck Surg. 2008;139:460–2.

36. Cherry JD, Mundi J, Shapiro NL. Rhinosinusitis. In: Cherry JD, Harrison GJ, Kaplan SL, Steinbach WJ, Hotez PJ, editors. Feigin and Cherry's textbook of pediatric infectious diseases, vol. 1. 7th ed. Philadelphia: Elsevier; 2014. p. 193–203.
37. Edvinsson M, Asplund MS, Hjelm E, Nystrom-Rosander C. Chlamydophila pneumoniae in chronic rhinosinusitis. Acta Otolaryngol. 2006;126:952–7.
38. Cultrara A, Goldstein NA, Ovchinsky A, Reznik T, Roblin PM, Hammerschlag MR. The role of Chlamydia pneumoniae infection in children with chronic sinusitis. Archi Otolaryngol Head Neck Surg. 2003;129:1094–7.
39. Savolainen S, Jousimies-Somer H, Kleemola M, Ylikoski J. Serological evidence of viral or Mycoplasma pneumoniae infection in acute maxillary sinusitis. Eur J Clin Microbiol Infect Dis. 1989;8:131–5.
40. Lee RE, Kaza S, Plano GV, Casiano RR. The role of atypical bacteria in chronic rhinosinusitis. Otolaryngol Head Neck Surg. 2005;133:407–10.
41. Griffin JP, Klein EW. Role of sinusitis in primary atypical pneumonia. Clin Med. 1971;78:23–7.
42. Pitkaranta A, Starck M, Savolainen S, Poyry T, Suomalainen I, Hyypia T, Carpen O, Vaheri A. Rhinovirus RNA in the maxillary sinus epithelium of adult patients with acute sinusitis. Clin Infect Dis. 2001;33:909–11.
43. Goytia VK, Giannoni CM, Edwards MS. Intraorbital and intracranial extension of sinusitis: comparative morbidity. J Pediatr. 2011;158:486–91.
44. Hicks CW, Weber JG, Reid JR, Moodley M. Identifying and managing intracranial complications of sinusitis in children: a retrospective series. Pediatr Infect Dis J. 2011;30:222–6.
45. McKinley SH, Yen MT, Miller AM, Yen KG. Microbiology of pediatric orbital cellulitis. Am J Ophthalmol. 2007;144:497–501.
46. Teul I, Lorkowski J, Lorkiewicz W, Nowakowski D. Sinusitis in people living in the medieval ages. Adv Exp Med Biol. 2013;788:133–8.
47. Marom T, Alvarez-Fernandez PE, Jennings K, Patel JA, McCormick DP, Chonmaitree T. Acute bacterial sinusitis complicating viral upper respiratory tract infection in young children. Pediatr Infect Dis J. 2014;33:803–8.
48. Vaz LE, Kleinman KP, Raebel MA, Nordin JD, Lakoma MD, Dutta-Linn MM, Finkelstein JA. Recent trends in outpatient antibiotic use in children. Pediatrics. 2014;133:375–85.
49. Ueda D, Yoto Y. The ten-day mark as a practical diagnostic approach for acute paranasal sinusitis in children. Pediatr Infect Dis J. 1996;15:576–9.
50. McLean DC. Sinusitis in children. Lessons from twenty-five patients. Clin Pediatr. 1970;9:342–5.
51. Revai K, Dobbs LA, Nair S, Patel JA, Grady JJ, Chonmaitree T. Incidence of acute otitis media and sinusitis complicating upper respiratory tract infection: the effect of age. Pediatrics. 2007;119:e1408–12.
52. Low DE, Desrosiers M, McSherry J, et al. A practical guide for the diagnosis and treatment of acute sinusitis. Can Med Assoc J. 1997;156 Suppl 6:S1–14.
53. Leo G, Triulzi F, Incorvaia C. Sinus imaging for diagnosis of chronic rhinosinusitis in children. Curr Allergy Asthma Rep. 2012;12(2):136–43.
54. Slavin RG, Spector SL, Bernstein IL, et al. American Academy of Allergy, Asthma and Immunology, American College of Allergy, Asthma and Immunology, Joint Council of Allergy, Asthma and Immunology. The diagnosis and management of sinusitis: a practice parameter update. J Allergy Clin Immunol. 2005;116(6 Suppl):S13–47.
55. Oxford LE, McClay J. Complications of acute sinusitis in children. Otolaryngol Head Neck Surg. 2005;133:32–7.
56. Herrmann BW, Forsen Jr JW. Simultaneous intracranial and orbital complications of acute rhinosinusitis in children. Int J Pediatr Otorhinolaryngol. 2004;68:619–25.
57. Sultész M, Csákányi Z, Majoros T, Farkas Z, Katona G. Acute bacterial rhinosinusitis and its complications in our pediatric otolaryngological department between 1997 and 2006. Int J Pediatr Otorhinolaryngol. 2009;73(11): 1507–12.
58. Chow AW, Benninger MS, Brook I, Brozek JL, Goldstein EJ, Hicks LA, Pankey GA, Seleznick M, Volturo G, Wald ER, File TM Jr, Infectious Diseases Society of America. IDSA clinical practice guideline for acute bacterial rhinosinusitis in children and adults. Clin Infect Dis. 2012;54:e72–112.
59. Wald ER, Applegate KE, Bordley C, Darrow DH, Glode MP, Marcy SM, Nelson CE, Rosenfeld RM, Shaikh N, Smith MJ, Williams PV, Weinberg ST, American Academy of Pediatrics. Clinical practice guideline for the diagnosis and management of acute bacterial sinusitis in children aged 1 to 18 years. Pediatrics. 2013;132:e262–80.
60. Bradley JS, Kauffman RE, Balis DA, Duffy CM, Gerbino PG, Maldonado SD, Noel GJ. Assessment of musculoskeletal toxicity 5 years after therapy with levofloxacin. Pediatrics. 2014;134:e146–53.
61. Pichichero ME. A review of evidence supporting the American Academy of Pediatrics recommendation for prescribing cephalosporin antibiotics for penicillin-allergic patients. Pediatrics. 2005;115:1048–57.
62. Pichichero ME, Casey JR. Safe use of selected cephalosporins in penicillin-allergic patients: a meta-analysis. Otolaryngol Head Neck Surg. 2007;136:340–7.
63. Fenoll A, Gimenez MJ, Robledo O, Aguilar L, Tarrago D, Granizo JJ, Gimeno M, Coronel P. In vitro activity of oral cephalosporins against pediatric isolates of Streptococcus pneumoniae non-susceptible to penicillin, amoxicillin or erythromycin. J Chemother. 2008;20:175–9.

64. Fenoll A, Gimenez MJ, Robledo O, Aguilar L, Tarrago D, Granizo JJ, Martin-Herrero JE. Influence of penicillin/amoxicillin non-susceptibility on the activity of third-generation cephalosporins against Streptococcus pneumoniae. Eur J Clin Microbiol Infect Dis. 2008;27:75–80.
65. Jenkins SG, Farrell DJ. Increase in pneumococcus macrolide resistance, United States. Emerg Infect Dis. 2009;15:1260–4.
66. Harrison CJ, Woods C, Stout G, Martin B, Selvarangan R. Susceptibilities of Haemophilus influenzae, Streptococcus pneumoniae, including serotype 19A, and Moraxella catarrhalis paediatric isolates from 2005 to 2007 to commonly used antibiotics. J Antimicrob Chemother. 2009;63:511–9.
67. Falagas ME, Karageorgopoulos DE, Grammatikos AP, Matthaiou DK. Effectiveness and safety of short vs. long duration of antibiotic therapy for acute bacterial sinusitis: a meta-analysis of randomized trials. Br J Clin Pharmacol. 2009;67:161–71.
68. Wang YH, Yang CP, Ku MS, Sun HL, Lue KH. Efficacy of nasal irrigation in the treatment of acute sinusitis in children. Int J Pediatr Otorhinolaryngol. 2009;73:1696–701.
69. Meltzer EO, Gates D, Bachert C. Mometasone furoate nasal spray increases the number of minimal-symptom days in patients with acute rhinosinusitis. Ann Allergy Asthma Immunol. 2012;108:275–9.
70. Barlan IB, Erkan E, Bakir M, Berrak S, Basaran MM. Intranasal budesonide spray as an adjunct to oral antibiotic therapy for acute sinusitis in children. Ann Allergy Asthma Immunol. 1997;78:598–601.
71. Manning S. Surgical intervention for sinusitis in children. Curr Allergy Asthma Rep. 2001;1(3):289–96.
72. Mair EA, Bolger WE, Breisch EA. Sinus and facial growth after pediatric endoscopic sinus surgery. Arch Otolaryngol. 1995;121(5):547–52.
73. Ramadan HH, Terrell AM. Balloon catheter sinuplasty and adenoidectomy in children with chronic rhinosinusitis. Ann Otol Rhinol Laryngol. 2010;119(9):578–82.
74. Thottam PJ, Haupert M, Saraiya S, Dworkin J, Sirigiri R, Belenky WM. Functional endoscopic sinus surgery (FESS) alone versus balloon catheter sinuplasty (BCS) and ethmoidectomy: a comparative outcome analysis in pediatric chronic rhinosinusitis. Int J Pediatr Otorhinolaryngol. 2012;76(9):1355–60.
75. Ahmed J, Pal S, Hopkins C, Jayaraj S. Functional endoscopic balloon dilation of sinus ostia for chronic rhinosinusitis. Cochrane Database Syst Rev. 2011;7.
76. Lindstrand A, Bennet R, Galanis I, Blennow M, Ask LS, Dennison SH, et al. Sinusitis and pneumonia hospitalization after introduction of pneumococcal conjugate vaccine. Pediatrics. 2014;134(6):e1528–36.
77. Duse M, Caminiti S, Zicari AM. Rhinosinusitis: prevention strategies. Pediatr Allergy Immunol. 2007;18:S71–4.
78. Wang LF, White DR, Andreoli SM, Mulligan RM, Discolo CM, Schlosser RJ. Cigarette smoke inhibits dynamic ciliary beat frequency in pediatric adenoid explants. Otolaryngol Head Neck Surg. 2012;146:659–63.
79. Goldstein-Daruech N, Cope EK, Zhao KQ, Vokovic K, Kofonow JM, Doghramji L, et al. Tobacco smoke mediated induction of sinonasal biofilms. PLoS One. 2011;6, e15700.
80. Merenstein D, Whittaker C, Chadwell T, Wegner B, D'Amico F. Are antibiotics beneficial for patients with sinusitis complains? A randomized double-blind clinical trial. J Fam Pract. 2005;54:144–51.
81. Van Buchem FL, Knottnerus JA, Schrijnemaekers VJ, Peeters MF. Primary-care based randomised placebo-controlled trial of antibiotic treatment in acute maxillary sinusitis. Lancet. 1997;349:683–7.
82. Wald ER, Nash D, Eickhoff J. Effectiveness of amoxicillin/clavulanate potassium in the treatment of acute bacterial sinusitis in children. Pediatrics. 2009;124:9–15.
83. Wald ER, Chiponis D, Ledesma-Median J. Comparative effectiveness of amoxicillin and amoxicillin-clavulanate potassium in acute paranasal sinus infections in children: a double-blind, placebo-controlled trial. Pediatrics. 1986;77:795–800.

Chapter 8
Complications of Sinusitis

Lucila Marquez, Matthew Sitton, Jennifer Dang, Brandon H. Tran, and Deidre R. Larrier

Anatomy

Complications of sinusitis can be divided into extra and intra cranial complications.

Extracranial complications of sinusitis include orbital complications and osteomyelitis/subperiosteal abscess of the frontal bone (Pott's puffy tumor). The orbit is separated from the ethmoid sinus air cells by a thin bony plate called the lamina papyracea. This "plate" has naturally occurring bony dehiscences, which contribute to the spread of infection from sinus to orbit.

Orbital complications are broadly divided into two groups based on their location in relation to the orbital septum. The orbital is a natural barrier made up of connective tissue attaching peripherally to the periosteum of the orbit and centrally attaching near the lid margins. It lies just deep to the orbicularis oculi and separates the lid (preseptal) component from the orbital (postseptal) component.

L. Marquez, M.D., M.P.H.
Department of Pediatrics, Sections of Pediatric Infectious Diseases and Pediatric Hospital Medicine, Baylor College of Medicine, 6621 Fannin, Houston, TX 77030, USA
e-mail: lm043062@bcm.edu

M. Sitton, M.D.
Department of Otolaryngology, Baylor College of Medicine, Houston, TX, USA

Texas Children's Hospital, Houston, TX, USA
e-mail: mssitton@texaschildrens.org

J. Dang, M.D.
Department of Otolaryngology, Baylor College of Medicine, Houston, TX, USA

B.H. Tran, M.D.
Neuroradiology Section, Baylor College of Medicine, Houston, TX, USA
e-mail: brandontran10@yahoo.com

D.R. Larrier, M.D. (✉)
Bobby Alford Department of Otolaryngology Head and Neck Surgery, Baylor College of Medicine, 6701 Fannin St Ste 640.00, Houston, TX 77030, USA
e-mail: drlarrie@texaschildrens.org

T.A. Valdez, J.G. Vallejo (eds.), *Infectious Diseases in Pediatric Otolaryngology*,
DOI 10.1007/978-3-319-21744-4_8

Frontal sinuses generally begin developing around age 7 or 8 and complete pneumatization in adolescence/early adulthood. The veins of Breschet, which are diploic veins, drain the mucosa of the frontal sinus. These veins are valve-less allowing a route for infection to spread through the anterior or posterior table of the frontal sinus.

Microbiology

Complications of sinusitis are largely polymicrobial involving any combination of Streptococci, *Staphylococcus aureus*, oral-gram negatives, and oral anaerobes.

Several case series of pediatric patients with complications of sinusitis have noted the *Streptococcus anginosus* group (which includes *S. anginosus, S. intermedius, and S. constellatus*) as a leading pathogen occurring in 15–28 % of cases of complicated sinusitis [1, 2]. Additionally, one case series identified greater morbidity, including increased severity of infection, need for neurosurgical intervention, and long-term neurologic deficits, in patients in whom the *Streptococcus anginosus* group was identified as a pathogen [2]. Of note, the Streptococcus group works synergistically with anaerobes to produce abscess formation [2].

The *Strep. anginosus* group is largely susceptible to penicillin. However, intermediate susceptibility to penicillin and cephalosporins can occur and resistance to penicillin has been reported [3]. In a large case series of infections in children, 89 % of isolates were susceptible to penicillin, though 11 % had intermediate susceptibility [3]. Additionally, 3 % had intermediate susceptibility to cefotaxime. Resistance to clindamycin was observed in 3 % of isolates. All were susceptible to vancomycin.

The role of *Staphylococcus aureus* in complications of sinusitis has been well documented. A case series of 94 children with orbital cellulitis found *Staphylococcus aureus* to be the second most frequent pathogen after the *Streptococcus anginosus* group [1]. Methicillin-resistant infections must also be considered in cases of complicated sinusitis. A study from Houston, TX of surgical sinus cultures in children between 2005 and 2008 noted that 21 % of isolated *S. aureus* were methicillin-resistant [4].

Streptococcus pneumoniae has been variably reported as a pathogen in complicated sinusitis. A large retrospective series of Canadian pediatric patients with intracranial extension identified *Streptococcus pneumoniae* in 20 % of cases [2].

Anaerobes have been identified in over two thirds of patients with intracranial complications. Pathogens in this category include Prevotella species, Fusobacterium species, and Peptostreptococcus [5].

Occasionally, gram negative pathogens are isolated. These can include pathogens associated with uncomplicated sinusitis, such as *Haemophilus influenzae* and *Moraxella catarrhalis*. In some case series, gram-negative enterics such as *E. coli* and Pseudomonas have been reported.

Extracranial Complications

Pathophysiology/Etiology for Extracranial Complications

The close proximity of the orbit to the sinuses makes orbital complications the most common complication of sinusitis. Any of the sinuses may cause orbital complications, yet the ethmoid sinuses are the most common source. Infection may spread to the orbit by (1) direct extension through the lamina papyracea, (2) congenital or acquired defects, (3) thrombophlebitis via valveless veins and (4) osteitis of the bone.

Pott's puffy tumor is a subperiosteal abscess of the frontal bone associated with osteomyelitis [6]. The most common cause of this is frontal sinusitis and trauma. It may occur from either direct bony erosion of the anterior table of the frontal sinus or by way of diploic veins. Pott's puffy tumor is more common in teenagers than any other age group. This is likely because of the lack of frontal sinus development in children and decreased diploic veins in adults [7].

Classification of Orbital Complications

In 1970, Chandler's classification was created, dividing orbital complications from sinusitis into: *preseptal cellulitis, orbital cellulitis, subperiosteal abscess, orbital abscess, and cavernous sinus thrombosis* [8]. Chandler's classification does not imply a chronologic progression of symptoms. Preseptal cellulitis, class 1, is inflammatory edema limited to the eyelid. Preseptal infections are nine times more common than postseptal infections [9, 10]. Chandler's class 2–5 are postseptal infections. *Orbital Cellulitis*, class 2, is inflammatory edema that involves orbital components posterior to the orbital septum. *Subperiosteal Abscess*, class 3, is a purulent collection between the periorbital and bony orbital wall. *Orbital Abscess*, class 4, is a purulent collection within the orbit. *Cavernous sinus thrombosis*, class 5, is a retrograde phlebitis extending to the cavernous sinus (Fig. 8.1).

Specimen Collection

Nasal swabs are unreliable for identifying a pathogen associated with sinusitis, as bacteria that colonize the respiratory tract may not be the causative agent of a suppurative infection [1, 11].

Studies that have utilized proper methods for recovery of anaerobes have identified these pathogens in an overwhelming majority of abscesses [12]. In one study, 90 % of intracranial abscess cultures revealed anaerobes [12]. Lack of proper technique in collecting and/or processing anaerobic cultures is felt to be responsible for the poor yield observed in many operative cultures [13]. In order to maximize recovery, it is imperative that if collected in a syringe the sample is immediately sealed or is transported in anaerobic media and that samples are promptly delivered to the microbiology laboratory [14].

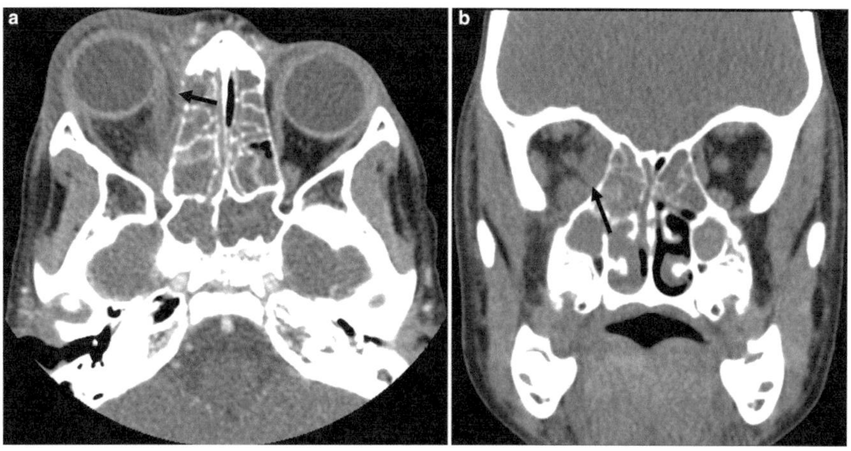

Fig. 8.1 Orbital cellulitis. Contrast CT (**a**) axial (**b**) coronal. *Black arrow* demonstrating fat stranding and edema involving the medial and inferior recti muscle on the right with no abscess collection

Medical Management of Extracranial Complications

Empiric therapy for orbital infections must include drugs with activity against the expected pathogens including Streptococci, *Staphylococcus aureus*, oral-gram negatives, and oral anaerobes. Local patterns with regard to the frequency of methicillin-resistant *Staphylococcus aureus* infections should be considered. Commonly used antibiotics with activity against Streptococcal species and oral-gram negatives include ampicillin-sulbactam and third-generation cephalosporins. Clindamycin and vancomycin have activity against methicillin-resistant *Staphylococcus*. Ampicillin-sulbactam and clindamycin provide good coverage of oral anaerobes whereas vancomycin is only active against gram-positive anaerobes. If MRSA is not suspected, monotherapy with ampicillin-sulbactam can be considered [14].

A retrospective review of cases of sinogenic orbital infections from a large tertiary pediatric hospital noted that the mean parenteral and total duration of antibiotics was 12 and 24 days, respectively [15]. Abscesses that have not required surgical intervention may warrant longer parenteral therapy. In patients with normal visual acuity, some providers may elect to initiate treatment with IV antibiotics for 24–48 h prior to obtaining imaging. Imaging is then obtained if there is no improvement of signs and symptoms [16].

Surgical Management of Extracranial Complications

Preseptal cellulitis is caused by sinusitis in 15 % of cases [10]. Other causes of preseptal cellulitis are localized skin infection, local trauma, insect bites, animal bites, foreign bodies, or acute dacryocystitis. Classic physical exam findings demonstrate eyelid swelling and erythema with normal eye movement and no evidence of chemosis. Imaging is not initially necessary for patients demonstrating classic physical exam findings, but may be necessary for patient failing to improve after 24–48 h of treatment. Children older than 1 year with mild preseptal cellulitis and no signs of toxicity may be treated as outpatient with close follow-up. Other patients should be treated as inpatient with IV antibiotics. If there is concern that sinusitis is the causative mechanism, treatment also may include nasal decongestant, i.e., oxymetazoline, nasal steroids, and nasal saline.

Patients with *postseptal infection* typically present with fever. In one study, 94 % of patients with postseptal infections vs. 47 % of patients with preseptal infections demonstrated a fever [9]. Postseptal infections are preceded by sinus disease in 90 % of cases. Patients with a suspected postseptal infection should have an ophthalmology and otolaryngology consultation.

Patients with *orbital cellulitis* may have ophthalmoplegia, pain with eye movement or diplopia (Fig. 8.1). They will have periorbital erythema, edema and chemosis. An ophthalmology consult is warranted to assess for changes in visual acuity and intraocular pressure. Imaging in these cases is a debated topic as the goal of imaging is to identify a drainable abscess [17]. Provided that there is no compromise in visual acuity, some clinicians elect to initiate treatment with IV antibiotics for 24–48 h prior to obtaining imaging. The imaging modality commonly obtained is contrasted CT scan of the sinuses, although MRI may be considered particularly if there is concern for intracranial involvement. Imaging followed by surgery should be performed urgently if decreased vision is a concern. Treatment for uncomplicated orbital cellulitis consists of IV antibiotics, nasal decongestant, nasal steroid, and nasal saline.

Signs and symptoms of *subperiosteal abscess* are similar to orbital cellulitis except patients with a subperiosteal abscess may have proptosis and inhibition of extraocular movement (Fig. 8.2). Patients may complain of diplopia, but visual acuity is typically normal. If visual acuity is normal, treatment may be initiated prior to imaging and imaging obtained if improvement is not observed in 24–48 h or if symptoms worsen. Subperiosteal abscesses along the medial wall, <1 cm in width, and in patients

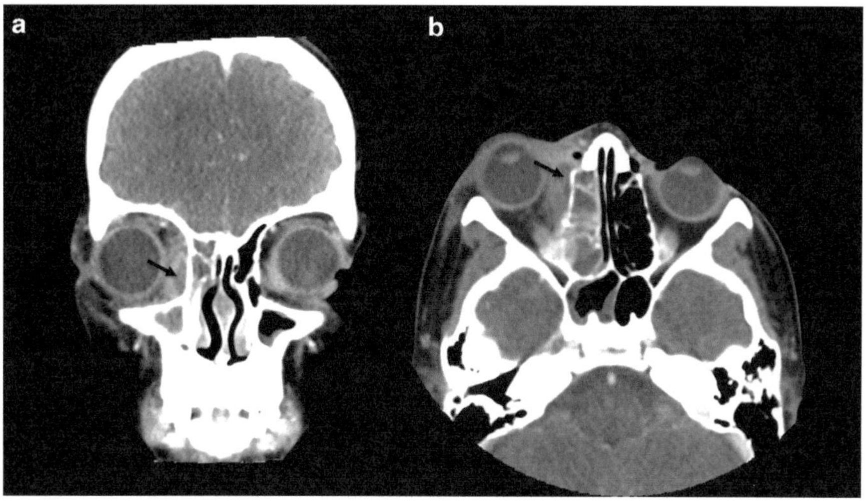

Fig. 8.2 Subperiosteal abscess. Contrast CT scan (**a**) coronal (**b**) axial. *Black arrow* shows evidence of peripherally enhancing small subperiosteal abscess collection in the extra-conal space of the right orbit with moderate surrounding edema and mass effect on the adjacent medial rectus muscle. There is fluid opacification in the right ethmoid and maxillary sinuses

younger than 9 years of age have a higher likelihood of responding to medical management alone [18–21]. Surgical approaches can be external, endoscopic, or combined. Most medial or inferior wall abscesses are amendable to drainage via a transnasal endoscopic approach. Lateral or superior abscess require an external approach [22].

Patients with an *orbital abscess* typically exhibit the same signs as orbital cellulitis plus proptosis and visual acuity changes. Imaging should be obtained in patients with a suspected orbital abscess. Treatment consists of IV antibiotics and in most institutions an oculoplastic surgery consult for drainage of the abscess through an external approach.

Cavernous sinus thrombosis is a life threatening condition (Fig. 8.3). It should be suspected if the contralateral eye is also affected. Signs and symptoms which may be observed are ptosis (CNIII), extraocular eye movement impairment (CNIII, IV, VI), numbness of forehead or midface (CNV1 and V2), headache, and loss of vision (CNII). Magnetic resonance venography should be obtained. Treatment consists of IV antibiotics. Anticoagulation may be used with the aim to inhibit propagation of the thrombus and promote recanalization of the sinus.

Pott's Puffy Tumor

Pott's puffy tumor is osteomyelitis/subperiosteal abscess of the frontal bone from frontal sinusitis (Fig. 8.4). Patients present with forehead or scalp swelling and tenderness over the forehead. Treatment involves aspiration and/or drainage of forehead abscess and treatment of the sinusitis. Management of the underlying frontal sinusitis should be with IV antibiotics +/– surgical drainage of the frontal sinus. Surgical drainage may be achieved by an external approach (trephination), combined external and endoscopic approach, or endoscopic approach [23].

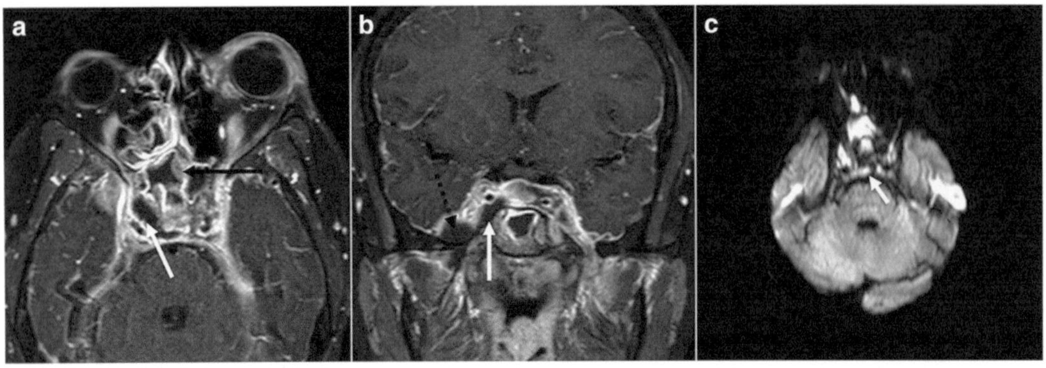

Fig. 8.3 Cavernous sinus thrombosis. (**a**) MRI contrast axial T1 (**b**) MRI contrast coronal T1 (**c**) MR axial DWI. There is evidence of complicated sphenoiditis with right subtemporal epidural abscess and associated right cavernous sinus thrombosis. Note of decreased enhancement in the right cavernous sinus when compared to the contralateral side. Evidence of restricted diffusion is noted in the involved sphenoid sinus and cavernous sinus. *Black arrow* shows marked sphenoiditis; *white arrow* shows right cavernous sinus thrombosis with decreased enhancement; *dashed black arrow* shows peripherally enhancing epidural abscess in the right sub-temporal region with accompanying dural enhancement

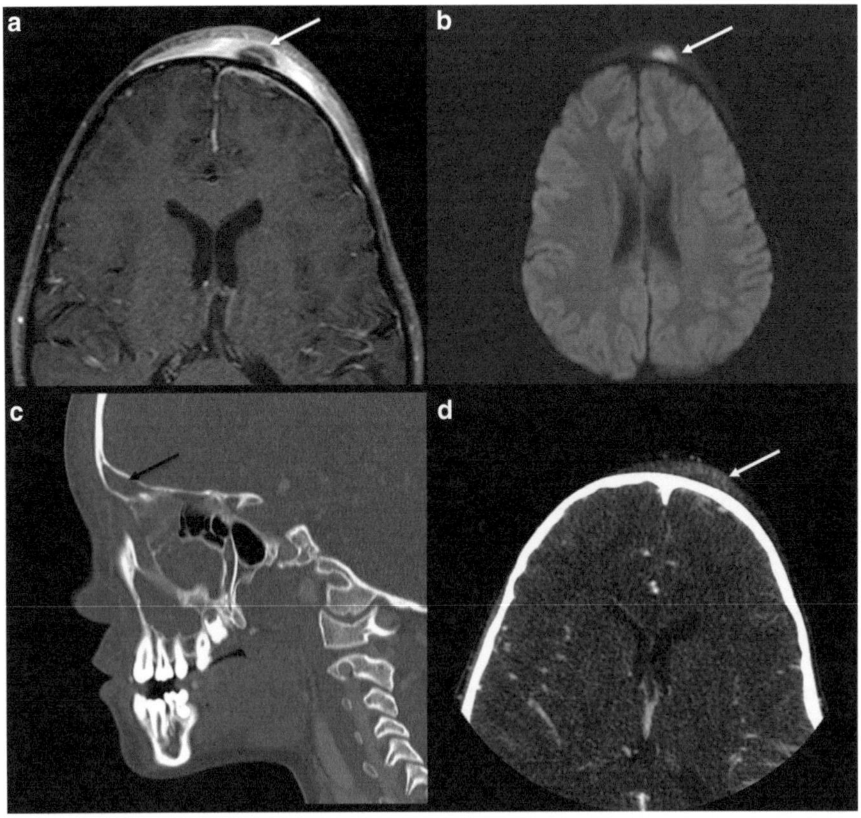

Fig. 8.4 Pott's Puffy Tumor. (**a**) MRI post axial T1 (**b**) MRI axial DWI (**c**) contrast CT sagittal (**d**) contrast CT axial. There is peripherally enhancing subperiosteal abscess in the left anterior frontal area with marked adjacent scalp edema. There is associated dural thickening and enhancement in the left frontal convexity and interhemispheric fissure. *White arrow* shows restricted diffusion in the abscess. *Black arrow* shows acute frontal sinusitis with complete fluid opacification

Intracranial Complications

Pathophysiology of Intracranial Complications

The frontal sinuses are most commonly associated with intracranial complications, followed by the ethmoid, sphenoid and maxillary sinuses. Intracranial spread of infections is believed to occur mainly by progression of septic thrombi through the valveless diploic veins of the skull base that penetrate dura [24]. Less commonly, it can occur via direct extension of osteomyelitis of the bony sinus walls or via penetration through existing bony defects (e.g., congenital or posttraumatic) [5]. The frontal skull is particularly vulnerable to spread of infection, likely because of its rich network of diploic veins. It has been postulated that the rapid growth of the frontal sinuses and their blood supply account for the high association of intracranial complications in adolescent males [25]. Intraparenchymal brain abscesses are seeded by the hematogenous route, and therefore, can be found in all regions of the brain.

Classification of Intracranial Complications

Intracranial complications of sinusitis are less common than orbital infections, but may lead to significant morbidity and mortality. The incidence of intracranial complications has been reported to be 3–17 % [26–28]. They include meningitis, epidural or subdural empyema and abscess, venous sinus thrombosis and intraparenchymal abscesses. Subdural empyema is the most common intracranial complication, comprising 33–85 % of all intracranial complications of sinusitis [29]. Sinus infection may progress to intracranial infection despite adequate IV antibiotic therapy. Maintaining a high index of suspicion is key in the prevention of potential lifelong disability. Intracranial complications should be suspected in a patient who presents with fevers, severe headache, photophobia, seizures, or other focal neurologic findings. Rhinorrhea and nasal congestion are not always observed. Diagnostic evaluations often include imaging studies such as CT and MRI. CT has the superior ability to demonstrate bony detail and anatomy, which are critical in guiding Endoscopic Sinus Surgery. MRI is obtained when intracranial extension is suspected, due to its ability to discriminate brain and meningeal inflammation as well as fluid collections [30]. Examples of an epidural abscess and subdural abscess are shown in Figs. 8.5 and 8.6, respectively.

Medical Management of Intracranial Complications

Empiric therapy in suspected or confirmed intracranial infections should always begin with vancomycin, a third-generation cephalosporin, and metronidazole. Alternatively, vancomycin and ampicillin-sulbactam can be considered. Vancomycin is active against gram-positive bacteria including Staphylococcal and Streptococcal species and gram-positive anaerobes. Clindamycin has poor CNS penetration and should not be used as an anti-staphylococcal antibiotic for CNS infections. Third-generation cephalosporins are active against most of the gram-negative bacilli associated with complicated sinusitis. Metronidazole has anaerobic coverage, especially against gram-negative anaerobes.

Antibiotics can be tailored according to culture results, albeit caution must be used given that improper specimen handling may yield false negatives, especially for anaerobes.

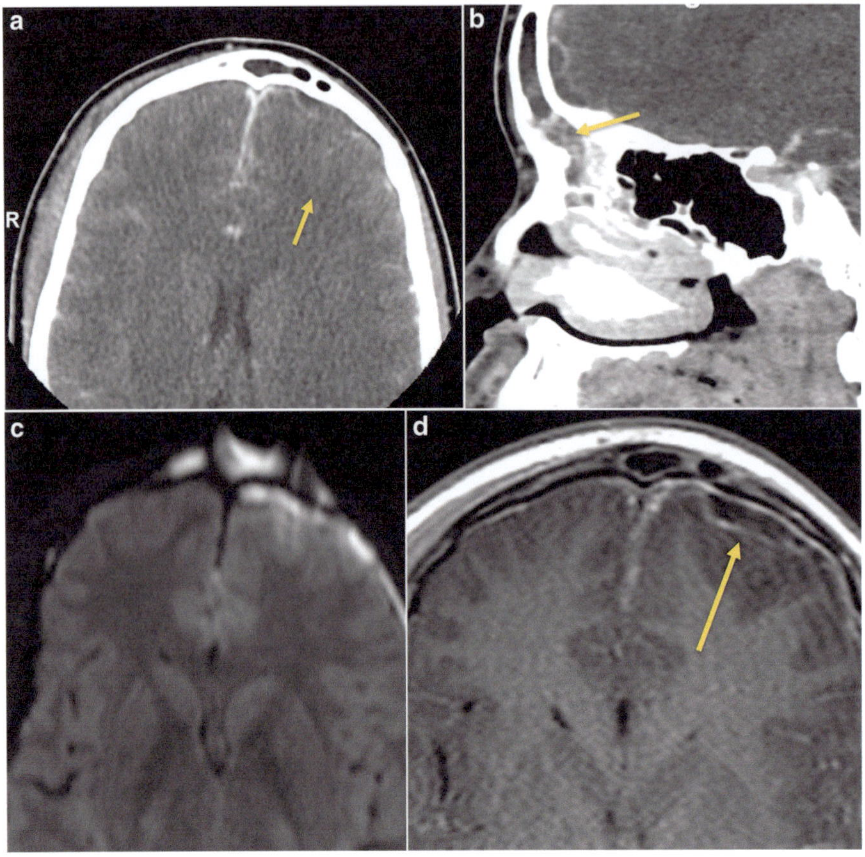

Fig. 8.5 Subdural empyema. (**a**) Axial and (**b**) sagittal post contrast CT images show a peripherally enhancing subdural empyema in the left anterior frontal convexity secondary to complicated acute sinusitis from the frontal sinus. (**c**) Axial MRI diffusion (DWI) sequence and (**d**) post-axial T1 showing left frontal subdural empyema and anterior frontal lobe cerebritis secondary to frontal sinus abscess with restricted diffusion. Restricted diffusion is also noted in the abscess. There is associated dural thickening and enhancement in the contralateral frontal convexity and interhemispheric fissure

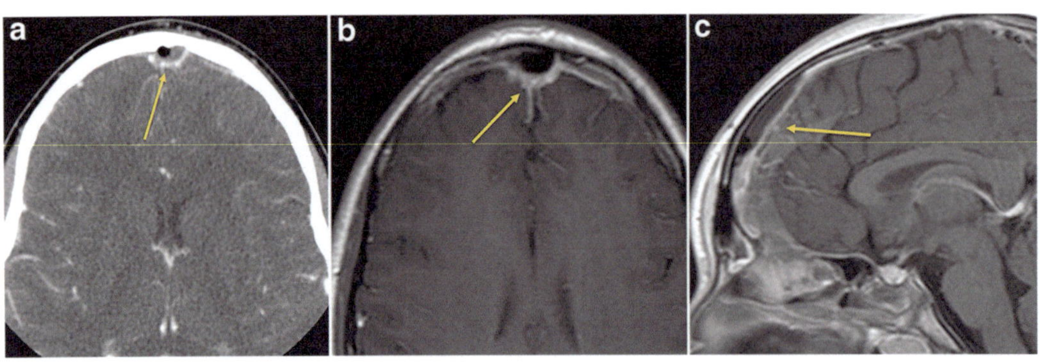

Fig. 8.6 Epidural empyema. (**a**) Contrast axial CT image shows peripherally enhancing epidural empyema in the mid-frontal area with focal air bubble within it. There is associated adjacent dural thickening and enhancement. (**b**) Post-contrast axial and (**c**) sagittal T1 MRI shows peripheral enhancing epidural empyema with adjacent fluid opacification and mucosal thickening in the frontal sinus

The total duration of antibiotics for intracranial extension of sinusitis has not been studied systematically. In general, 4–6 weeks of intravenous therapy is recommended, however, clinical course should dictate duration. A retrospective review of cases of intracranial extension from a large tertiary pediatric hospital noted that the mean total duration of intravenous antibiotics was 36 days [15]. Given poor CSF penetration of oral antibiotics, parenteral antibiotics should be utilized. Follow-up imaging prior to discontinuing antibiotics is recommended. Persistence of a sizeable intracranial collection may warrant extending therapy further.

Surgical Management of Intracranial Complications

Treatment is both medical and surgical. Surgical management requires coordination with otolaryngology and neurosurgery services [30]. Surgical drainage of the affected sinuses via endoscopic sinus surgery by the otolaryngologist should be performed as soon as possible. Medical management requires high dose, aggressive, culture directed IV antibiotics with adequate CSF fluid penetration. Thus, early consultation with Infectious Disease is also critical.

Allergic Fungal Sinusitis

Pathophysiology/Etiology for Allergic Fungal Sinusitis

Allergic fungal sinusitis (AFS) is a distinct subtype of eosinophilic chronic rhinosinusitis marked by 5 major criteria: Type 1 hypersensitivity (by history, skin tests, or serology), nasal polyposis, characteristic computed tomography findings, eosinophilic mucus, presence of fungal elements of the tissue removed during surgery without evidence of fungal tissue invasion [31]. The etiologic basis of AFS is the abnormally robust immunologic response elicited by an allergy to ubiquitous fungal species. AFS accounts for 7–12 % of patients with CRS who undergo sinus surgery in the United States [32, 33]. The onset of AFS is typically a protracted, indolent process. Children report a slow onset of nasal airway obstruction and production of large, dark-colored nasal debris. Because of the gradual onset and progression, patients may develop facial dysmorphia with proptosis and/or telecanthus. If pain is a presenting symptom, it generally indicates a concomitant bacterial infection. If endoscopy is tolerated, the examiner should examine the nasal cavities bilaterally for evidence of allergic mucin, polypoid edema, or polyposis [31]. However, in children this may not be well tolerated. Thus, imaging findings, along with history, are helpful towards diagnosing AFS. CT scan images reveal opacification of the paranasal sinuses bilaterally and a combination of osseous expansion and/or erosion (Fig. 8.7). The definitive diagnosis, however, relies on surgical and histopathological tissue findings. Histopathologic analysis of resected tissue demonstrates distinct mucinous material containing eosinophils, Charcot-Leyden crystals and fungal hyphae. One study identified *Curvularia*, *Aspergillus*, *Alternaria* and *Bipolaris* as the most common pathogens in their cohort of allergic fungal sinusitis [34].

Management of Allergic Fungal Sinusitis

The treatment of AFS is both medical and surgical. With increasing awareness of the pathogenesis of the disease and its relationship with eosinophilic inflammatory cascade, a paradigm shift has led to medical therapies aimed at suppressing inflammation rather than eradicating fungal pathogens.

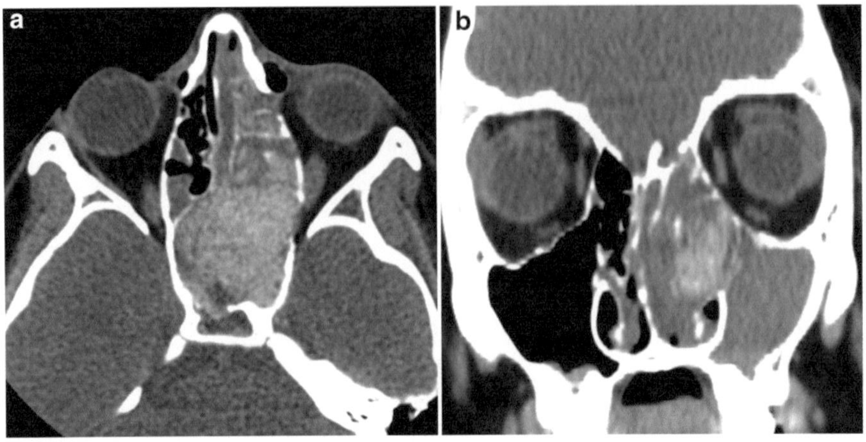

Fig. 8.7 Allergic fungal sinusitis. (**a**) Non-contrast axial and (**b**) coronal CT images show complete opacification of the sphenoid, left ethmoid and maxillary sinuses with expansion of the left ethmoid and sphenoid sinuses . Additionally, there are multifocal hyperattenuation within the opacified sinuses and polypoid soft tissue opacification within the left nasal cavity. On axial view, there is rarefaction and dehiscence of the bony septations and the walls of the sphenoid and ethmoid sinuses

Functional endoscopic sinus surgery continues to remain the intervention of choice, as nearly all cases of AFS will require some form of surgical management. Surgery, while representing an important arm (removal of mechanical obstruction, clearance of sinus contents and creation of adequate outflow tracts while maintaining the functional capacity of the lining mucosa), does not obviate the need for adjuvant medical therapy [35].

Both systemic and nasal corticosteroids appear to have benefit, though toxicity from systemic steroids must be considered. Systemic steroids have been shown to decrease the inflammatory response and are typically used in an initial burst pre-operatively and with a taper in the post-operative period [34]. Long-term treatment includes suppressive therapy, topical steroid treatment and irrigations, and serial endoscopic evaluations in post-operative AFS patients. The disease process has a high chance of recurrence (79 % recurrence rate in one study [34]), and therefore requires both medical management and surgical intervention for long-term, continuous treatment.

Other investigators have postulated that decreasing the fungal antigen load in the sinonasal cavities with either systemic or topical antifungal agents may be useful [36]. There are limited data on the use of antifungals for allergic fungal sinusitis in children. The Infectious Diseases Society of America recommends that itraconazole be considered in adults with allergic Aspergillus sinusitis as the benefits outweigh potential from toxicity [37]. Of note, itraconazole has been shown to have a steroid-sparing effect. Other antifungals have not been studied specifically for allergic fungal sinusitis, though in a similar clinical entity, allergic bronchopulmonary aspergillosis, voriconazole and posaconazole are considered second-line agents. Because of the potential side-effects of systemic therapy, interventions that warrant further study include antifungals via topical or nebulized formulations.

References

1. Seltz LB, Smith J, Durairaj VD, Enzenauer R, Todd J. Microbiology and antibiotic management of orbital cellulitis. Pediatrics. 2011;127:e566–72.
2. Deutschmann MW, Livingstone D, Cho JJ, Vanderkooi OG, Brookes JT. The significance of Streptococcus anginosus group in intracranial complications of pediatric rhinosinusitis. JAMA Otolaryngol Head Neck Surg. 2013;139(2):157–60.

3. Belko J, Goldman D, Macone A, Zaidi A. Clinically significant infections with organisms of the Streptococcus milleri group. Pediatr Infect Dis J. 2002;21(8):715–23.
4. Whitby CR, Kaplan SL, Mason EO, Carrillo-Marquez M, Lamberth LB, Hammerman WA, et al. Staphylococcus aureus sinus infections in children. Int J Pediatr Otorhinolaryngol. 2011;75:118–21.
5. Brook I. Microbiology and antimicrobial treatment of orbital and intracranial complications of sinusitis in children and their management. Int J Pediatr Otorhinolaryngol. 2009;73:1183–6.
6. Blackshaw G, Thomson N. Pott's puffy tumour reviewed. J Laryngol Otol. 1990;104:574–7.
7. Younis RT, Lazar RH, Anand VK. Intracranial complications of sinusitis: a 15-year review of 39 cases. Ear Nose Throat J. 2002; 81: 636–8, 640–2, 4.
8. Chandler JR, Langenbrunner DJ, Stevens ER. The pathogenesis of orbital complications in acute sinusitis. Laryngoscope. 1970;80(9):1414–28.
9. Botting AM, McIntosh D, Mahadevan M. Paediatric pre- and post-septal peri-orbital infections are different diseases. A retrospective review of 262 cases. Int J Pediatr Otorhinolaryngol. 2008;72(3):377–83.
10. Ambati BK, Ambati J, Azar N, Stratton L, Schmidt EV. Periorbital and orbital cellulitis before and after the advent of Haemophilus influenzae type B vaccination. Ophthalmology. 2000;107(8):1450–3.
11. Chow AW, Benninger MS, Brook I, Brozek JL, Goldstein EJC, Hicks LA, et al. IDSA clinical practice guideline for acute bacterial rhinosinusitis in children and adults. Clin Infect Dis. 2012;54(8):e72–112.
12. Brook I. Microbiology of intracranial abscesses and their associated sinusitis. Arch Otolaryngol Head Neck Surg. 2005;131(11):1017–9.
13. Osborn MK, Steinberg JP. Subdural empyema and other suppurative complications of paranasal sinusitis. Lancet Infect Dis. 2007;7(1):62–7.
14. DeMuri GP, Wald ER. Complications of acute bacterial sinusitis in children. Pediatr Infect Dis J. 2011;30(8):701–2.
15. Goytia VK, Giannoni CM, Edwards MS. Intraorbital and intracranial extension of sinusitis: comparative morbidity. J Pediatr. 2011;158(3):486–91.
16. Howe L, Jones NS. Guidelines for the management of periorbital cellulitis/abscess. Clin Otolaryngol Allied Sci. 2004;29(6):725–8.
17. Rudloe TF, Harper MB, Prabhu SP, Rahbar R, Vanderveen D, Kimia AA. Acute periorbital infections: who needs emergent imaging? Pediatrics. 2010;125(4):e719–26.
18. Harris GJ. Subperiosteal abscess of the orbit. Age as a factor in the bacteriology and response to treatment. Ophthalmology. 1994;101(3):585–95.
19. Greenberg MF, Pollard ZF. Medical treatment of pediatric subperiosteal orbital abscess secondary to sinusitis. J AAPOS. 1998;2(6):351–5.
20. Oxford LE, McClay J. Medical and surgical management of subperiosteal orbital abscess secondary to acute sinusitis in children. Int J Pediatr Otorhinolaryngol. 2006;70(11):1853–61.
21. Garcia GH, Harris GJ. Criteria for nonsurgical management of subperiosteal abscess of the orbit: analysis of outcomes 1988–1998. Ophthalmology. 2000;107(8):1454–6.
22. Tanna N, Preciado DA, Clary MS, Choi SS. Surgical treatment of subperiosteal orbital abscess. Arch Otolaryngol Head Neck Surg. 2008;134(7):764–7.
23. Parida PK, Surianarayanan G, Ganeshan S, Saxena SK. Pott's puffy tumor in pediatric age group: a retrospective study. Int J Pediatr Otorhinolaryngol. 2012;76(9):1274–7.
24. Kuczkowski J, Narozny W, Mikaszewski C. Suppurative complications of frontal sinusitis in children. Clin Pediatr. 2005;44(8):675–82.
25. Hakim E, Malik AC, Aronyk K. The prevalence of intracranial complications in pediatric frontal sinusitis. Int J Pediatr Otorhinolaryngol. 2006;70(8):1383–7.
26. Clayman GL, Adams GL, Paugh DR. Intracranial complications of paranasal sinusitis: a combined institutional review. Laryngoscope. 1991;101(3):234–9.
27. Lerner DH, Choi SS, Zalzal GH. Intracranial complications of sinusitis in childhood. Ann Otol Rhinol Laryngol. 1995;104(4 Pt 1):288–93.
28. Johnson DL, Markle BM, Wiedermann BL. Treatment of intracranial abscesses associated with sinusitis in children and adolescents. J Pediatr. 1988;113(1 Pt 1):15–23.
29. Giannoni C, Sulek M, Friedman EM. Intracranial complications of sinusitis: a pediatric series. Am J Rhinol. 1998;12:173–8.
30. Germiller JA, Monin DL, Sparano AM. Intracranial complications of sinusitis in children and adolescents and their outcomes. Arch Otolaryngol Head Neck Surg. 2006;132(9):969–76.
31. Thorp BD, McKinney KA, Rose AS. Allergic fungal sinusitis in children. Otolaryngol Clin North Am. 2012;45(3):631–42.
32. Ence BK, Gourley DS, Jorgensen NL. Allergic fungal sinusitis. Am J Rhinol. 1990;4(5):169–78.
33. Granville L, Chirala M, Cernoch P. Fungal sinusitis: histologic spectrum and correlation with culture. Hum Pathol. 2004;35:474–81.

34. Kupferberg SB, Bent JP, Kuhn FA. Prognosis for allergic fungal sinusitis. Otolaryngol Head Neck Surg. 1997;117:35–41.
35. Bent JP, Kuhn FA. Diagnosis of allergic fungal sinusitis. Otolaryngol Head Neck Surg. 1994;111(5):580–8.
36. Kuhn FA, Javer AR. Allergic fungal sinusitis: a four year follow-up. Am J Rhinol. 2000;14:149–56.
37. Walsh TJ, Anaissie EJ, Denning DW, Herbrecht R, Kontoyiannis DP, Marr KA, Infectious Diseases Society of America, et al. Treatment of aspergillosis: clinical practice guidelines of the Infectious Diseases Society of America. Clin Infect Dis. 2008;46(3):327–60.

Chapter 9
Sinus Disease in Cystic Fibrosis

Melanie S. Collins, Thomas S. Murray, and Mark D. Rizzi

Introduction

Cystic fibrosis (CF) is an autosomal recessive disease that most commonly affects Caucasians (approximately 1:3500) but can affect individuals of any race or ethnicity. There are 70,000 individuals with CF worldwide and more than 30,000 of those reside in the US [1]. The signs and symptoms of CF are caused by a genetic defect in the Cystic Fibrosis Transmembrane Regulatory (CFTR) protein that impairs sodium and chloride transport across cell membranes. In the United States and many other countries, mandated universal newborn screening for CF results in diagnosis at an early age and improved access to care. Seventy-five percent of patients in the United States with CF are diagnosed by age 2 [1]. There are more than 1800 different mutations in the CFTR gene that result in defective CFTR function thus newborn screening and genetic testing are not considered definitive diagnostic tests. The gold standard for diagnosing CF is the sweat chloride test [2]. A sweat chloride test must be performed at a CF Foundation Accredited Sweat Laboratory. A sweat chloride level greater than 60 mmol/L is diagnostic of CF.

CFTR mutations are grouped in five different classes based on the functional result of the mutation (summarized in Table 9.1). Regardless of the mutation, the end result of defective CFTR activity is the production of viscous secretions, impairment of mucociliary clearance, creation of a proinflammatory milieu and increased susceptibility to bacterial colonization and infection of both the upper and

M.S. Collins, M.D. (✉)
Department of Pediatric Pulmonary Medicine, Connecticut Children's Medical Center, Hartford, CT, USA

University of Connecticut School of Medicine, Farmington, CT, USA
e-mail: Mcollin@connecticutchildrens.org

T.S. Murray, M.D., Ph.D.
Department of Medical Sciences, Frank H. Netter MD School of Medicine at Quinnipiac University, 275 Mount Carmel Ave, Hamden, CT 06518-1908, USA

Department of Pediatric Infectious Disease, Connecticut Children's Medical Center, Hartford, CT, USA
e-mail: Thomas.murray2@quinnipiac.edu; tscotmurray@gmail.com

M.D. Rizzi, M.D.
Department of Otolaryngology, The Children's Hospital of Philadelphia, 3400 Civic Center Blvd Wood Building, 1st Floor, Philadelphia, PA 19104, USA
e-mail: RIZZIM@email.chop.edu

T.A. Valdez, J.G. Vallejo (eds.), *Infectious Diseases in Pediatric Otolaryngology*,
DOI 10.1007/978-3-319-21744-4_9

Table 9.1 Brief summary of CFTR mutation classes

Class I—No CFTR protein produced
Class II—CFTR protein is degraded in the cell before reaching the plasma membrane
Class III—CFTR protein reaches the plasma membrane; however, is unable to be activated
Class IV—CFTR protein reaches the plasma membrane and is activated; however, it does not properly conduct ion flow
Class V—CFTR protein produced in decreased amounts

Table 9.2 Brief summary evidence of affected organ systems with CF (JPeds 2008)

Upper airway
– Chronic rhinosinusitis
– Nasal polyps (highly suggestive of CF-sweat test should be performed)
Lower airway
– Chronic cough
– Recurrent pneumonia/infection with “CF specific” bacteria-*P. Aeruginosa*, Methicillin Resistant *S. Aureus*, non-typeable *H. Influenzae*; *S. maltophilia*, *B. cepacia*
– Radiographic abnormalities (bronchiectasis, mucus plugging)
– Evidence of airway obstruction on pulmonary function testing or clinical examination
– Digital clubbing
Pancreas/GI tract
– Failure to thrive, steatorrhea (due to malabsorption secondary to pancreatic insufficiency)
– Elevated liver function tests, abnormal bile transport
– Deficiency of fat soluble vitamins (Vitamin A, D, E and K)
Reproductive tract
– Absence of vas deferens

lower airways. While pulmonary manifestations are a primary cause of morbidity and mortality, CF also affects the pancreas, liver, GI and reproductive tracts (see Table 9.2). Due to earlier diagnosis and aggressive medical and surgical management of CF related disease, survival has significantly improved with more than 50 % of patients with CF surviving into adulthood. In fact, a recent study showed that children born with CF can have a median life expectancy of greater than 50 years [3] with the majority of children with CF in the US maintaining normal lung function through age 18 [4].

Epidemiology of Sinus Disease in CF

Several studies have highlighted the lack of nasal sinus symptoms in individuals with CF. Therefore, estimates of the incidence of nasal sinus disease vary, with figures as high as 71–100 % [5]. To address concerns about the accuracy of estimates of sinus disease in CF patients, many experts advocate using questionnaires such as the Sinonasal Outcome Test-22 (SNOT-22) to improve both the ability to diagnose sinus disease and more objectively quantify the response to therapies/surgical intervention [6]. However, these scoring systems have not been well validated in patients with CF [7]. A recent study in the Journal of Cystic Fibrosis [8] demonstrated that sinus disease is more severe in patients with class I–III mutations. This was based on CT scan findings, endoscopy and a symptom scoring system providing support for a previously hypothesized relationship between CFTR genotype and sinus disease phenotype.

Relevant Anatomy and Pathophysiology

The paranasal sinuses are a series of paired mucosa-lined bony chambers that surround and drain into the nose. They are named for the bones into which they have pneumatized: maxillary, ethmoid, frontal and sphenoid. The maxillary and ethmoid sinuses are present though diminutive at birth. The maxillary sinuses expand from their initial outpouching of the middle meatus at birth and continue to grow into early adulthood. The anterior ethmoids emerge from the middle meatus as well and expand into the ethmoid bone throughout childhood and into early adulthood. The frontal sinuses eventually extend as an outgrowth of the anterior ethmoids into the frontal bone. They are not usually radiographically evident until age 6–7 years; their growth continues into adulthood. The sphenoid sinuses are usually not visible on radiographs until about age 1 year. They form through marrow degeneration within the sphenoid body and they fully develop fully by late adolescence [9]. Each sinus generates mucus, which it drains via a characteristic drainage pathway into the nose. This mucociliary clearance occurs through the action of ciliated epithelial cells that line the nose and sinuses. An understanding of these pathways is important, as their obstruction is felt to be a key factor in the pathogenesis of chronic rhinosinusitis (CRS).

The frontal, maxillary and anterior ethmoid sinuses share a common pathway of drainage into the middle meatus through an anatomical region known as the ostiomeatal complex. The posterior ethmoid and sphenoid sinuses drain into the superior meatus via the sphenoethmoidal recess. Ultimately, the products of the sinonasal mucus-producing cells are swept posteriorly into the pharynx and swallowed. A healthy adult nose generates up to 1 L of mucus per day. In the healthy state, the amount, viscosity and composition of mucus allow it to be effortlessly circulated through the nose.

The increased viscosity of mucus produced in patients with CF can lead to mechanical obstruction of sinus ostia and mucus stasis. Consequently, local infection and tissue hypoxia then develop and generate additional inflammation which perpetuates a vicious cycle that compounds the impairment of mucociliary clearance and is a fertile environment for subsequent bacterial colonization within these regions of diminished blood supply [10]. Another consequence of obstructed mucus flow is mucocele formation, whereupon an expanding collection of mucus exerts pressure on the bony confines by which it is trapped. Mucoceles have the ability to erode into neighboring structures such as the orbit or cranium (Fig. 9.1).

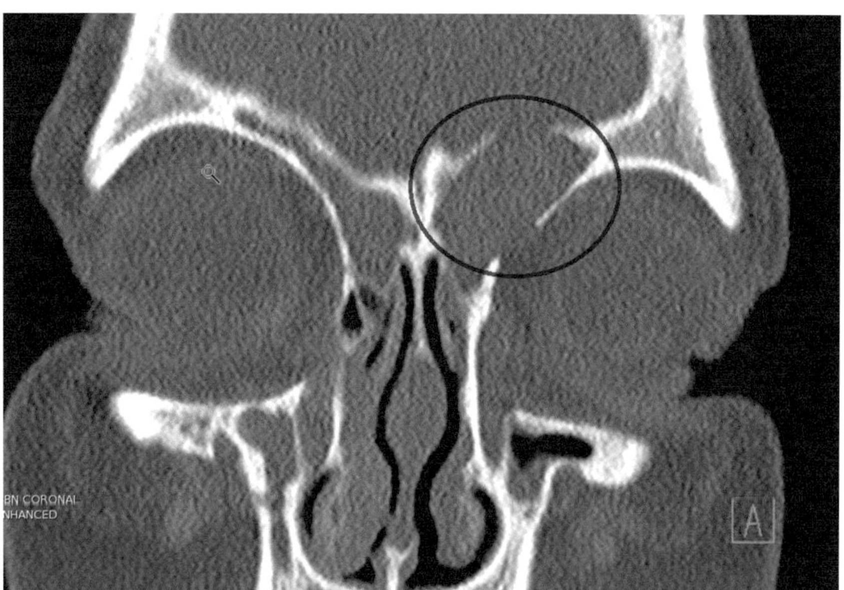

Fig. 9.1 The black oval highlights a left expansile frontoethmoidal mucocele which is eroding into the orbit and intracranially

Nasal polyps (NP) are present in up to 50 % of CF patients and their prevalence is highest during adolescence [11–13]. Since polyps are otherwise rare in children, their presence should alert clinicians to the possibility of CF being present. Conversely, many CF patients do not have polyps, underscoring the need for vigilance on the part of clinicians to suspect CF when appropriate (Table 9.2) even if polyps are absent. The pathogenesis of sinonasal polyposis is unknown although the presence of chronic inflammation clearly plays a role. The inflammatory cellular milieu associated with NP appears to be different in patients with CF when compared with non-CF patients who have polyposis associated with chronic rhinosinusitis (CRSwNP). In patients with CF, polyps are more often associated with a neutrophilic infiltrate whereas eosinophilic associated inflammation is more commonly seen in patients with CRSwNP [11]. Nevertheless, NP are grossly identical in CF and non-CF patients as are their effects of nasal obstruction and impedance of normal mucus flow.

Radiographically, the classic sinonasal anatomic aberrance associated with CF is hypoplastic sinuses with medialization of the lateral nasal walls from expansile polyps within the maxillary antra [14–21] (Fig. 9.2). The maxillary and ethmoid sinuses are commonly smaller than in non-CF patients and the frontal and sphenoid sinuses are sometimes absent (Fig. 9.3). The mechanism for this developmental hypoplasia is not fully elucidated and there is controversy as to whether it develops as a consequence of a patient's genetic abnormality or from chronic infection itself. It has been stated that normal developmental pneumatization is impaired as a result of chronic inflammation and reduced ventilation alone as is seen in the temporal bone in patients who suffer early chronic otitis media [13]. However, Kim et al. [9] noted that patients with chronic rhinosinusitis without CF did not suffer from the same degree of sinonasal hypoplasia that is seen in CF patients. In a study examining the correlation of genotype with the degree of sinus hypoplasia, Woodworth et al. [22] found that homozygosity for the delta F508 mutation of the CFTR, the most common genotype, was predictive of more severe hypoplasia. A mechanism by which such a mutation would generate this phenotype remains unidentified. Externally, the skeletal changes that can occur due to expansile polyp formation can lead to externally visible stigmata, such as hypertelorism or proptosis [23].

Fig. 9.2 Bilaterally maxillary polyps with overall small maxillary sinuses and medialized infundibula (*black arrows*)

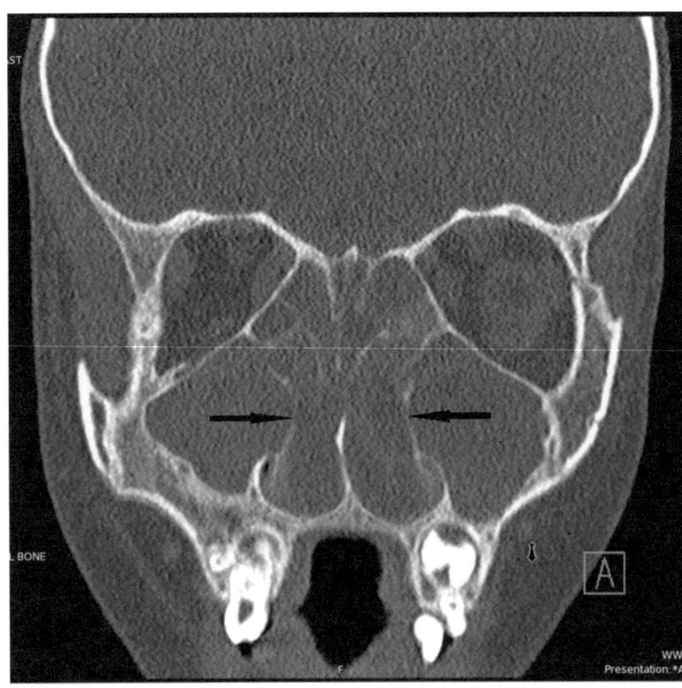

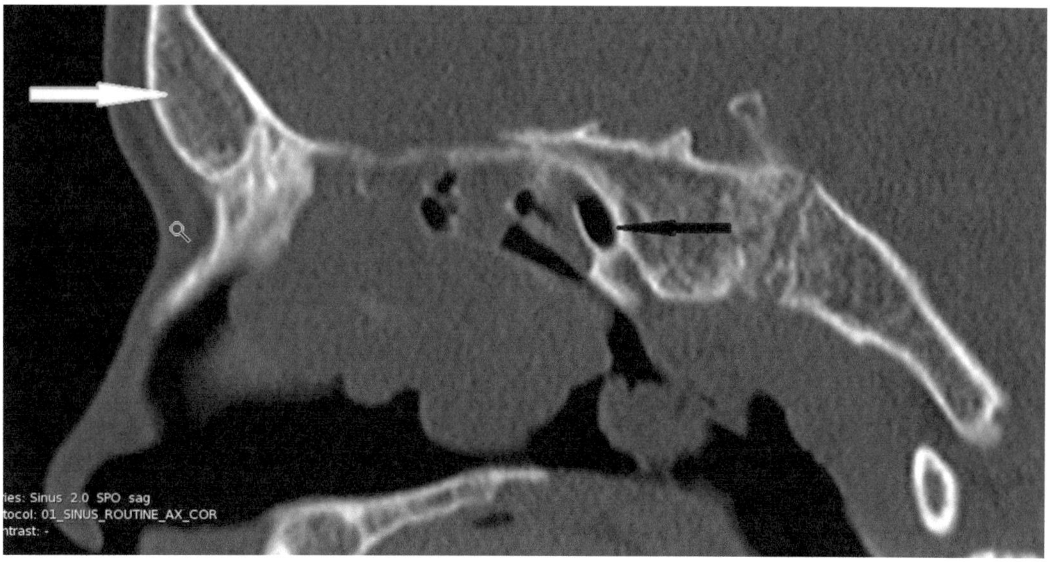

Fig. 9.3 Absent frontal (*white arrow*) and hypoplastic sphenoid (*black arrow*) in this 15 year-old patient with CF

Clinical Presentation

As mentioned previously, sinus disease symptoms are not always elicited on routine history taking. However, reported symptoms include nasal congestion (81 %), rhinorrhea (>50 %), headache (51 %), difficulties with smell/taste (27–66 % depending on the study), morning cough and constant throat clearing [24].

Physical Examination

Chronic rhinosinusitis in CF has been defined as inflammation of nose/paranasal sinuses for >12 weeks with (two or more symptoms): nasal blockage, obstruction, congestion, nasal discharge, facial pain/pressure, and/or reduction in olfaction [25]. One must additionally have at least one of the following finding on examination-nasal polyps, mucopurulent discharge, edema/mucosal obstruction or mucosal changes. Nasal examination begins with simple observation of the patient and should be accompanied by a complete head and neck exam. Patients should be observed for evidence of nasal obstruction such as open mouth or stertorous breathing. Hypertelorism or subtle proptosis suggests underlying expansile mucocele or polyps. Intranasal exam begins with anterior rhinoscopy, which can be accomplished using an otoscope fitted with a wide (>4 mm) speculum or by using a nasal speculum. Polyps, if present, are usually evident through this method (Fig. 9.4). Attention should be directed to the middle meatus from which polyps typically arise. Mucopurulent discharge seen in this region suggests active sinonasal infection. Nasal endoscopy can provide further information about the presence of polyps, purulence and the degree of apparent inflammation present within the nasal cavity. Note that while a polyp is a protuberant growth of solid tissue that arises from nasal mucosa and is visible; a mucocele is a sequestered collection of mucus within a sinus, without a drainage route and therefore is not visible on exam. Their presence is detected either coincidentally on imaging or because infection of their contents causes acute symptoms or external signs (like proptosis). Nasal

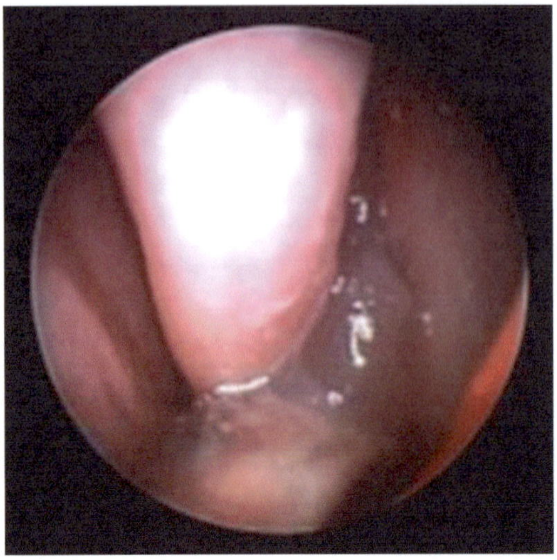

Fig. 9.4 Nasal polyps emanating from the left middle meatus

endoscopy may not be well tolerated in young children but can be accomplished with minimal discomfort. Use of child life specialist or distraction techniques will significantly aid in cooperation with this examination.

Radiographic Studies

CT imaging is considered the gold standard imaging modality for evaluating the paranasal sinuses due to its unparalleled resolution of air, bone and soft tissue. However, since CF patients essentially always have abnormalities on sinonasal CT and since these abnormalities do not predictably correlate with symptoms, CT is of little value when performed simply to establish the presence or absence of sinusitis. Since CT, particularly when performed in children, may increase future risk of leukemia and brain cancer [26], clinicians must consider their likelihood for improved management prior to obtaining them. CT scans should be performed for preoperative evaluation prior to endoscopic sinus surgery, after the decision to proceed with surgery has been reached clinically. Non-contrast images with reconstructed coronal views should be ordered. Requesting contiguous 1 mm axial images is prudent since this degree of resolution and method of scan acquisition is necessary for image guided surgery. Additionally, CT imaging is indicated in patients in whom a complication of acute exacerbated sinusitis, such as orbital or intracranial extension of infection, is suspected. In these cases, the addition of IV contrast is necessary to assess for such a complication.

Microbiology of the CF Sinus

Chronic rhinosinusitis of infectious etiology in the CF patient is due predominately to bacterial pathogens with few reports of disease due to fungi such as *Aspergillus species*. Recent data support the hypothesis that colonization and infection of the sinuses by bacteria is a reservoir for colonization of the lower airway and pulmonary infection [27]. It is also possible that bacteria from the lower airway can move anterograde and infect the sinuses as well. Evidence for this close relationship between bacteria chronically colonizing the sinuses and lower airway infection results from studies that compare bacteria cultured from the sinuses with cultures from the lower airway of the same patient. While the organisms recovered vary depending on the study and the individual patient, a consistent finding is that the traditional CF bacterial pathogens of the lower respiratory tract are commonly found in the sinuses as well [27–31]. For example, two of the most common organisms found in the sinuses of CF patients are *Staphylococcus aureus*, ranging from 46 % of studied patients [28] to 71 % [27], and *Pseudomonas aeruginosa*, 27 % in one study [27] and 57 % in another [28] (including mucoid strains). The recovery of *Haemophilus influenzae*, *Streptococcus pneumoniae* and other pathogens of the lower respiratory tract is also reported [27–31].

Bacteria not necessarily implicated in sinus disease such as viridans group streptococci and *Neisseria sp.* can still be present in sinuses from both CF and healthy patients. A more detailed genotypic/phenotypic examination of *P. aeruginosa* strains recovered from the sinuses and lungs of the same patient with CF demonstrate similar adaptive mutations and phenotypes in both the sinuses and the lung despite differences in the microenvironment [10, 31]. While *P. aeruginosa* form biofilms in the lungs and sinuses, lung infection is associated with a robust neutrophil response, while in the sinuses a strong IgA response blunts neutrophil recruitment. Despite these differences, *P. aeruginosa* recovered from both the lungs and sinuses exhibited decreased motility and protease activity compared with environmental strains [31]. After lung transplant, lower respiratory infection with strains present prior to transplant is reported, again arguing that bacteria from the upper airway are a source of lower airway disease.

More recently, deep DNA sequencing molecular techniques have been applied to characterize the bacterial populations that live in different ecological niches of the human body (the human microbiome). Results from multiple studies demonstrate that bacterial culture is an insensitive technique to adequately capture the microbial diversity that colonizes the human body, including the bacterial population in the sinuses. Many organisms, especially anaerobes, do not grow well under standard conditions in the clinical microbiology laboratory leading to an underestimate of the numbers and types of these organisms present. While comprehensive data are lacking, molecular evidence is emerging that sinuses of CF patients are populated with anaerobes such *Propionibacterium acnes* [27]. Since these organisms can also be found in sinus samples from non-CF patients, the contribution of these uncultivated organisms to pathogenesis and sinus disease in CF patients remains unclear. It does raise the interesting possibility that unrecognized pathogens exist in the CF sinus that contribute to disease but currently little data exists to support this hypothesis.

Initial Therapeutic Options

Nasal irrigations are commonly used to treat nasal sinus symptoms in patients with CF to remove thick secretions and improve mucociliary clearance of the nasal passages. Saline irrigation solutions may be composed of isotonic or hypertonic with/without bicarbonate solutions to provide optimum "clearance". Devices vary from squeeze bottle to neti pot to even home electronic irrigation devices. There are no large randomized controlled trials in CF patients to support this approach. However, it is a widely accepted method of maintaining good sinus health both pre/post-surgical intervention.

Topical nasal steroids have also been used in CF to decrease nasal inflammation and decrease size of nasal polyps. There is a single randomized controlled trial of betamethasone which demonstrated both decrease in polyp size as well as nasal symptoms during treatment [32]. In clinical practice, some have combined both topical nasal steroids (i.e. budesonide) mixed into saline irrigation to maximize lasting topical benefit but large supporting clinical trial data have not been obtained.

Another therapy currently under investigation is dornase alfa which enzymatically degrades extracellular DNA (a large component of the debris in CF mucus). Inhaled into the lower airway, Dornase alfa is an effective medication for maintaining lower airway function and decreasing the frequency of pulmonary exacerbations in individuals with CF. It is a recommended daily therapy in both the US and Europe for patients over the age of 6 [33]. Several studies have suggested dornase alfa can improve upper airway function and sinus disease based on symptoms as well as endoscopic evaluation. Furthermore, a recent study by Mainz et al, demonstrated significant improvements in pulmonary function as well [34]. This method of aerosoling dornase alfa by intranasal nebulization to deliver medication the sinuses is not widely available in the US currently.

The latest in therapy for patients with CF are a variety of medications that work as correcting the underlying molecular defect. These drugs, known as correctors and potentiators, are mutation specific. The most widely known drug, ivacaftor, corrects the defect associated with class III mutations. There are several case reports of patients who have significant improvement in their upper airway symptoms and sinus CT once starting the medication [35, 36].

Antimicrobial Therapy for Bacterial Sinusitis in CF Patients

An implication of the hypothesis that the sinuses are a reservoir for lung infection is that aggressive treatment of bacterial rhinosinusitis may prevent or at least delay the onset of pulmonary exacerbations in children with CF. However, multiple courses of intravenous antibiotics for pulmonary infections that cover common sinus pathogens fail to eradicate the bacteria in the sinuses in the vast majority of patients once infection is established. Therefore any antibiotic therapy should be supplemental to additional therapies such as topical saline irrigation. Topical antibiotic therapy with tobramycin is reported to be effective at clearing or reducing the bacterial load of *P. aeruginosa*. A recent report with small numbers of patients used a vibrating irrigation system to deliver the drug to the paranasal sinuses leading to decreased recovery of *P. aeruginosa* and improved SNOT-22 scores in patients receiving tobramycin compared with those receiving placebo [37]. Vibration has the potential to disrupt bacterial biofilms making the microbes more susceptible to the antibiotic. An aggressive therapeutic regimen post sinus surgery for CF patients is reported to not only eradicate sinus colonization with *P. aeruginosa* but also reduce lower airway infections in patients not yet chronically infected [38]. This regimen included 2 weeks of intravenous antibiotic therapy and 6 months of topical colistimethate sodium (adjusted when necessary based on bacterial susceptibility) in addition to nasal irrigation and topical steroids.

For sinus symptoms, as described, topical tobramycin and colistimethate sodium have the potential to be effective with fewer adverse systemic effects than systemic antibiotic therapies [39]. Oral therapy with ciprofloxacin, an anti-pseudomonal fluoroquinolone, is often used to treat pulmonary infection to avoid intravenous antibiotic therapy, but evidence that it clears *P. aeruginosa* from the sinuses is lacking [25]. Furthermore, anti-pseudomonal intravenous antibiotics including ceftazidime and meropenem also fail to eradicate *P. aeruginosa* from the sinuses as well. Macrolide administration (e.g. azithromycin) as an anti-inflammatory rather than as an anti-microbial has been shown to improve symptoms and reduce nasal polyps [25].

There are little current data regarding the use of anti-staphylococcal drugs for sinusitis in CF patients. The topical agent mupirocin has been delivered via nasal irrigation with short-term success in non-CF patients with chronic rhinosinusitis refractory to surgery [40]. Unfortunately, there are no data for its use in the CF population. For methicillin susceptible *S. aureus* (MSSA) cephalexin is a first line oral therapy. For methicillin resistant *S. aureus* (MRSA) oral choices include clindamycin and trimethoprim/sulfamethoxazole. These drugs also have activity against MSSA and may be used in patients allergic to β-lactam antibiotics. Intravenous therapies of choice directed against MSSA include oxacillin/nafcillin, or cefazolin. Vancomycin provides excellent coverage against MRSA. Again, there is a paucity of data supporting intravenous antibiotics as therapy for *S. aureus* sinusitis in the CF population. Inhaled vancomycin is currently being studied for MRSA pulmonary infections in CF patients and may be adaptable as a topical therapy for the sinuses in the future [41].

Since molecular methods have only recently identified anaerobic bacterial populations in the sinuses of CF patients, a role for anti-microbial therapy directed against anaerobes remains to be determined. Most importantly, antimicrobial therapy should be guided by antibiotic susceptibility of pathogens cultured directly from the sinuses whenever possible.

Surgical Management of Chronic Rhinosinusitis in CF Patients

Endoscopic sinus surgery (ESS) is a safe and well established treatment modality for medically refractory CRS in children [42–45]. In patients with CF, it has been shown to improve symptoms and quality of life [46, 47]. The goals of endoscopic sinus surgery in general are to provide improved ventilation of the paranasal sinuses by widening and relieving obstruction of the natural ostia through which they drain into the nose. Sequestered infection, polyps and diseased bone and mucosa can be removed from these regions and from the sinuses themselves. Such treatment allows for improved drainage of the sinuses, acquisition of inspissated exudate for culture, access for debridement in the office and facilitates access of topical nasal irrigants, antibiotics and anti-inflammatory medicines. A commonly cited, though poorly defined, a requisite for proceeding to surgery is failure of maximal medical therapy. It is generally accepted that such treatment includes more than one round of systemic antibiotics, each lasting 3–6 weeks in conjunction with topical or occasionally systemic corticosteroid treatment [48]. Unfortunately, evidence based protocols for proceeding to surgery in patients with CRS are lacking in the literature and they are essentially absent for the subset of CRS patients with CF. In CF, mucosal disease and mucociliary clearance abnormalities are not cured by ESS alone, and the underlying disease process inevitably persists. Additionally, while nearly all patients with CF exhibit radiological abnormalities consistent with CRS, few actually complain of manifestations of these findings [11]. Patient selection for surgery must therefore focus on the degree to which sinonasal inflammatory disease is impacting patient health and quality of life. Commonly described indications for surgical intervention in CF patients include: nasal obstruction, symptomatic polyps, pulmonary exacerbations that correlate with episodes of rhinosinusitis and declining pulmonary function tests. A systematic review by Macdonald et al., showed that nasal obstruction, olfaction, rhinorrhea, facial pain and headache all appear to be significantly alleviated by ESS in CF patients; although pulmonary function tests are not consistently improved [49]. There is a decreased rate of hospitalization for pulmonary exacerbation in the 6 months following sinus surgery [50] and ESS has been shown to be beneficial in patients with medically refractory CRS post lung transplant [51].

Unfortunately, revision sinus surgery is frequently necessary in patients with CF. The degree of sinonasal disease present at the outset of surgery may predict the need for patients to undergo revision procedures. A study in 2010 showed that 58 % of a subset of patients with extensive polyposis required revision surgery [52]. A benefit of ESS in CF patients is facilitated access for the application of antibiotic rinses [53] which may decrease the need for revision procedures. The overall trend in ESS in CF patients has been toward more aggressive surgical opening of the sinuses [54]. The need for repeat surgery may be lower with such therapy [55]. The modified endoscopic medial maxillectomy (MEMM) may be associated with improved outcomes in patients with CF in whom standard maxillary antrostomy has failed to adequately alleviate symptoms. In this procedure, the standard maxillary antrostomy is extended to remove the entire lateral nasal wall including the middle third of the inferior turbinate. The proposed benefits of this procedure are the allowance of more gravity dependent drainage of the maxillary sinuses and enhanced access for topical medicines. A recent study showed that MEMM significantly improved sinonasal symptom scores, and Lund Kennedy endoscopic scores [56]. A drawback of this study was the lack of a control group comparing patients who underwent MEMM with those who underwent less invasive procedures.

Postoperatively, patients are typically maintained on systemic antibiotics, preferably directed by sinonasal cultures. The duration of such treatment is not supported by evidence based guidelines and is best individualized to a patient's overall degree of infection and medical condition. High volume saline rinses can be initiated on the first post-operative day. Such irrigations facilitate mucus clearance, debride the sinonasal cavities of crusts and debris and are widely accepted as standard care in post ESS patients. Patients are typically seen in the office 1–2 weeks post operatively. Debridement of crusts and absorbable packing should be performed in tolerant patients. Further debridement may be necessary in the months following surgery. As stated above, the care of patients with CRS has been evolving to emphasize topical based therapies. Such treatment is greatly facilitated by ESS, wherein sinonasal ostia are widened to allow access of therapeutic agents. These include antibiotics, such as mupirocin and tobramycin as well as steroids such as mometasone or budesonide.

Major complications from ESS are fortunately rare and include cerebrospinal fluid leak, brain injury, orbital injury potentially leading to permanent diplopia or blindness, retro orbital hematoma, meningitis, loss of sense of smell and hemorrhage. There are no reports of increased surgical risk in patients with CF. Revision surgery, need to enter the frontal sinus, presence of polyps, or significant active sinonasal inflammation all increase the difficulty and potential risks of surgery. Utilizing image guidance may decrease the risk of complications in these scenarios. Minor complications such as mild epistaxis, crusting or intranasal synechiae are more common and are ameliorated by meticulous, mucosal sparing technique and by post operative irrigations and debridements as possible. Persistence of the underlying disease and risk of recurrence is ubiquitous in the CF population.

Conclusions

Sinus disease is present in almost all individuals with CF, and perhaps more severe in those individuals with class I–III mutations. The pathophysiology of CF creates a unique anatomic and microbiologic environment of the sinuses. Early and aggressive recognition of nasal sinus symptoms is key to maintenance of both upper and lower airway function. Use of nasal irrigations and topical medications can help improve symptoms and improve the efficacy of both antimicrobial and surgical intervention.

Lastly, ESS in CF patients is safe and effective for relief of sinonasal symptoms and appears to be helpful to minimize pulmonary exacerbations for patients in whom sinonasal infections are worsening overall disease status. Evidence based guidelines pertaining to the timing or degree of surgical intervention are lacking. Physicians must therefore individualize these decisions and should focus on the effect of CRS on quality of life and overall health rather than on the basis of radiological abnormalities or the presence of polyps alone.

References

1. About CF: causes, signs & symptoms of cystic fibrosis | CF foundation [Internet]. 2014. http://www.cff.org/AboutCF/. Accessed 16 Nov 2014.
2. Farrell PM, Rosenstein BJ, White TB, Accurso FJ, Castellani C, Cutting GR, Durie PR, Legrys VA, Massie J, Parad RB, Rock MJ, Campbell PW 3rd; Cystic Fibrosis Foundation. Guidelines for diagnosis of cystic fibrosis in newborns through older adults: cystic fibrosis foundation consensus report [Internet]. J Pediatr. 2008. http://www.sciencedirect.com/science/article/pii/S0022347608003983. Accessed 12 Nov 2014.
3. Dodge JA, Lewis PA, Stanton M, Wilsher J. Cystic fibrosis mortality and survival in the UK: 1947–2003 [Internet]. Eur Respir J. 2007;29(3):522–6. http://www.ncbi.nlm.nih.gov/pubmed/17182652. Accessed 14 Nov 2014.
4. Report AD. Patient Registry. 2010

5. Babinski D, Trawinska-Bartnicka M. Rhinosinusitis in cystic fibrosis: not a simple story [Internet]. Int J Pediatr Otorhinolaryngol. 2008;72(5):619–24. http://www.ncbi.nlm.nih.gov/pubmed/18294702. Accessed 17 Dec 2014.
6. Illing EA, Woodworth BA. Management of the upper airway in cystic fibrosis [Internet]. Curr Opin Pulm Med. 2014;20(6):623–31. http://www.ncbi.nlm.nih.gov/pubmed/25250804. Accessed 6 Nov 2014.
7. VanDevanter DR, Southern KW. The challenge of improving outcomes for patients with CF sinonasal disease [Internet]. J Cyst Fibros; 2014;13(4):361–2. http://www.ncbi.nlm.nih.gov/pubmed/24890305. Accessed 12 Nov 2014.
8. Berkhout MC, Van Rooden CJ, Aalbers RC, El Bouazzaoui LH, Fokkens WJ, Rijntjes E, et al. Temporal bone pneumatization in cystic fibrosis: a correlation with genotype? [Internet]. Laryngoscope. John Wiley and Sons Inc.; 2014;124(7):1682–6. http://www.ncbi.nlm.nih.gov/pubmed/24374715. Accessed 11 Nov 2014.
9. Kim HJ, Friedman EM, Sulek M, Duncan NO, Mccluggage C. Paranasal sinus development in chronic sinusitis, cystic fibrosis, and normal comparison population: a computerized tomography correlation study. Am J Rhinol. 1997;11(4):275–81.
10. Hansen SK, Rau MH, Johansen HK, Ciofu O, Jelsbak L, Yang L, et al. Evolution and diversification of Pseudomonas aeruginosa in the paranasal sinuses of cystic fibrosis children have implications for chronic lung infection. ISME J. 2012;6(1):31–45.
11. Mainz JG, Koitschev A. Pathogenesis and management of nasal polyposis in cystic fibrosis. Curr Allergy Asthma Rep. 2012;12(2):163–74.
12. Koitschev A, Wolff A, Koitschev C, Preyer S, Ziebach R, Stern M. Routine otorhinolaryngological examination in patients with cystic fibrosis. HNO. 2006;54:361–4, 366, 368.
13. Gysin C, Alothman GA, Papsin BC. State of the Art sinonasal disease in cystic fibrosis: clinical characteristics, diagnosis, and management. Pediatr Pulmonol. 2000;30(6):481–9.
14. Krzeski A, Kapiszewska-Dzedzej D, Jakubczyk I, Jedrusik A, Held-Ziółkowska M. Extent of pathological changes in the paranasal sinuses of patients with cystic fibrosis: CT analysis [Internet]. Am J Rhinol. 2001;15(3):207–10. http://www.ncbi.nlm.nih.gov/pubmed/11453510. Accessed 13 Nov 2014.
15. Eggesbø HB, Søvik S, Dølvik S, Eiklid K, Kolmannskog F. CT characterization of developmental variations of the paranasal sinuses in cystic fibrosis. Acta Radiol. 2001;42:482–93.
16. Eggesbø HB, Eken T, Eiklid K, Kolmannskog F. Hypoplasia of the sphenoid sinuses as a diagnostic tool in cystic fibrosis. Acta Radiol. 1999;40:479–85.
17. Eggesbø HB, Søvik S, Dølvik S, Eiklid K, Kolmannskog F. Proposal of a CT scoring system of the paranasal sinuses in diagnosing cystic fibrosis. Eur Radiol. 2003;13:1451–60.
18. Eggesbø HB, Dølvik S, Stiris M, Søvik S, Storrøsten OT, Kolmannskog F. Complementary role of MR imaging of ethmomaxillary sinus disease depicted at CT in cystic fibrosis. Acta Radiol. 2001;42:144–50.
19. Eggesbo HB, Sovik S, Dolvik S, Kolmannskog F. CT characterization of inflammatory paranasal sinus disease in cystic fibrosis [Internet]. Acta Radiol. 2002;43:21–8. http://www.ncbi.nlm.nih.gov/pubmed/11972457
20. Kim HJ, Friedman EM, Sulek MS, Duncan NO, McCluggage C. Paranasal sinus development in chronic sinusitis, cystic fibrosis, and normal comparison population: a computerized tomography correlation study [Internet]. Am J Rhinol. 1997;(11): 275-281. 2. Hansen SK, Rau. https://search.yahoo.com/search;_ylt=AtshGcQY481R03td5izpRdKbvZx4?p=1.+Kim+HJ,+Friedman+EM,+Sulek+MS,+Duncan+NO,+McCluggage+C.+Paranasal+sinus+development+in+chronic+sinusitis,+cystic+fibrosis,+and+normal+comparison+population:+a+computerized+tomography+correlation+study.+Am+J+Rhinol.+1997+(11):+275-281.+2.+Hansen+SK,+Rau+MH,+Johansen+HK,+et+al.+Evolution+and+diversification+of+Pseudomonas+aeruginosa+in+the+paranasal+sinuses+of+cystic+fibrosis+children+have+implications. Accessed cited 10 Nov 2014.
21. Brihaye P, Clement PAR, Dabb I, Desprechin B. Pathological-changes of the lateral nasal wall in patients with cystic-fibrosis (Mucoviscidosis). Int J Pediatr Otorhinolaryngol. 1994;28:141–7.
22. Woodworth B a., Ahn C, Flume P a., Schlosser RJ. The delta F508 mutation in cystic fibrosis and impact on sinus development [Internet]. Am J Rhinol. 2007;21(1):122–7. http://openurl.ingenta.com/content/xref?genre=article&issn=1050-6586&volume=21&issue=1&spage=122. Accessed 11 Nov 2014.
23. Hui Y, Gaffney R, Crysdale WS. Sinusitis in patients with cystic fibrosis. Eur Arch Otorhinolaryngol. 1995;252:191–6.
24. Robertson JM, Friedman EM, Rubin BK. Nasal and sinus disease in cystic fibrosis [Internet]. Paediatr Respir Rev. 2008;9(3):213–9. http://www.ncbi.nlm.nih.gov/pubmed/18694713. Accessed 20 Oct 2014.
25. Chaaban MR, Kejner A, Rowe SM, Woodworth BA. Cystic fibrosis chronic rhinosinusitis: a comprehensive review. Am J Rhinol Allergy. 2013;27(5):387–95.
26. Pearce MS, Salotti JA, Little MP, McHugh K, Lee C, Kim KP, et al. Radiation exposure from CT scans in childhood and subsequent risk of leukaemia and brain tumours: a retrospective cohort study [Internet]. Lancet. Elsevier Ltd; 2012380(9840):499–505. http://www.pubmedcentral.nih.gov/articlerender.fcgi?artid=3418594&tool=pmcentrez&rendertype=abstract. Accessed 10 Jul 2014.
27. Rudkjøbing VB, Aanaes K, Wolff TY, von Buchwald C, Johansen HK, Thomsen TR. An exploratory study of microbial diversity in sinus infections of cystic fibrosis patients by molecular methods. J Cyst Fibros. 2014;13(6): 645–52.

28. Digoy GP, Dunn JD, Stoner JA, Christie A, Jones DT. Bacteriology of the paranasal sinuses in pediatric cystic fibrosis patients. Int J Pediatr Otorhinolaryngol. 2012;76(7):934–8. Elsevier Ireland Ltd.
29. Godoy JM, Godoy AN, Ribalta G, Largo I. Bacterial pattern in chronic sinusitis and cystic fibrosis. Otolaryngol Head Neck Surg. 2011;145(4):673–6.
30. Lavin J, Bhushan B, Schroeder JW. Correlation between respiratory cultures and sinus cultures in children with cystic fibrosis. Int J Pediatr Otorhinolaryngol. 2013;77(5):686–9. Elsevier Ireland Ltd.
31. Ciofu O, Johansen HK, Aanaes K, Wassermann T, Alhede M, von Buchwald C, et al. P. aeruginosa in the paranasal sinuses and transplanted lungs have similar adaptive mutations as isolates from chronically infected CF lungs. J Cyst Fibros. 2013;12(6):729–36.
32. Hadfield PJ, Rowe-Jones JM, Mackay IS. A prospective treatment trial of nasal polyps in adults with cystic fibrosis [Internet]. Rhinology. 2000;38(2):63–5. http://www.ncbi.nlm.nih.gov/pubmed/10953842. Accessed 16 Nov 2014.
33. Mogayzel PJ, Naureckas ET, Robinson KA, Mueller G, Hadjiliadis D, Hoag JB, et al. Cystic fibrosis pulmonary guidelines. Chronic medications for maintenance of lung health [Internet]. Am J Respir Crit Care Med. 2013;187(7):680–9. http://www.ncbi.nlm.nih.gov/pubmed/23540878. Accessed 7 Aug 2014.
34. Mainz JG, Schien C, Schiller I, Schädlich K, Koitschev A, Koitschev C, et al. Sinonasal inhalation of dornase alfa administered by vibrating aerosol to cystic fibrosis patients: a double-blind placebo-controlled cross-over trial [Internet]. J Cyst Fibros. 2014;13(4):461–70. http://www.ncbi.nlm.nih.gov/pubmed/24594542. Accessed 12 Nov 2014.
35. Hayes D, McCoy KS, Sheikh SI. Improvement of sinus disease in cystic fibrosis with ivacaftor therapy [Internet]. Am J Respir Crit Care Med. 2014;190(4):468. http://www.ncbi.nlm.nih.gov/pubmed/25127305. Accessed 10 Nov 2014.
36. Chang EH, Tang XX, Shah VS, Launspach JL, Ernst SE, Hilkin B, et al. Medical reversal of chronic sinusitis in a cystic fibrosis patient with ivacaftor [Internet]. Int Forum Allergy Rhinol. 2014; 5(2):178-81. http://www.ncbi.nlm.nih.gov/pubmed/25363320. Accessed 16 Nov 2014.
37. Mainz J, Schädlich K, Schien C, Michl R, Schelhorn-Neise P, Koitschev A, Koitschev C, Keller PM, Riethmüller J, Wiedemann B, Beck JF. Sinonasal inhalation of tobramycin vibrating aerosol in cystic fibrosis patients with upper airway Pseudomonas aeruginosa colonization: results of a randomized, double-blind, placebo-controlled pilot study. Drug Des Devel Ther. 2014;8:209–17.
38. Aanaes K, Eickhardt S, Johansen HK, von Buchwald C, Skov M, Høiby N, et al. Sinus biofilms in patients with cystic fibrosis: is adjusted eradication therapy needed? [Internet] Eur Arch Otorhinolaryngol. 2014. http://www.ncbi.nlm.nih.gov/pubmed/25297534. Accessed 11 Oct 2014.
39. Lim M, Citardi MJ, Leong J-L. Topical antimicrobials in the management of chronic rhinosinusitis: a systematic review. Am J Rhinol. 2014;22(4):381–9.
40. Solares CA, Batra PS, Hall GS, Citardi MJ. Treatment of chronic rhinosinusitis exacerbations due to methicillin-resistant Staphylococcus aureus with mupirocin irrigations. Am J Otolaryngol. 2006;27(3):161–5.
41. Jennings MT, Boyle MP, Weaver D, Callahan KA, Dasenbrook EC. Eradication strategy for persistent methicillin-resistant Staphylococcus aureus infection in individuals with cystic fibrosis—the PMEP trial: study protocol for a randomized controlled trial [Internet]. Trials. 2014;15(1):223. http://www.pubmedcentral.nih.gov/articlerender.fcgi?artid=4068380&tool=pmcentrez&rendertype=abstract. Accessed 17 Dec 2014.
42. Hebert RL, Bent JP. Meta-analysis of outcomes of pediatric functional endoscopic sinus surgery. Laryngoscope. 1998;108:796–9.
43. Siedek V, Stelter K, Betz CS, Berghaus A, Leunig A. Functional endoscopic sinus surgery—a retrospective analysis of 115 children and adolescents with chronic rhinosinusitis. Int J Pediatr Otorhinolaryngol. 2009;73:741–5.
44. Rudnick EF, Mitchell RB. Long-term improvements in quality-of-life after surgical therapy for pediatric sinonasal disease [Internet]. Otolaryngol Head Neck Surg. 2007;137(6):873–7. http://www.ncbi.nlm.nih.gov/pubmed/18036413. Accessed 13 Nov 2014
45. El Sharkawy AA, Elmorsy SM, Eladl HM. Functional endoscopic sinus surgery in children: predictive factors of outcome [Internet]. Eur Arch Otorhinolaryngol. 2012;269:107–11. http://www.ncbi.nlm.nih.gov/pubmed/21706318
46. Nishioka GJ, Barbero GJ, König P, Parsons DS, Cook PR, Davis WE. Symptom outcome after functional endoscopic sinus surgery in patients with cystic fibrosis: a prospective study. Otolaryngol Head Neck Surg. 1995;113:440–5.
47. Jones JW, Parsons DS, Cuyler JP. The results of functional endoscopic sinus (FES) surgery on the symptoms of patients with cystic fibrosis. Int J Pediatr Otorhinolaryngol. 1993;28:25–32.
48. Rizzi MD, Kazahaya K. Pediatric chronic rhinosinusitis: when should we operate? [Internet] Curr Opin Otolaryngol Head Neck Surg. 2014;22(1):27–33. http://www.ncbi.nlm.nih.gov/pubmed/24300841. Accessed 11 Nov 2014.
49. Macdonald KI, Gipsman A, Magit A, Fandino M, Massoud E, Witterick IJ, et al. Endoscopic sinus surgery in patients with cystic fibrosis: a systematic review and meta-analysis of pulmonary function [Internet]. Rhinology. 2012;50(4):360–9. http://www.ncbi.nlm.nih.gov/pubmed/23181249. Accessed 13 Nov 2014.
50. Rosbe KW, Jones DT, Rahbar R, Lahiri T, Auerbach AD. Endoscopic sinus surgery in cystic fibrosis: do patients benefit from surgery? Int J Pediatr Otorhinolaryngol. 2001;61(2):113–9.

51. Vital D, Hofer M, Boehler A, Holzmann D. Posttransplant sinus surgery in lung transplant recipients with cystic fibrosis: a single institutional experience [Internet]. Eur Arch Otorhinolaryngol. 2013;270(1):135–9. http://www.ncbi.nlm.nih.gov/pubmed/22460525. Accessed 13 Nov 2014.
52. Rickert S, Banuchi VE, Germana JD, Stewart MG, April MM. Cystic fibrosis and endoscopic sinus surgery: relationship between nasal polyposis and likelihood of revision endoscopic sinus surgery in patients with cystic fibrosis. Arch Otolaryngol Head Neck Surg. 2013;136(10):988–92.
53. Fokkens WJ, Lund VJ, Mullol J, Bachert C, Alobid I, Baroody F, et al. EPOS 2012: European position paper on rhinosinusitis and nasal polyps 2012. A summary for otorhinolaryngologists [Internet]. Rhinology. 2012;50(1):1–12. http://www.ncbi.nlm.nih.gov/pubmed/22469599. Accessed 16 Nov 2014.
54. Crosby DL, Adappa ND. What is the optimal management of chronic rhinosinusitis in cystic fibrosis? [Internet]. Curr Opin Otolaryngol Head Neck Surg. Lippincott Williams & Wilkins, 530 Walnut St, Philadelphia, Pa 19106-3621 Usa; 2014;22(1):42–6. http://apps.webofknowledge.com.ezproxy.library.ubc.ca/full_record.do?product=WOS&search_mode=Refine&qid=19&SID=3DwtSxMaoz7v425ZsaI&page=1&doc=3. Accessed 11 Nov 2014.
55. Shatz A. Management of recurrent sinus disease in children with cystic fibrosis: a combined approach [Internet]. Otolaryngol Head Neck Surg. 2006;135(2):248–52. http://www.ncbi.nlm.nih.gov/pubmed/16890077. Accessed 11 Nov 2014.
56. Virgin FW, Rowe SM, Wade MB, Gaggar A, Leon KJ, Young KR, et al. Extensive surgical and comprehensive postoperative medical management for cystic fibrosis chronic rhinosinusitis [Internet]. Am J Rhinol Allergy. 2014;26(1):70–5. http://www.pubmedcentral.nih.gov/articlerender.fcgi?artid=3622282&tool=pmcentrez&rendertype=abstract. Accessed 11 Nov 2014.

Part III
Oral Cavity, Oropharynx and Upper Airway

Chapter 10
Tonsillitis and Peritonsillar Abscess

Luis A. Castagnini, Meha Goyal, and Julina Ongkasuwan

Abbreviations

AAO-HNS	American Academy of Otolaryngology—Head and Neck Surgery
ARF	Acute rheumatic fever
ASO	Anti-streptolysin-O
CMV	Cytomegalovirus
CN	IX Cranial nerve IX
CT	Computed tomography
EBV	Epstein-Barr virus
GABHS	Group A β-hemolytic streptococcus
HSV	Herpes simplex virus
IDSA	Infectious Disease Society of America
NSAID	Non-steroidal anti-inflammatory
PCR	Polymerase chain reaction
PFAPA	Periodic fevers, aphthous stomatitis, pharyngitis, and adenitis
PSGN	Post-streptococcal glomerulonephritis
RADT	Rapid antigen detection test
SDB	Sleep disordered breathing

L.A. Castagnini, M.D., M.P.H.
Department of Pediatrics, Baylor College of Medicine, 315 N San Saba, San Antonio, TX 78207, USA
e-mail: lcastagnini@me.com; castagni@bcm.edu

M. Goyal, B.B.A.
Department of Otolaryngology - Head and Neck Surgery, Baylor College of Medicine, 6501 Fannin St, Houston, TX 77030, USA
e-mail: mehag89@gmail.com

J. Ongkasuwan, M.D. (✉)
Department of Otolaryngology—Head and Neck Surgery, Baylor College of Medicine, Texas Children's Hospital, 6701 Fannin, Suite 640, Houston, TX 77030, USA
e-mail: julinao@bcm.edu

T.A. Valdez, J.G. Vallejo (eds.), *Infectious Diseases in Pediatric Otolaryngology*,
DOI 10.1007/978-3-319-21744-4_10

Anatomy

Tonsils are lymphoid organs found in the nasopharynx and oropharynx. There are three main sets of tonsils: pharyngeal tonsils, lingual tonsils and palatine tonsils. The pharyngeal tonsils are more commonly referred to as the adenoids and reside midline in the nasopharynx. The lingual tonsils are found on the posterior one-third of the tongue. The palatine tonsils are nestled in the tonsillar fossa, defined by the tonsillar pillars of the oropharynx. The anterior pillar is comprised of the palatoglossus muscle, whereas the palatopharyngeus muscle makes up the posterior pillar. These tonsils are encapsulated by a specialized portion of the pharyngobasilar fascia. They are the most commonly infected set of tonsils and will be henceforth referred to as the "tonsils."

Neurovascular Supply

Numerous blood vessels supply the tonsils, all branches of the external carotid artery. These arteries include branches of ascending pharyngeal, dorsal lingual, facial, and maxillary arteries, with the tonsillar branch of the facial artery being the greatest contributor.

Venous drainage of the tonsils is via the lingual and pharyngeal veins. Lymphatic drainage of the tonsils is primarily via the jugulodigastric system [1, 2].

Sensory innervation to the region is via the glossopharyngeal nerve (CN IX).

Relationship to Surrounding Structures

Carotid Artery

The external branch of the carotid artery is located just lateral to the tonsillar fossa. The internal carotid artery is about 2 cm posterolateral to the deep portion of the tonsillar fossa. These structures can be compromised by acute processes or as a result of interventions taken in the tonsillar region (Fig. 10.1).

Pterygoid Muscles

The capsule of the tonsil is separated from the superior constrictor muscle by loose connective tissue. Lateral to the superior constrictor muscle lies the parapharyngeal space. The lateral border of the parapharyngeal space consists of the medial pterygoid muscle which can get irritated and inflamed in the event of parapharyngeal irritation or infection, resulting in trismus.

Crypts

The tonsils are not smooth; instead they have numerous crypts or pits where food can get caught. Food accumulated within these crypts forms small stone-like structures known as tonsilliths which can then lead to inflammation and chronic throat pain.

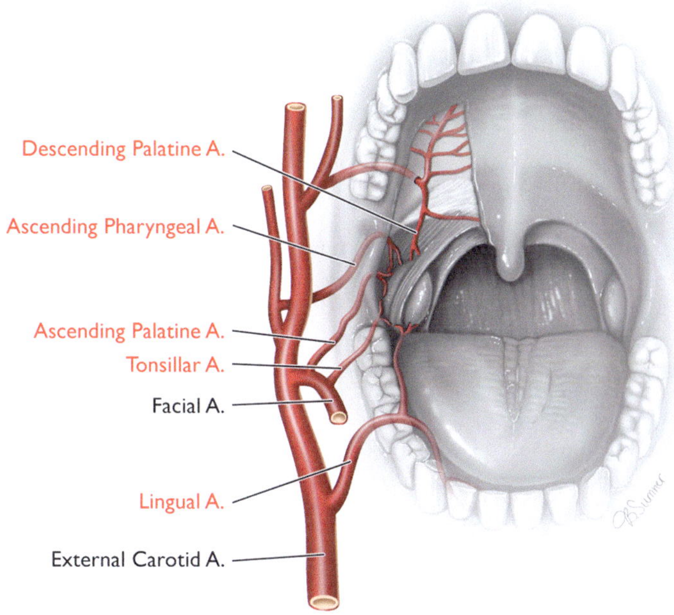

Fig. 10.1 Vascular anatomy of the tonsil (Printed with permission from Texas Children's Hospital)

Immunologic Function of Tonsils

The tonsils are lymphoepithelial organs that function as secondary lymphoid organs. They contain specialized epithelial M cells that capture and transport antigens entering through the mouth and nose to extrafollicular regions or lymphoid follicles. The lymphoid follicles then release antibody-expressing memory B cells or plasma cells that migrate to the tonsils and produce antibodies. These antibodies are subsequently released into the tonsillar crypt lumen. All five isotypes of immunoglobulins are produced in the tonsil. The most important of these isotypes is IgA which functions as an important component of the mucosal immune system of the upper airway [3].

The tonsils are at their largest size during the most active immunologic activity, which is estimated to be between the ages of 3 and 10 years. After this period they display spontaneous age-depended involution [3]. Chronic or recurrent tonsillitis alters the tonsillar immune system by causing shedding of the M cells and the tonsillar immunologic response to antigens weakens. The clinical significance of this dysfunction is controversial. There are no data demonstrating significant change in the systemic immune system after tonsillectomy [3].

Tonsillitis

Tonsillitis is inflammation of the tonsils, specifically the palatine tonsils.

Epidemiology

Acute pharyngitis is one of the most common illnesses seen in the primary care setting accounting for up to 1.2 % of all emergency department visits and up to 6 % of office visits for children and adolescents [4, 5]. Most cases in children are observed during winter and early spring when respiratory viruses are more common. During the summer months enteroviruses are responsible for the majority of cases [6]. Tonsillitis caused by Group A β-hemolytic streptococcus (GABHS) most commonly occurs in children 5–15 years old, affecting less than 15 % of children younger than 3 years old, 24 % of children less than 5 years old, and 37 % of school-aged children [7]. The financial burden of GABHS tonsillitis is estimated to be between $224 and $539 million per year with more than half being associated to non-medical costs [8]. *Neisseria gonorrhoeae* is an important pathogen in sexually active individuals or in victims of sexual abuse [6]. Repeated episodes of all-cause tonsillitis is reported in 0.9 % of children less than 1 year old and 5.3 % of children between the ages of 1 and 4 years old [9].

Microbiology

Tonsillitis may be caused by a viral or bacterial infection of the tonsils, most commonly the palatine tonsils. Viral etiologies are the most common cause of tonsillitis in the pediatric population. Common viral pathogens include enteroviruses, particularly coxsackie virus, respiratory viruses (e.g. adenovirus, rhinovirus, influenza virus, coronavirus, parainfluenza virus and respiratory syncytial virus), and viruses of the herpesviridae family like Epstein-Barr Virus (EBV), cytomegalovirus (CMV) and herpes simplex virus (HSV) [7]. The most common bacterial pathogen implicated in acute tonsillitis is GABHS, accounting for up to 30 % of all episodes of acute pharyngotonsillitis in children. Less frequent bacterial causes include *Staphylococcus aureus*, *Streptococcus pneumoniae*, Group C streptococcus, *Mycoplasma pneumoniae*, *Chlamydophila pneumoniae*, *Corynebacterium diphtheriae*, *Arcanobacterium haemolyticum*, *Neisseria gonorrhea*, *Francisella tularensis*, *Yersinia enterocolitica*, and mixed anaerobic flora from the oral cavity [7]. *Fusobacterium necrophorum*, a gram-negative aerobic bacilli, and the most common cause of Lemierre's syndrome, has been cultured from adolescents and young adults with uncomplicated tonsillitis [10].

Symptoms

Patients with tonsillitis present with a variety of symptoms that include sore throat, fever, chills, odynophagia, cervical adenopathy, trismus, halitosis, erythematous and exudative tonsils and tonsillar pillars (Fig. 10.2). The presence of conjunctivitis, coryza, cough, stomatitis, diarrhea and hoarseness strongly suggest a viral etiology. Children younger than 3 years of age may have an atypical presentation of GABHS infection called streptococcosis, which is characterized by fever, mucopurulent or serous rhinitis, and adenopathy, followed by irritability, loss of appetite and lethargy. Exudative tonsillitis is rare in this age group. On physical exam, it is often difficult to distinguish between viral and bacterial tonsillitis, but some clinical findings may provide important clues of the etiologic agent. For example, HSV typically presents with stomatitis, EBV may include lymphadenitis and coxsackie virus infections may present with throat ulcers (herpangina) or as part of hand-foot-mouth disease.

Complications

Complications of tonsillitis can be suppurative or non-suppurative in nature. Suppurative complications include peritonsillar abscess, parapharyngeal or retropharyngeal space abscess, and suppurative cervical lymphadenitis. Acute airway compromise, rheumatic fever, glomerulonephritis, and scarlet

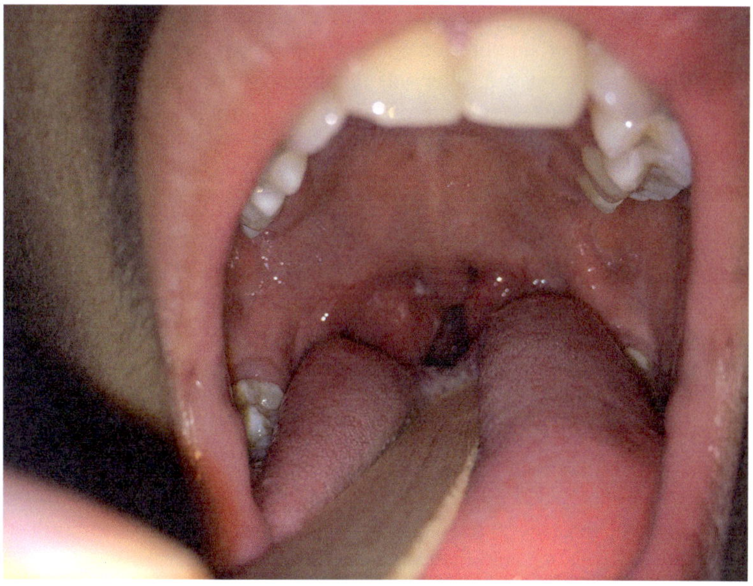

Fig. 10.2 Tonsillitis with suppuration (Photo courtesy of Dr. Daniel P. Fox)

fever are non-suppurative complications of tonsillitis caused by GABHS. Streptococcal toxic shock syndrome, an uncommon but rapidly progressive disease, can complicate cases of pharyngitis caused by a toxic-producing strain of GABHS [11].

Diagnosis

Tonsillitis is primarily a clinical diagnosis. Supportive tests include throat cultures, GABHS rapid antigen test, and anti-streptolysin-O (ASO), anti-deoxyribonuclease B (anti-Dnase B), anti-hyaluronidase and anti-streptokinase antibody titers [12]. Other tests may be helpful based on clinical suspicion, for example, EBV specific serology or Monospot (heterophile antibody) test, EBV polymerase chain reaction (PCR) or HSV PCR as needed. The monospot test is particularly insensitive in young children, with only 25–50 % of children under the age of 12 years infected with EBV having a positive Monospot test [13]. Specific EBV serology to detect antibodies against viral capsid antigens (VCA) that includes VCA-IgG and VCA-IgM in conjunction with antibodies against Epstein-Barr nuclear antigen or EBNA are the preferred diagnostic method in this age group. A real-time EBV PCR assay is helpful in patients with immunocompromising conditions and to confirm the diagnosis in patients with negative serology but strong clinical suspicion of infection [14].

The most important step in diagnosis is distinguishing between viral and GABHS tonsillitis as anti-bacterial agents are not effective in the treatment viral tonsillitis. Furthermore, with a few rare exceptions (e.g. *Arcanobacterium haemolyticum*, *Neisseria gonorrhoeae* and *Fusobacterium* spp.) anti-microbial treatment is not beneficial for bacterial causes of tonsillitis except GABHS given that there is not a significant reduction in the rate of complications or in duration of clinical symptoms [7]. Seventy percent of patients presenting with sore throat are treated with antibiotics while only 20–30 % have documented GABHS tonsillitis. Antibiotic treatment may be associated with adverse drug events that range from mild diarrhea to severe allergic reactions. Thus, the utility of these drugs must be determined in order to avoid potential selection of resistant organisms, exposure to adverse events associated with anti-microbial use, and extra cost. Treatment of GABHS is instrumental in preventing the potentially long-term and life-threatening complications associated with this pathogen, specifically and most importantly, ARF. Treatment also aids in the control of acute signs and symptoms, prevention of suppurative complications, and decreased transmission of GABHS to close contacts [7]. Throat pain and fever self-resolve by 1 week and 3–5 days, respectively, after onset if left untreated; if treated, both symptoms resolve within 3 days [15]. The organisms are eradicated from the pharynx after 10 days of treatment. ARF can be prevented even if therapy is initiated after 9 days of onset [11]. Of note, treatment does not prevent the development of PSGN [7].

The Infectious Disease Society of America (IDSA) recommends testing for GABHS unless a patient presents with symptoms strongly suggestive of a viral etiology; examples of such symptoms include cough, coryza, rhinorrhea, stomatitis or hoarseness. Testing for GABHS is also not indicated in children less than 3 years old. Children in this age group do not present with classic symptoms of GABHS tonsillitis and the incidence of ARF is rare, affecting approximately 0.2 % of children [7, 9]. Testing for GABHS in these children should only be pursued in the presence of other risk factors such as school-aged sibling with documented infection by GABHS, close household contact with diagnosis of symptomatic disease, or with personal or family history of a GABHS complication (ARF) [7].

One of the most commonly used in-office diagnostic tests for GABHS is the Rapid Antigen Detection Test (RADT). This test is done via throat swab of the surface of either tonsil or tonsillar fossa and posterior pharyngeal wall. Swabs of other areas of the oropharynx or oral cavity may lead to false negatives. An enzyme immunoassay test with turn-around times as little as 5 min is then done. It is 95 % specific and 70–90 % sensitive based on the type or manufacturer of RADT used. In the case of a positive RADT, children should be treated with antibiotics. In the case of a negative RADT, the IDSA recommends a throat culture be done during the same office visit. Due to the variability in sensitivity of RDTA based on manufacturer, the high rate of GABHS in children and implications of complications, a throat culture is recommended in order to capture any false negatives. The rapid turnaround time for RADT makes it useful for rapid identification and treatment of GABHS. Rapid treatment decreases the risk of spread of GABHS among close contacts, the amount of time missed from school or work for caregivers, and the duration and severity of acute signs and symptoms of GABHS tonsillitis [7].

Throat cultures are recommended in children in the case of negative RADT prior to the administration of antibiotics in order to avoid false negative results. A single throat swab has a 90–95 % sensitivity rate when done correctly. A throat swab similar to the RADT test is done and is then either processed in an in-office laboratory or sent to a microbiology laboratory. If the cultures are grown in-office, specific instructions must be followed. The swab is processed on a sheep's blood agar plate and incubated at 35–37 °C for 18–24 h. While treatment decisions can be made based on growth patterns at 24 h, a plate with no growth should be re-examined at 48 h to ensure a correct diagnosis. Two major disadvantages of using throat cultures for diagnostic purposes are the training and cost associated with accurate testing as well as delayed diagnosis due to processing time. However, even a delayed diagnosis can be beneficial. Studies show that treatment of GABHS tonsillitis can be delayed up to 9 days from the onset of symptoms and still effectively prevent complications such as ARF [7, 16, 17]. Therefore, regardless of the delay in treatment, throat cultures should be done in children with negative RADT [7].

Other testing options include anti-streptococcal antibody titers; however, these titers are not helpful in the diagnosis of acute GABHS tonsillitis. Rather, they are indicative of previous infection. Antibody titers become positive 3–8 weeks after an acute infection and may persist for up to a year after the resolution of the infection. Thus, they may be useful in determining the etiology of complications [7, 17, 18].

Children with recurrent tonsillitis are sometimes chronic carriers of GABHS with superimposed viral infections. Up to 20 % of asymptomatic school aged children can be carriers of GABHS in the winter and spring months [7, 19]. The IDSA does not recommend identification or treatment of these chronic carriers for several reasons. Distinguishing chronic carriers from recurrent acutely infected children is not possible with the current diagnostic modalities, chronic carriers of GABHS are unlikely to spread bacteria to close contacts and they are at minimal to no risk of developing complications of GABHS [7]. Moreover, eradication of GABHS from colonized tonsils and adenoids is much more difficult than treatment of acute GABHS tonsillitis. However, certain specific circumstances do call for treatment of chronic carriers of GABHS [7]. These indications, along with treatment options, are discussed below in the section entitled "Treatment of Tonsillitis."

Routine post-treatment RADT or throat cultures to confirm eradication of GABHS are not recommended. Post-treatment testing can be pursued in the case of a patient at high risk for developing ARF (personal or family history of ARF) or recurrent classic symptoms of GABHS tonsillitis shortly after the completion of treatment. Testing or treatment of asymptomatic household contacts is not recommended as it has not been shown to decrease the incidence of subsequent GABHS tonsillitis [7].

Treatment

Treatment of viral tonsillitis primarily consists of supportive measures including bed rest, hydration, analgesics, and oral hygiene. Most cases of viral tonsillitis self-resolve in 3–4 days. Recommended analgesics include acetaminophen and non-steroidal anti-inflammatory drugs (NSAIDs). Aspirin should be avoided due to the risk of Reye's syndrome, a rare severe illness characterized by rapidly progressive encephalopathy with liver dysfunction and a mortality rate of up to 40 % in children and adolescents suffering from a viral infection, especially varicella-zoster or influenza, in association with the use of salicylates [20]. Other NSAIDs such as ibuprofen or diclofenac can be used. NSAIDs and acetaminophen not only provide pain control but also act to reduce fever. Corticosteroids have proven beneficial in the reduction of the duration and severity of other signs and symptoms, but they do not affect pain levels. Thus, they are not recommended for symptomatic control in acute tonsillitis [7, 21].

Acute bacterial tonsillitis is treated with anti-microbial therapy in addition to the supportive measures listed above. Penicillins target the most commonly implicated pathogen, GABHS. They are narrow spectrum drugs with the greatest safety profile and provide the highest efficacy at a lower cost than other alternatives. Furthermore, there have been no documented cases of penicillin resistant GABHS. A ten-day course of oral penicillin or amoxicillin or a one-time dose of intramuscular benzathine penicillin G is the treatment of choice. An amoxicillin suspension is preferred for younger children due to once a day dosing and better taste that facilitates improved compliance. While a clinical response should be achieved within 24–48 h of beginning antibiotic therapy, a 10 day course of antibiotics has been shown to achieve the maximum rates of pharyngeal eradication of bacteria [7].

Patients with previous non-anaphylactic allergic reactions to penicillin can be treated with first generation cephalosporins for 10 days. Narrow spectrum first generation cephalosporins such as cefadroxil and cephalexin are preferred over broad spectrum cephalosporins such as cefaclor, cefuroxime, cefixime, cefdinir, and cefpodoxime. Approximately 10 % of patients allergic to penicillins will also be allergic to cephalosporins. These patients can be treated with a 10 day course of clindamycin, clarithromycin or a 5 day course of azithromycin. Erythromycin should be reserved for treatment resistant infections due to its high rate of gastrointestinal side effects. Rate of GABHS antibiotic resistance in the United States are approximately 1 % to clindamycin and 5–8 % to macrolides [7, 22].

Ampicillin and oral penicillin-based antibiotics can cause a generalized papular rash in the setting of infectious mononucleosis. Thus, if infectious mononucleosis is suspected, treatment with antibiotics is not recommended.

The IDSA discourages the use of several antibiotics for the treatment of GABHS tonsillitis. Given the high prevalence of resistant strains of GABHS, tetracyclines are not recommended and trimethoprim-sulfamethoxazole does not effectively eradicate GABHS in acute tonsillitis. Newer fluoroquinolones such as levofloxacin and moxifloxacin have proven active against GABHS in vitro but no in vivo efficacy has been documented. Fluoroquinolones are also expensive, broad-spectrum antibiotics with emerging resistance to *Streptococcus pneumoniae* worldwide and are not recommended in children 18 years of age or younger due to their potential for joint and cartilage toxicity [7, 23, 24].

Recurrent tonsillitis can be treated with penicillin, cephalosporins, macrolides, or clindamycin. If tonsillitis recurs shortly after the completion of a course of antibiotics, intramuscular penicillin should be considered. Alternatively, a 3–6 week course of a penicillin coupled with a beta lactamase inhibitor such as amoxicillin plus clavulanate has been shown to be effective in treatment of recurrent tonsillitis [7].

As discussed previously, routine treatment of chronic carriers of GABHS is not recommended. However, there are a few specific indications for treatment. According to the IDSA and the American Academy of Pediatrics, chronic carriers should be treated in the following circumstances: (1) during a local outbreak of ARF, PSGN, or invasive GABHS infection, (2) outbreaks of GABHS pharyngitis in a closed community, (3) personal or family history of ARF, (4) excessive family or caregiver anxiety about a GABHS infection, or (5) if tonsillectomy is being considered only on the basis of chronic carriage of GABHS. Patients meeting any of the above criteria should be treated with oral clindamycin, oral penicillin plus rifampin, oral amoxicillin plus clavulanate, or intramuscular penicillin plus oral rifampin [7, 11].

Tonsillectomy should be considered for patients suffering from chronic or recurrent tonsillitis whose frequency of infection does not decrease despite appropriate antibiotic treatment and with no other explanation for tonsillitis. Specific indications for tonsillectomy are further discussed in the section entitled "Tonsillectomy."

Peritonsillar Abscess

Peritonsillar abscess is one of the most common deep space head and neck infections in children. This collection of pus is thought to be formed most commonly as a result of spread of infection from the tonsils or the minor salivary glands of Weber, found on the superior tonsillar pole. The abscess forms deep to the tonsillar capsule between the tonsil, the superior constrictor muscle, and the palatopharyngeus muscle. The most common location is superior and medial to the tonsil; however it can occur lateral to the tonsil or even inferior [3].

Epidemiology

Peritonsillar abscess comprises 30 % of all soft tissue head and neck infections. In patients younger than 20 years old, the incidence of peritonsillar abscess is 0.82–0.94 cases per 10,000 patients. It is most commonly diagnosed in adolescents and young adults, but can occur in any age group with an average age at diagnosis of 13.6 years old [25].

Microbiology

Peritonsillar abscesses are generally polymicrobial, representing the normal flora of the oral cavity and tonsillar area. Aerobes such as GABHS, *Streptococcus viridans*, *Staphylococcus aureus* and *Haemophilus influenza*, and anaerobes such as *Bacteroides* spp., *Fusobacterium necrophorum* and *Peptostreptococcus* spp. that make up normal oral flora are frequently reported [26]. The most commonly isolated pathogen is GABHS.

Clinical Presentation

Findings at presentation commonly include fever, odynophagia, trismus, erythema, bulging of the soft palate with deviation of the uvula, unilateral otalgia, drooling, and "hot potato" voice (Fig. 10.3). Trismus is a key finding in patients with peritonsillar abscess and is likely related to peritonsillar inflammation of the pterygoid muscles. Inability to swallow or significant odynophagia usually results in dehydration in younger patients.

Diagnosis and Imaging

The diagnosis of peritonsillar abscess is typically a clinical one; however, computed tomography (CT) can be utilized in atypical presentation such as when trismus limits the utility of a physical exam, or in uncooperative young children (Fig. 10.4). While the use of intra-oral ultrasound for diagnosis of peritonsillar abscess has been suggested, it is not yet widely used [27]. An elevated white blood cell count and C-reactive protein are commonly found. Throat culture and testing for infectious mononucleosis may be helpful to evaluate for other disease processes.

Complications

Complications of a peritonsillar abscess include airway distress, parapharyngeal or retropharyngeal abscess, aspiration pneumonia, and erosion into the carotid sheath. Lemierre's syndrome, a severe disease characterized by thrombophlebitis of the internal jugular vein with metastatic septic emboli as a result of an acute oropharyngeal infection, is another potential complication [28].

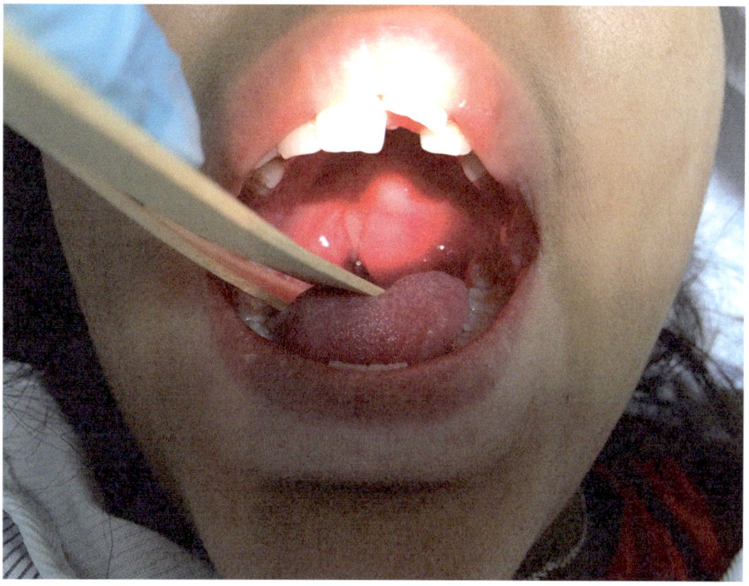

Fig. 10.3 Left peritonsillar abscess. Note the bulging soft palate (Photo courtesy of Dr. Amy L. Richter)

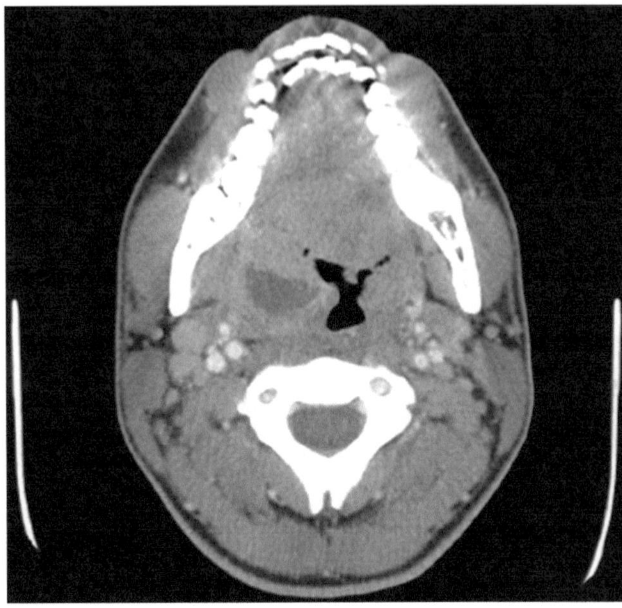

Fig. 10.4 CT scan of a right peritonsillar abscess

Management

Definitive treatment consists of incision and drainage or needle aspiration of abscess contents, antibiotics, and elective tonsillectomy after resolution of infection. In rare cases, Quinsy tonsillectomy at the time of infection can be considered. Indications for Quinsy tonsillectomy are discussed below in the section entitled "Quinsy tonsillectomy."

Drainage of the abscess leads to immediate improvement in pain and hastens recovery. Drainage can be done with local anesthesia in the cooperative awake patient or in the operating room. Children are more likely to undergo drainage in the operating room. When performing awake, transoral drainage, a pre-procedure dose of an opioid can be helpful with patient tolerance and the degree of trismus. Needle aspiration or incision and drainage appear to have equal efficacy [29]. Purulent material should be sent for aerobic and anaerobic culture.

Complications of drainage include bleeding, airway obstruction, and possible puncture of the carotid artery. Ten to twenty percent of children undergoing incision and drainage or needle aspiration of a recurrent peritonsillar abscess will require a subsequent tonsillectomy for persistent symptoms or residual abscess contents [3, 30, 31]. Peritonsillar abscesses recur 9–22 % of the time depending on the definition of recurrence which varies by practitioner and system [29, 32].

The use of tonsillectomy as a treatment for peritonsillar abscess remains controversial. It is favored by some practitioners in the setting of recurrent peritonsillar abscesses. A tonsillectomy at the time of infection (Quinsy tonsillectomy) can be considered in rare cases (see section entitled "Quinsy tonsillectomy"). An interval tonsillectomy 4–6 weeks after the resolution of infection may be performed in patients with recurrent tonsillitis.

Antimicrobials

Antimicrobials are used as adjunctive therapy for peritonsillar abscess. Combination therapy with penicillin and metronidazole is 98–99 % effective [32]. First generation cephalosporins can be used in patients with a non-anaphylactic penicillin allergy. Patients with previous anaphylactic reactions to penicillin can be treated with clindamycin, clarithromycin or azithromycin. Supportive therapy with hydration, pain control, and corticosteroids should also be administered [29, 30, 32, 33].

Tonsillectomy

Epidemiology

Tonsillectomy is one of the most common ambulatory surgeries performed in the pediatric population. Recent studies show that 530,000 tonsillectomies are performed per year in children less than 15 years old in the United States [3]. A bimodal distribution of tonsillectomies is observed with the two most frequent age groups being 5–8 years old and 17–21 years old [31]. A tonsillectomy entails the removal of the palatine tonsils with their capsule from the tonsillar fossa.

Indications

The indications for tonsillectomy include recurrent infection and sleep disordered breathing (SDB). The American Academy of Otolaryngology—Head and Neck Surgery (AAO-HNS) recommends that children that suffered from greater than seven infections in the last year or greater than five infections per year in the last 2 years or greater than three infections per year in the last 3 years and fulfilled one or more of the following criteria should undergo a tonsillectomy with or without an adenoidectomy: temperature greater than 38.3 °C, cervical adenopathy, tonsillar exudate, or positive test for GABHS. Children that do not meet these criteria but have multiple antibiotic allergies or intolerances or suffer from periodic fevers, aphthous stomatitis, pharyngitis and adenitis (PFAPA syndrome) or with a history of peritonsillar abscesses may also be considered candidates for tonsillectomy. A significant amount of missed school or work for patients and/or caregivers due to SDB or recurrent infections should also be considered when creating a treatment plan [3]. The AAO-HNS emphasizes that children that do not meet this criteria may not significantly benefit from undergoing a tonsillectomy. Guidelines suggest close observation and recording of frequency of episodes and symptoms instead of invasive intervention.

The use of tonsillectomy as treatment of PFAPA is still controversial. The AAO-HNS recommends consideration of tonsillectomy in these cases depending on the frequency of symptomatic illness, severity of infection and the patient's response to medical management, commonly steroid therapy [3]. Two randomized control trials showed statistically significant benefit of tonsillectomy to treat PFAPA [34, 35].

Tonsillectomy is recommended in the case of SDB if caused by hypertrophic tonsils and there is significant possibility of improvement of other co-morbidities caused by SDB. Examples of such co-morbidities include growth retardation, poor school performance, and behavioral problems. The decision to undergo surgery must be made in close communication with the child's caregiver(s) [3].

Complications

Complications of a tonsillectomy include throat pain, post-operative nausea and vomiting, dehydration due to delayed oral intake, post-obstructive pulmonary edema, velopharyngeal insufficiency and nasopharyngeal stenosis in the case of concurrent adenoidectomy, hemorrhage and death.

The most common morbidity of tonsillectomy is throat pain. Treatment includes over the counter analgesics and hydration. Commonly used analgesics include acetaminophen and acetaminophen plus hydrocodone. The use of non-steroidal anti-inflammatory drugs (NSAIDs) is generally not recommended due to a potential risk of post-operative bleeding. However, several studies show that NSAIDs do not significantly increase the number of post-tonsillectomy bleeds requiring surgical or non-surgical intervention and that they decrease the incidence of post-operative vomiting [36]. Other studies show that while aspirin is associated with increased risk of post-tonsillectomy bleeding, non-aspirin NSAIDs do not significantly increase this risk with one exception [37]. Intravenous ketorolac has been associated with post-tonsillectomy hemorrhage rates as high as 17 % [3, 38].

Studies show that post-tonsillectomy pain in children is undertreated by caregivers, primarily due to caregiver attempt at balancing pain control with overtreatment [39]. The AAO-HNS guidelines state that no specific medication or dosing interval (as needed versus scheduled) has been proven superior. It is most important that caregivers assess and re-assess a child's pain level even when the child does not spontaneously complain of pain [3].

Post-tonsillectomy hemorrhage is a much less common but the most concerning complication of tonsillectomy. It is the most common complication brought to the attention of medical personnel. Post-tonsillectomy hemorrhage is stratified based on time after surgery in order to help delineate the cause of bleeding. Primary hemorrhage is bleeding occurring within the first 24 h after tonsillectomy and occurs in 0.2–2.2 % of patients. The most common cause is surgical technique or reopening of blood vessels. Secondary hemorrhage is bleeding that occurs more than 24 h after surgery, most commonly on post-operative days 5–10. Secondary hemorrhage is most commonly due to sloughing of the eschar as the tonsillar bed heals and occurs in 0.1–3 % of patients [40]. The incidence of post-tonsillectomy hemorrhage has been noted to range significantly due to the definition of clinically significant bleeding and the consideration of primary or secondary hemorrhage only. The use of specific surgical techniques to reduce the incidence of post-tonsillectomy hemorrhage is still under investigation [40]. Bleeding following a tonsillectomy requires clinical evaluation and profuse bleeding may be treated with cauterization, inpatient observation, transfusion, or surgery.

The rate of mortality associated with tonsillectomy has been cited as less than 1 in 20,000 [41]. The most common causes of tonsillectomy-associated death include bleeding and opioid related respiratory depression [31].

Quinsy Tonsillectomy

A Quinsy tonsillectomy is done at the time of tonsillar infection. While tonsillectomy is generally recommended after the resolution of infection, it can be considered at the time of infection in a select few cases. Indications include peritonsillar abscess in younger children; recurrent or unresponsive cases of peritonsillar abscess or in the setting of previous history of deep neck abscess, and peritonsillar abscess presenting with severe airway compromise [42]. Due to the inflammation in an infected field, the risk of intraoperative, and potentially post-operative, bleeding is increased. Thus, candidates for Quinsy tonsillectomy must be carefully and selectively chosen.

Conclusion

Tonsillitis and peritonsillar abscess are frequently seen in the pediatric population. Antimicrobial management should be directed by RADT or positive throat cultures. In the case of peritonsillar abscess, acute drainage of the pus is the definitive treatment in addition to the use of adjunctive antimicrobial therapy. Quinsy tonsillectomy can lead to bleeding complications and is typically reserved for rare cases.

References

1. DelGaudio J, Chen A. Oral cavity and oropharynx. In: Wood W, Staley C, Skandalakis J, editors. Anatomic basis of tumor surgery. 2nd ed. Heidelberg: Springer; 2010.
2. Drake R, Vogl W, Mitchell A. Gray's anatomy for students. 2nd ed. Philadelphia, PA: Churchill Livingstone/ Elsevier; 2010.
3. Baugh RF, Archer SM, Mitchell RB, Rosenfeld RM, Amin R, Burns JJ, et al. Clinical practice guideline: tonsillectomy in children. Otolaryngol Head Neck Surg. 2011;144(1 Suppl):S1–30.
4. National Hospital Ambulatory Medical Care Survey: 2011 Emergency Department Summary Tables. 2011. http:// www.cdc.gov/nchs/ahcd.htm. Accessed 12 Oct 2014.
5. Nash DR, Harman J, Wald ER, Kelleher KJ. Antibiotic prescribing by primary care physicians for children with upper respiratory tract infections. Arch Pediatr Adolesc Med. 2002;156(11):1114–9.
6. Arnold J, Nizet V. Pharyngitis. In: Long S, Pickering L, Prober C, editors. Principles and practice of pediatric infectious diseases. Philadelphia, PA: Elsevier Saunders; 2012. p. 200.
7. Shulman ST, Bisno AL, Clegg HW, Gerber MA, Kaplan EL, Lee G, et al. Clinical practice guideline for the diagnosis and management of group A streptococcal pharyngitis: 2012 update by the Infectious Diseases Society of America. Clin Infect Dis. 2012;55(10):1279–82.
8. Pfoh E, Wessels MR, Goldmann D, Lee GM. Burden and economic cost of group A streptococcal pharyngitis. Pediatrics. 2008;121(2):229–34.
9. Hardy AM. Incidence and impact of selected infectious diseases in childhood. Vital Health Stat. 1991; 10(180):1–22.
10. Jensen A, Hagelskjaer Kristensen L, Prag J. Detection of Fusobacterium necrophorum subsp. funduliforme in tonsillitis in young adults by real-time PCR. Clin Microbiol Infect. 2007;13(7):695–701.
11. American Academy of Pediatrics. In: Pickering L, Baker C, Kimberlin D, Long S, editors. Red Book: 2012 Report of the Committee on Infectious Diseases. Elk Grove Village, IL: American Academy of Pediatrics; 2012. p. 668.
12. Breda L, Nozzi M, De Sanctis S, Chiarelli F. Laboratory tests in the diagnosis and follow-up of pediatric rheumatic diseases: an update. Semin Arthritis Rheum. 2010;40(1):53–72.
13. Luzuriaga K, Sullivan JL. Infectious mononucleosis. N Engl J Med. 2010;362(21):1993–2000.
14. Pitetti RD, Laus S, Wadowsky RM. Clinical evaluation of a quantitative real time polymerase chain reaction assay for diagnosis of primary Epstein-Barr virus infection in children. Pediatr Infect Dis J. 2003;22(8):736–9.
15. Spinks A, Glasziou PP, Del Mar CB. Antibiotics for sore throat. Cochrane Database Syst Rev. 2013;11, CD000023.
16. Catanzaro FJ, Stetson CA, Morris AJ, Chamovitz R, Rammelkamp Jr CH, Stolzer BL, et al. The role of the streptococcus in the pathogenesis of rheumatic fever. Am J Med. 1954;17(6):749–56.
17. Gerber MA, Baltimore RS, Eaton CB, Gewitz M, Rowley AH, Shulman ST, et al. Prevention of rheumatic fever and diagnosis and treatment of acute Streptococcal pharyngitis: a scientific statement from the American Heart Association Rheumatic Fever, Endocarditis, and Kawasaki Disease Committee of the Council on Cardiovascular Disease in the Young, the Interdisciplinary Council on Functional Genomics and Translational Biology, and the Interdisciplinary Council on Quality of Care and Outcomes Research: endorsed by the American Academy of Pediatrics. Circulation. 2009;119(11):1541–51.
18. Johnson DR, Kurlan R, Leckman J, Kaplan EL. The human immune response to streptococcal extracellular antigens: clinical, diagnostic, and potential pathogenetic implications. Clin Infect Dis. 2010;50(4):481–90.
19. Martin JM, Green M, Barbadora KA, Wald ER. Group A streptococci among school-aged children: clinical characteristics and the carrier state. Pediatrics. 2004;114(5):1212–9.
20. Auriel E, Regev K, Korczyn AD. Nonsteroidal anti-inflammatory drugs exposure and the central nervous system. Handb Clin Neurol. 2014;119:577–84.
21. Bulloch B, Kabani A, Tenenbein M. Oral dexamethasone for the treatment of pain in children with acute pharyngitis: a randomized, double-blind, placebo-controlled trial. Ann Emerg Med. 2003;41(5):601–8.
22. Tanz RR, Shulman ST, Shortridge VD, Kabat W, Kabat K, Cederlund E, et al. Community-based surveillance in the united states of macrolide-resistant pediatric pharyngeal group A streptococci during 3 respiratory disease seasons. Clin Infect Dis. 2004;39(12):1794–801.
23. Bradley JS, Jackson MA. The use of systemic and topical fluoroquinolones. Pediatrics. 2011;128(4):e1034–45.
24. Leibovitz E. The use of fluoroquinolones in children. Curr Opin Pediatr. 2006;18(1):64–70.
25. Novis SJ, Pritchett CV, Thorne MC, Sun GH. Pediatric deep space neck infections in U.S. children, 2000–2009. Int J Pediatr Otorhinolaryngol. 2014;78(5):832–6.
26. Brook I. Microbiology and management of peritonsillar, retropharyngeal, and parapharyngeal abscesses. J Oral Maxillofac Surg. 2004;62(12):1545–50.
27. Schraff S, McGinn JD, Derkay CS. Peritonsillar abscess in children: a 10-year review of diagnosis and management. Int J Pediatr Otorhinolaryngol. 2001;57(3):213–8.
28. Syed MI, Baring D, Addidle M, Murray C, Adams C. Lemierre syndrome: two cases and a review. Laryngoscope. 2007;117(9):1605–10.

29. Johnson RF, Stewart MG, Wright CC. An evidence-based review of the treatment of peritonsillar abscess. Otolaryngol Head Neck Surg. 2003;128(3):332–43.
30. Herzon FS, Martin AD. Medical and surgical treatment of peritonsillar, retropharyngeal, and parapharyngeal abscesses. Curr Infect Dis Rep. 2006;8(3):196–202.
31. Herzon FS, Harris P. Mosher Award thesis. Peritonsillar abscess: incidence, current management practices, and a proposal for treatment guidelines. Laryngoscope. 1995;105(8 Pt 3 Suppl 74):1–17.
32. Powell J, Wilson JA. An evidence-based review of peritonsillar abscess. Clin Otolaryngol. 2012;37(2):136–45.
33. Baldassari C, Shah RK. Pediatric peritonsillar abscess: an overview. Infect Disord Drug Targets. 2012;12(4): 277–80.
34. Garavello W, Romagnoli M, Gaini RM. Effectiveness of adenotonsillectomy in PFAPA syndrome: a randomized study. J Pediatr. 2009;155(2):250–3.
35. Renko M, Salo E, Putto-Laurila A, Saxen H, Mattila PS, Luotonen J, et al. A randomized, controlled trial of tonsillectomy in periodic fever, aphthous stomatitis, pharyngitis, and adenitis syndrome. J Pediatr. 2007;151(3):289–92.
36. Lewis SR, Nicholson A, Cardwell ME, Siviter G, Smith AF. Nonsteroidal anti-inflammatory drugs and perioperative bleeding in paediatric tonsillectomy. Cochrane Database Syst Rev. 2013;7, CD003591.
37. Krishna S, Hughes LF, Lin SY. Postoperative hemorrhage with nonsteroidal anti-inflammatory drug use after tonsillectomy: a meta-analysis. Arch Otolaryngol Head Neck Surg. 2003;129(10):1086–9.
38. Judkins JH, Dray TG, Hubbell RN. Intraoperative ketorolac and posttonsillectomy bleeding. Arch Otolaryngol Head Neck Surg. 1996;122(9):937–40.
39. Barraclough J, Anari S. Tonsillectomy for recurrent sore throats in children: indications, outcomes, and efficacy. Otolaryngol Head Neck Surg. 2014;150(5):722–9.
40. Windfuhr JP, Chen YS, Remmert S. Hemorrhage following tonsillectomy and adenoidectomy in 15,218 patients. Otolaryngol Head Neck Surg. 2005;132(2):281–6.
41. Shay S, Shapiro NL, Bhattacharyya N. Revisit rates and diagnoses following pediatric tonsillectomy in a large multistate population. Laryngoscope. 2015;125(2):457–61.
42. Page C, Chassery G, Boute P, Obongo R, Strunski V. Immediate tonsillectomy: indications for use as first-line surgical management of peritonsillar abscess (quinsy) and parapharyngeal abscess. J Laryngol Otol. 2010;124(10):1085–90.

Chapter 11
Laryngeal Infections

Amy L. Hughes, Nicholas Karter, and Douglas S. Swanson

Introduction

Laryngeal infections are caused primarily by viruses and bacteria and have important implications on the ability to swallow, phonate, and breathe. A high suspicion and timely diagnosis is important in these patients as in the most serious of circumstances airway inflammation can progress to airway obstruction; with epiglottitis being the best example of this.

The following chapter will focus on the clinical evaluation of patients with a laryngeal infection as well as the differential diagnosis, specific diagnostic tools and treatment options for each infection.

General Approach to the Clinical Evaluation

The presentation of laryngeal inflammation and infection in the pediatric patient differs drastically from that of the adult. The adult larynx has more space to accommodate inflammation while the pediatric airway is proportionally smaller and therefore more susceptible to edema and inflammation. This can lead to a rapidly progressive clinical course in children, highlighted by the presence of obstructive symptoms and impending airway compromise. The assessment of a patient with a suspected laryngeal infection should include a prompt evaluation for airway compromise focusing on stridor, increased work of breathing with retractions and accessory muscle use, and cyanosis.

A.L. Hughes, M.D.
Department of Otolaryngology and Communication Disorders,
Boston Children's Hospital, Boston, MA, USA

N. Karter, M.D.
Department of Otolaryngology, University of Connecticut,
263 Farmington Ave, Farmington, CT 06030, USA

D.S. Swanson, M.D. (✉)
Department of Pediatrics, Children's Mercy Hospital, Kansas City, MO, USA

University of Missouri, Kansas City, MO, USA
e-mail: dswanson@cmh.edu; alawrason@gmail.com

T.A. Valdez, J.G. Vallejo (eds.), *Infectious Diseases in Pediatric Otolaryngology*,
DOI 10.1007/978-3-319-21744-4_11

If the patient's airway is in stable condition, the provider should complete a history and physical exam. Information on the duration of symptoms, associated symptoms, history of exposure to ill contacts, recent travel, and any possibility of foreign body aspiration should be obtained. Commonly associated symptoms include difficulty feeding, cough, and voice changes. After a complete history, a physical exam is performed including vital signs with a focus on the patient's respiratory status. As previously mentioned, the provider needs to first determine if the patient has a stable airway. This is determined by watching the child's work of breathing as well as by listening to their breathing. Should the patient have stridor, it is important to determine if it is inspiratory, expiratory or biphasic stridor as they are each associated with different levels of obstruction.

In the stable patient, flexible laryngoscopy may provide important diagnostic information about laryngeal involvement; however the provider should take caution as laryngoscopy can exacerbate laryngeal swelling and cause acute airway obstruction, especially in a patient with epiglottitis. Additional diagnostic tools that may be helpful include neck and chest radiographs and blood work including a white blood cell count to evaluate for infection.

In general if a patient with a laryngeal infection is suspected of having severe airway obstruction, the airway should be secured in a controlled manner, with the operating room often the best option. If significant obstruction is suspected, but the patient is stable, they should be admitted for continuous monitoring with treatment targeted towards the suspected cause.

Laryngitis

Laryngitis is inflammation of the larynx and generally occurs in older children. It is most commonly caused by a viral infection or vocal strain.

Infectious Etiology

Respiratory viruses, especially adenovirus and influenza, are the most common etiology (Table 11.1). Secondary bacterial infections from *Streptococcus pyogenes* (group A streptococcus) or *Staphylococcus aureus* may also occur. Fungal infections are rare, but can occur in immunocompromised children.

Clinical Features

The most common symptom in patients with laryngitis is dysphonia with hoarseness and a change in voice at presentation. Other respiratory viral symptoms, such as rhinorrhea, low-grade fever, sore throat, and cough may also be present. Although adenovirus and influenza can be associated with high fevers, if purulent exudate or progressive pain are present, a secondary bacterial infection should be considered.

Diagnostic Evaluation

No specific laboratory testing is usually needed; some clinicians obtain a rapid influenza test or adenoviral polymerase chain reaction (PCR) for highly febrile patients. A rapid strep test and bacterial culture should be obtained if the child has purulent exudate with progressive pain.

Table 11.1 Etiologies of laryngeal infections

Laryngitis
Common
Viruses: adenovirus, influenza
Less common
Viruses: parainfluenza, coronavirus, rhinovirus, RSV, enteroviruses, HSV
Bacteria: *Streptococcus pyogenes*, *Staphylococcus aureus*
Uncommon
Viruses: mumps, measles[a], CMV, EBV
Bacteria: *Corynebacterium diphtheriae*[a]
Fungi: *Candida albicans*[b]
Croup
Common
Viruses: parainfluenza (especially type 1)
Less common
Viruses: RSV, adenovirus, coronavirus, influenza, human metapneumovirus
Uncommon
Viruses: measles[a], rhinovirus, enteroviruses, HSV
Bacteria: *Mycoplasma pneumoniae*, *S. aureus*, *S. pyogenes*, *Streptococcus pneumonia*, *Corynebacterium diphtheriae*[a]
Fungi: *Candida* species[b]
Epiglottitis
Common
Bacteria: *Haemophilus influenzae* type b
Less common
Bacteria: *H. influenzae* non-type b, *H. parainfluenzae*, *S. pyogenes*, *S. pneumoniae*
Uncommon
Bacteria: *Pseudomonas aeruginosa*[b], *Klebsiella* species
Fungi: *Candida* species[b]

[a]Important in endemic areas, but not the USA
[b]Immunocompromised patients
RSV respiratory syncytial virus, *HSV* herpes simplex virus, *CMV* cytomegalovirus, *EBV* Epstein-Barr virus

Management

Acute laryngitis is typically a self-limited illness that can be treated symptomatically with oral hydration, voice rest, and over-the-counter pain medication. Treatment with antibiotics or steroids is not usually necessary, but antibiotics are indicated in cases of secondary bacterial infection, and steroids if there is considerable concern over airway edema.

Croup (Acute Laryngotracheitis)

Croup is edema and inflammation of the subglottic airway. It is the most common cause of airway obstruction in children aged 6 months to 6 years [1].

Infectious Etiology

Parainfluenza virus accounts for two-thirds of the cases, with less common causes including respiratory syncytial virus, influenza, rhinovirus, adenovirus, enterovirus and rarely measles virus or HSV (Table 11.1) [2].

Epidemiology

Croup mainly affects patients aged 6 months to 3 years, with a peak incidence in the second year of life [3]. It occurs more commonly in males, with a male to female preponderance of 1.4/1 [3]. Patients most often develop croup in the fall or early winter.

Clinical Features

Viral croup has an incubation period of 2–6 days and typically starts with a prodrome of rhinorrhea, congestion, and low grade fever [3]. Following the prodrome, patients develop the characteristic symptoms of barky cough, hoarseness, and inspiratory stridor. The cough usually resolves after 3 days.

Diagnostic Evaluation

The diagnosis of croup is typically made based on the history and physical exam, however, an anterior-posterior (AP) and lateral radiograph of the neck may help confirm the diagnosis. The typical finding on AP imaging of the neck is the "steeple sign" which occurs secondary to the subglottic edema [4]. The radiographic findings are neither sensitive nor specific, making clinical history the most reliable diagnostic tool [5].

Management

Treatment of viral laryngotracheobronchitis varies depending on the severity of the infection. Patients with a mild episode of croup are typically treated with a single dose of intramuscular (IM) or oral corticosteroids, usually dexamethasone [0.6 mg/kg (maximum dose of 10 mg)], or inhaled budesonide (2 mg) prior to discharge home. However, should a child present with more significant symptoms, they may be admitted for observation and treated with fluids, intravenous corticosteroids, nebulized racemic epinephrine (2.25 %; 0.5 mL in 2.5 mL of saline), and oxygen supplementation if the O_2 saturation is <92 %. Nebulized racemic epinephrine can be repeated every 15–20 min if indicated, but the clinical effect only lasts 1–2 h, so children should be carefully observed for symptom return.

The benefits of corticosteroids in the treatment of viral laryngotracheitis has been established in multiple randomized placebo controlled trials demonstrating a variety of benefits including an improvement in croup scores, decreased rates of return to the emergency department (ED) or health care provider, decreased rates of hospitalization, decreased length of hospital stays, and decreased need for respiratory support [6–9]. The majority of patients will respond to treatment within the first 6–12 h [9].

In the most severe cases of croup, patients may require direct laryngoscopy, bronchoscopy and intubation, although this is typically avoided as the endotracheal tube can contribute to the development of subglottic stenosis. Children with a history of multiple episodes of croup or who are under 6 months of age at the time of their first episode should undergo elective laryngoscopy and bronchoscopy when they are healthy to evaluate for a concomitant subglottic disease process (Fig. 11.1).

Epiglottitis

Acute bacterial laryngeal infections represent a relatively rare group of conditions in the pediatric population; however it is imperative that physicians are familiar with and recognize bacterial laryngitis due to its significant potential for morbidity and mortality.

Infectious Etiology

In the post-vaccination era the bacteriology of epiglottitis has changed. Although *Haemophilus influenzae* type b continues to be the most commonly implicated organism, other organisms are now increasingly found. There have been reports of β-hemolytic streptococci, Staphylococcus *aureus*, pneumococcus, nontypable *Haemophilus influenzae*, *H. parainfluenzae*, and *Klebsiella* species (Table 11.1) [10].

Epidemiology

Epiglottitis has historically been one of the most devastating pediatric bacterial laryngeal infections. It most commonly affects children between 2 and 7 years of age [5]. Prior to the introduction of the polysaccharide vaccine to *Haemophilus influenzae* type b in 1985, epiglottitis was routinely

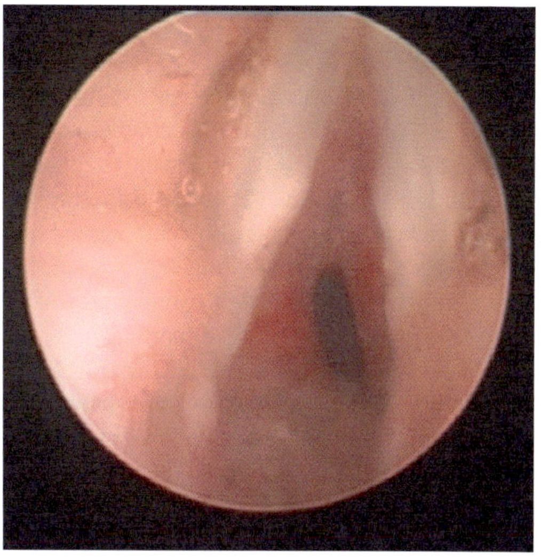

Fig. 11.1 Patient with a history of SGS and acute croup

encountered in the pediatric setting. Rates in the pre-vaccination era were reportedly between 4.9 and 6.1 cases per 100,000 children per year. These rates have dropped dramatically, and are now reported between 0.02 and 0.3 cases per 100,000 children per year [11]. Indeed, epiglottitis has become almost exclusively a condition of adults, and is often referred to as supraglottitis; however, diligence to identify epiglottitis in children remains necessary due to the potentially fatal outcomes. Contributing factors for continued *H. influenzae* type b infection are susceptibility of children under the age of 1 who have not completed their vaccination schedule, the increasing frequency of vaccination deferment, and the imperfect rate of immunity conferred by the vaccine.

Clinical Features

The classic teaching is that a child will present toxic appearing, assuming the tripod position (sitting upright, with the chin tilted upwards, and bracing themselves with an outstretched arm). There is typically a history of fever, severe odynophagia, drooling, and muffled speech. Inspiratory stridor is present at times, and signals almost complete airway obstruction. These symptoms tend to develop rapidly over the course of hours.

Diagnostic Evaluation

The diagnosis of epiglottitis is accomplished through history and a non-invasive clinical examination. The patients, having a combination of airway swelling and significant pooling of secretions, can be easily be pushed into airway collapse or laryngospasm. Anxiety provoking maneuvers should be avoided, including intraoral examination to reduce patient anxiety.

In a patient with no symptoms of airway compromise, radiographic imaging may be considered with the patient accompanied to the radiology department by an anesthesiologist or otolaryngologist. The imaging study of choice is a lateral soft tissue film of the neck. Classically patients will exhibit thickening and rounding of the epiglottis on lateral neck film, often referred to as the "thumb print" sign.

Management

The definitive treatment in patients with epiglottis is establishment of an airway, preferably in the operating room under controlled conditions. Reports from the pediatric literature indicate that institution of an artificial airway significantly reduces the number of deaths [12]. In the operating room open lines of communication between the anesthesia team and otolaryngologists is imperative. The patient should be kept spontaneously breathing and direct laryngoscopy and intubation should be performed either over a telescope or with a bronchoscope if possible (Fig. 11.2). After cannulation of the airway is accomplished, a thorough examination of the larynx takes place, cultures can be obtained, and blood may be drawn for any remaining tests. After the airway is established the patient remains intubated and is transferred to the ICU for intravenous antibiotics.

Multiple antibiotic regimens have been suggested. Traditionally chloramphenicol and ampicillin were used, but this has been replaced with third generation cephalosporins (i.e. ceftriaxone) or beta-lactamase resistant penicillins (i.e. ampicillin/sulbactam). The use of corticosteroids in reduction of airway edema is controversial. Their use has been advocated in the past; however no studies have reported any significant association with better outcome. Most data supporting their use is based on anecdotal reports [13]. Patients typically show significant improvement over the course of 2–3 days.

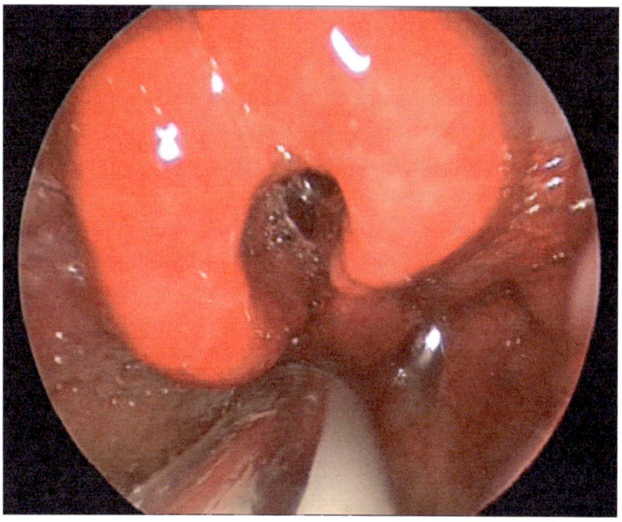

Fig. 11.2 Direct laryngoscopy findings in a 10-year-old presenting with epiglottitis

The patient is eligible for extubation when the ventilator is weaned to minimal settings and there is a free leak around an intact endotracheal tube cuff. The optimal location for extubation is the operating room, where direct laryngoscopy can be repeated prior to extubation to ensure that the inflammation has resolved. Once extubated, the patient should be monitored for an additional 24–48 h.

Recurrent Respiratory Papillomatosis

Recurrent respiratory papillomatosis (RRP) is a chronic disease caused by human papillomavirus (HPV) types 6 and 11. It is characterized by the benign growth of squamous papillomas in the aerodigestive tract and is the most common benign laryngeal neoplasm in children.

Infectious Etiology

HPV was confirmed as the causative agent in RRP in the 1990s and has been identified in nearly every case [14]. HPV 6 and HPV 11 are the most common subtypes identified in airway RRP and the disease severity and course vary depending on the identified subtype. In general, patients infected with HPV 11 have a more significant course with a higher incidence of airway obstruction, making them more likely to require a tracheotomy than those patients infected with HPV 6 [15, 16].

Epidemiology

The majority of patients (75 %) with RRP are diagnosed before their fifth birthday [17]. The youngest recorded patient to develop RRP is 1 day old, with the oldest being 84 [18]. Patients diagnosed before 3 years of age are 3.6 times more likely to require more than 4 procedures a year and 2 times more likely to have 2 anatomic sites affected [19].

The incidence of RRP in the United States is estimated to be 4.3 per 100,000 children, with between 80 and 1500 new cases of childhood-onset RRP diagnosed per year [18–20].

Clinical Features

RRP is the second most common cause of hoarseness in children, with the majority of patients presenting with hoarseness, as the vocal fold is usually the first site of lesions. The second most common presenting symptom is inspiratory stridor. Less common symptoms include cough, dyspnea, dysphagia, and acute respiratory distress. Extralaryngeal RRP is present in about 30 % of children and the oral cavity is the most common site, followed by the trachea and bronchi, and esophagus [18, 21].

RRP has a somewhat unpredictable clinical course. The majority of patients will have 1 year of symptoms prior to diagnosis [18]. Disease progression also varies greatly between patients. In some patients, the disease spontaneously regresses, while others may require surgical interventions and adjuvant therapies every few weeks to months.

Diagnostic Evaluation

RRP is diagnosed on endoscopy when the characteristic papillomatous type lesions are identified within the larynx. Once suspected, direct laryngoscopy, bronchoscopy and surgical removal with biopsy should be performed to evaluate the extent of the disease and to provide pathologic confirmation (Fig. 11.3). Histopathology demonstrates stratified squamous epithelium covering multiple finger-like projections with a central fibrovascular core. The tissue should also be sent for viral typing.

Management

The primary goal of treatment for RRP is to prevent airway obstruction while minimizing laryngeal scarring and complications. Microlaryngoscopy is performed and the papillomas are debulked using either cold steel, microdebrider, or a laser, most commonly CO2. The intervals between surgical interventions can vary greatly between patients. Adjuvant treatment is recommended in patients with four or more trips to the operating room per year, rapid regrowth of papillomas with airway compromise, or distal disease spread [14]. It is estimated that up to 20 % of patients require adjuvant treatments with intralesional cidofovir being the most widely used [21].

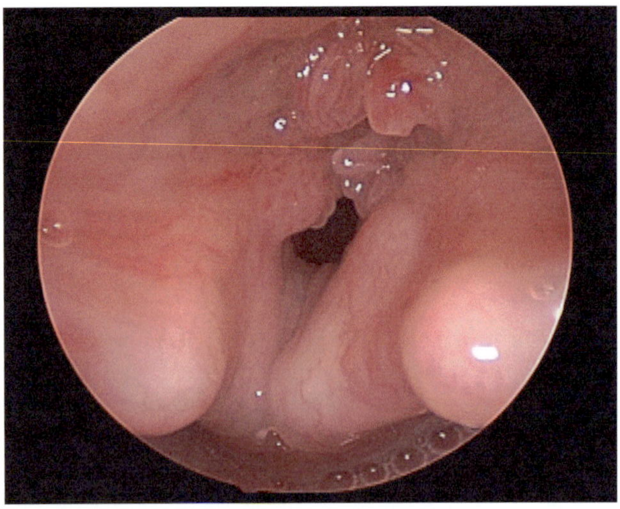

Fig. 11.3 Direct laryngoscopy on a 5-year-old patient with laryngeal recurrent respiratory papillomatosis affecting the true vocal folds

The most significant risk of surgical intervention in patients with RRP is airway stenosis. Patients with bilateral vocal cord disease extending toward the anterior or posterior commissure and patients requiring frequent surgical interventions are at the greatest risk. In some cases, complete removal should be avoided and debridement may be staged to avoid laryngeal web formation and scarring. Unless unavoidable, tracheotomy is not recommended due to the risk of disease spread into the lower airway.

Other Causes of Laryngeal Infection

There are several additional, however, less common causes of laryngeal infection that may present with airway symptoms. These include diphtheria, candidiasis, and tuberculosis.

Diphtheria

Diphtheria occurs globally and is endemic in many developing countries. It is caused by toxin-producing strains of *Corynebacterium diphtheriae*. Infected or colonized individuals transmit the organism to close contacts by respiratory droplets. Symptoms usually develop gradually, with mild fever, sore throat, and cervical lymphadenopathy. Initially, the pharynx is mildly erythematous. Up to three-fourths of patients progress to develop an adherent pseudomembrane that can involve any part of the respiratory tract.

The majority of diphtheria cases are exclusively tonsillopharyngeal. However, downward extension of infection can involve the larynx. Rarely, primary laryngeal diphtheria occurs without involvement of other anatomic sites, and presents as a nonspecific croup-like illness. A review of 1433 adult and pediatric cases from 1940 to 1950 in Los Angeles found that 276 cases (19 %) involved the larynx [22]. Twenty cases (1 %) were primary laryngeal diphtheria and all occurred in patients less than 20 years old. The mortality rate for non-laryngeal involvement was 4.7 % compared to 29.5 % for laryngeal involvement.

Diphtheria is diagnosed by culturing the nose, throat, and/or the pseudomembrane. Because special media is needed for bacterial growth, the microbiology laboratory should be notified that diphtheria is suspected. Samples should be promptly transported to the laboratory. Treatment consists of administration of antibiotics and antitoxin. Antitoxin should be administered based on clinical suspicion, and not delayed for culture results. It can be obtained from the Centers for Disease Control and Prevention (CDC) at 1-404-639-2889. Dose and frequency of antitoxin administration depends on the clinical presentation. The American Academy of Pediatrics has suggested 20,000–40,000 units for pharyngeal or laryngeal disease <48 h duration, 40,000–60,000 units for nasopharyngeal disease, and 80,000 to 120,000 units for diffuse neck swelling or extensive disease of ≥3 days duration [23]. Antibiotics stop toxin production, eradicates the infection, and reduces transmission. Recommended antibiotics include erythromycin (oral or intravenous) or penicillin G (intravenous or intramuscular) for 14 days. Repeat cultures should be obtained at 24 h intervals after completing antibiotics to confirm elimination of the organism from two consecutive negative cultures. Following treatment, patients should be immunized against diphtheria because disease does not assure immunity. The health department should be notified and close contacts identified, tested, and be considered for prophylactic antibiotics.

Candidiasis

Acute fungal infections of the larynx are uncommon among children. In the pediatric population, serious laryngeal candidiasis is seen almost exclusively in immune-compromised individuals, with only a few case reports in immune-competent children. [24]. Pediatric patients with serious laryngeal candidiasis most often present with odynophagia, dysphagia and hoarseness, however they may present as an airway emergency. A more mild clinical presentation of dysphonia has been reported among adolescents using steroid inhalers [25].

Diagnosis is made with flexible fiberoptic laryngoscopy and can be confirmed with biopsy and tissue culture. The typical appearance is erythematous and edematous mucosa with focal ulcerations and pseudomembrane-like white plaques. Exophytic lesions may also be seen, mimicking squamous cell carcinoma and respiratory papillomatosis. The lesions can involve the glottis, false cords, epiglottis, and surrounding tissue. Treatment is tailored to the individual patient depending on the underlying medical condition and extent of infection; intravenous amphotericin B, oral fluconazole, and topical nystatin have all been used. Oral antifungal agents, such as fluconazole, are the treatment of choice for laryngeal candidiasis associated with inhaled steroids [25].

Tuberculosis

Tuberculosis (TB) is a very rare laryngeal infection in the United States, and is caused by *Mycobacterium tuberculosis*. Patients typically present with severe pharyngitis with mucosal ulcerations and exudate. Patients with human immunodeficiency virus (HIV) infection are at increased risk for tuberculosis disease.

To diagnose laryngeal TB, patients must undergo a direct laryngoscopy and bronchoscopy with biopsies. The tissue is sent for culture and pathologic analysis and the diagnosis confirmed with the findings of acid-fast bacilli and caseating granulomas respectively. Due to the fastidiousness of mycobacteria, isolation by culture may take several weeks. PCR can be used to amplify the DNA and assist in diagnosis [5].

After establishment of a stable airway, laryngeal TB is treated with medical therapy with at least two antituberculous antibiotics for 6–12 months. The most commonly used antibiotics are isoniazid, rifampin, ethambutol, and pyrazinamide. In resistant cases, a 3–5 drug regimen and a longer course of therapy may be required.

References

1. Ewig JM. Croup. Pediatr Ann. 2002;31:125–30.
2. Denny F, Murphy T, Clyde W, Collier A, Henderson F. Croup: an 11-year study in a pediatric practice. Pediatrics. 1983;71:871–6.
3. Cressman WR, Myer III CM. Diagnosis and management of croup and epiglottitis. Pediatr Clin North Am. 1994;41:265–76.
4. Knutson D, Aring A. Viral croup. Am Fam Physician. 2004;69:535–42.
5. Sie KCY. Infectious and inflammatory disorders of the larynx and trachea in pediatric otolaryngology: principles and practice pathways. 2nd ed. New York: Thieme; 2012.
6. Ausejo M, Saenz A, Pham B, Kellner JD, Johnson DW, Moher D, et al. The effectiveness of glucocorticoids in treating croup: meta-analysis. Br Med J. 1999;319:595–600.
7. Osmond M. Croup. Clin Evid. 2002;7:297–306.
8. Rittichier KK, Ledwith CA. Outpatient treatment of moderate croup with dexamethasone: intramuscular versus oral dosing. Pediatrics. 2000;106:1344–8.

9. Russell K, Wiebe N, Saenz A, et al. Glucocorticoids for croup. Cochrane Database Syst Rev. 2004;1, CD001955.
10. Stroud RH, Friedman NR. An update on inflammatory disorders of the pediatric airway: epiglottitis, croup, and tracheitis. Am J Otolaryngol. 2008;22:268–75.
11. Mayo-Smith MF, Pinale JW, Donskey CJ, Yukawa M, Li RH, Schiffman FJ. Acute epiglottitis: an 18-year experience in Rhode Island. Chest. 1995;108:1640–7.
12. Cantrell RW, Bell RA, Morioka WT. Acute epiglottitis: intubation versus tracheostomy. Laryngoscope. 1978;88:994–1005.
13. Strom M, Jaffe B. Epiglottitis—individualized management with steroids. Laryngoscope. 1974;84:921–8.
14. Derkay CS, Wiatrak B. Recurrent respiratory papillomatosis: a review. Laryngoscope. 2008;118:1236–47.
15. Wiatrak BJ, Wiatrak DW, Broker TR, Lewis L. Recurrent respiratory papillomatosis: a longitudinal study comparing severity associated with human papilloma viral types 6 and 11 and other risk factors in a large pediatric population. Laryngoscope. 2004;114:1–23.
16. Rimell FL, Shoemaker DL, Pou AM, et al. Pediatric respiratory papillomatosis: prognostic role of viral typing and cofactors. Laryngoscope. 1997;107:915–8.
17. Cohn AM, Kos II JT, Taber LH, Adam E. Recurring laryngeal papilloma. Am J Otolaryngol. 1981;2:129–32.
18. Derkay C. Task force on recurrent respiratory papillomas. A preliminary report. Arch Otolaryngol Head Neck Surg. 1995;121:1386–91.
19. Armstrong LR, Prestor EJ, Reichert M, et al. Incidence and prevalence of recurrent respiratory papillomatosis among children in Atlanta and Seattle. Clin Infect Dis. 2000;31:107–9.
20. Armstrong LR, Derkay CS, Reeves WC. Initial results from the national registry for juvenile-onset recurrent respiratory papillomatosis. RRP Task Force. Arch Otolaryngol Head Neck Surg. 1999;125:743–8.
21. Schraff S, Derkay CS, Burke B, Lawson L. American Society of Pediatric Otolaryngology members' experience with recurrent respiratory papillomatosis and the use of adjuvant therapy. Arch Otolaryngol Head Neck Surg. 2004;130:1039–42.
22. Naiditich MJ, Bower AG. Diphtheria: a study of 1,433 cases observed during a ten-year period at the Los Angeles County Hospital. Am J Med. 1954;17:229–45.
23. American Academy of Pediatrics. Diphtheria. In: Pickering LK, Baker CJ, Kimberlin DW, Long SS, editors. Red book 2012: report of the Committee on Infectious Diseases. Elk Grove Village, IL: American Academy of Pediatrics; 2012. p. 307–11.
24. Wang JN, Liu CC, Huang TZ, Wu JM. Laryngeal candidiasis in children. Scand J Infect Dis. 1997;29(4):427–9.
25. Wong KK, Pace-Asciak P, Wu B, Morrison MD. Laryngeal candidiasis in the outpatient setting. J Otolaryngol Head Neck Surg. 2009;38(6):624–7.

Chapter 12
Tracheal Infections

Amal Isaiah, Kevin D. Pereira, and Armando G. Correa

Introduction

A plethora of epidemics, changes in immunization practices and endotracheal intubation have resulted in a better understanding of the pathogenesis of tracheal infections. Historic descriptions first appeared for croup; with the name derived from Anglo-Saxon root kropan referring to a child with a barking cough. This was first described in print as early as 1854 [1]. Much deliberation ensued concerning the treatment of this condition, with O'Dwyer being the first physician credited with treatment of acute croup either by insertion of a modified endotracheal tube [2] or a tracheostomy [3] in separate instances.

The first reported case of tracheitis was published in 1823 by Pierre Blaud [4]. An increase in incidence was observed during each influenza A virus pandemic—H1N1 during the great Spanish flu (1918), Asian flu caused by H2N2 (1957), Hong Kong flu resulting from H3N2 (1968), and more recently the pandemic H1N1 of 2009. Autopsies performed during the 2009 pandemic showed tracheal denudation, maceration, de-epithelialization and other pathologic changes consistent with tracheitis [5]. Bacterial tracheal infections still maintain a low level of presence in infants and children presenting with symptoms of airway obstruction, requiring ICU admission and potentially endotracheal intubation.

Different diagnostic terms have been used for conditions that affect the larynx and trachea. Although it is useful to distinguish between supraglottic and subglottic laryngitis, this distinction is often difficult

A. Isaiah, M.D., D.Phil. (Oxon.)
Department of Otorhinolaryngology—Head and Neck Surgery, University of Maryland School of Medicine, 16 S Eutaw St Ste 500, Baltimore, MD 21201, USA

K.D. Pereira, M.D., M.S. (✉)
Department of Otorhinolaryngology—Head and Neck Surgery, University of Maryland School of Medicine, 16 S Eutaw St Ste 500, Baltimore, MD 21201, USA

Department of Pediatric Otolaryngology, University of Maryland School of Medicine, 16 S Eutaw St Ste 500, Baltimore, MD 21201, USA

A.G. Correa, M.D.
Department of Pediatrics, Baylor College of Medicine, 6701 Fannin St; Suite 1540, Houston, TX 77030, USA

Texas Children's Hospital, Houston, TX, USA

T.A. Valdez, J.G. Vallejo (eds.), *Infectious Diseases in Pediatric Otolaryngology*, DOI 10.1007/978-3-319-21744-4_12

when the child is first seen. Laryngotracheitis or croup syndrome is a useful preliminary descriptive diagnosis until more definitive information is available [6]. "Croup syndrome" also has been used to emphasize the variety of possible causes and location of laryngotracheal disease. In this chapter, "croup" is used to refer to subglottic laryngitis or laryngotracheitis, presumably viral. "Epiglottitis" is an imprecise term often used in place of the better "supraglottitis" as the epiglottis may be minimally involved in some cases in which most of the swelling is in the aryepiglottic folds. Preferred terms for tracheal infections are (with the usual terms in parentheses): croup, supraglottitis (epiglottitis), and suppurative tracheitis, laryngotracheitis, laryngotracheobronchitis, or laryngotracheobronchopneumonitis (bacterial tracheitis), depending on the extent of the bacterial superinfection [6].

Epidemiology

Tracheal infections have a significantly lower incidence compared to infections of the upper respiratory tract, with 1–5 % of all children requiring outpatient evaluation for viral croup within the first 3 years of life. Croup also requires hospital admission in about 1.3–5.6 % of all children evaluated for the same in emergency settings [7, 8].

Viral croup has the highest incidence in the second year of life and is virtually non-existent in the first 3 months. The incidence is slightly higher in male children (odds ratio = 1.43), and is highest in late fall and early winter [7]. A time-series analysis performed from a large number of children admitted with a principal diagnosis of croup in Ontario suggested a strong component of seasonality, with a biennial mid-autumn peak and annual summer trough [9]. Of interest, the overall number of hospitalizations has continued to decrease in the last 20 years, given the improvement in diagnosis and treatment. Marx et al. [10] from the Centers for Disease Control (CDC) studied the overall burden of croup and showed that the mean annual number of croup hospitalizations is about 41,000 (range, 27,000–62,000/year) in the U.S. Ninety-one percent of hospitalizations occur among children <5 years of age. The authors also reported that minor peaks in croup hospitalizations occurred each year in February, and major peaks occurred in October of odd-numbered years, which coincides with peak parainfluenza type 1 activity.

Supraglottitis, in contrast, has no seasonal peak. This disease, almost always caused by *Haemophilus influenzae* type b and accompanied by bacteremia, has been virtually eradicated by widespread immunization during infancy. While the peak age frequency for croup is 1–3 years, supraglottitis occurs in older children, with a peak between 3 and 6 years. Suppurative tracheobronchitis also tends to be a disease of preschool and school-age children [6].

The reported incidence for bacterial tracheitis in the literature is about 0.1/100,000 [11]. This estimate was based on the combined experience of four pediatric intensive care units. The incidence of tracheal infections caused by other pathogens such as fungal or mycobacterial origin is exceedingly low. Over the last two decades, the availability of nebulized epinephrine as well as injectable corticosteroids have changed the landscape of serious, life-threatening tracheal infections, with the re-emergence of bacterial tracheitis. Currently, bacterial tracheitis has three times the risk of respiratory failure associated with it than epiglottitis and viral croup combined [4].

Etiology

Acute laryngotracheitis, considered to be the most common cause for croup, is almost exclusively caused by viral organisms. Both bacteria and viruses may be responsible for infections with collateral components, such as laryngotracheobronchitis, and the more general laryngotracheobronchopneumonitis. In 1958, the first evidence for association between croup and two newly isolated myxoviruses, parainfluenza virus types 1 and 2, resulted in separation of two categories of cases—mild, requiring only outpatient follow up, and severe, requiring hospitalization [12]. Parainfluenza is a RNA paramyxovirus that actively replicates in respiratory epithelial cells and is comprised of four major serotypes. Parainfluenza type 3, more commonly associated with bronchiolitis or bronchopneumonia, can also produce severe croup in an endemic pattern, while type 4 is rarely seen. Parainfluenza 1 and 2, account for >65 % of all causes of croup. A large series studied 6165 instances of lower respiratory tract infections (LRIs) wherein approximately 75 % of all isolates were identified as parainfluenza viruses. Of these, parainfluenza type 1 accounted for about 60 %. Conversely, the propensity of the various organisms to produce symptoms of croup reached 60 % for both parainfluenza 1 and 2. For parainfluenza type 3, the number dropped to about 30 %, whereas all the other microorganisms accounted for about 5–15 %. Thus, parainfluenza viruses were the most common cause for all age groups; whereas respiratory syncytial virus (RSV) caused croup in infants and the influenza viruses and *M. pneumoniae* were significant causes of croup only in children older than 5 years of age. Summertime croup may be due to enteroviruses, adenovirus, or parainfluenza type 3.

Among other important viral pathogens causing tracheal infections, RSV was studied in isolates from sentinel practices in England and Wales from 1975 to 1990, during which an increase in mortality, by as much as 60–80 %, was observed in comparison with parainfluenza and influenza viruses [13]. Prematurity is associated with an increased risk for mortality, with factors such as a decrease in gestational age, increased perinatal oxygen requirements and discharge within 3 months of the RSV season increasing the likelihood for hospitalization [14]. Among the rare viral causes, measles, by virtue of immunosuppression, leads to a bacterial superinfection that results in a condition termed measles-associated bacterial tracheitis (MABT), which carries an increased risk for need of artificial airway and intensive care admission [15].

Bacterial tracheitis is much less common when compared to that of viral origin. Previous reports have shown that the most consistent organism is *S. aureus*, followed by *S. pneumoniae* and *M. catarrhalis* [4]. Due to the universal immunization against *H. influenzae* type b, the incidence has dropped significantly. Similarly, immunization against *C. diphtheriae* has restricted the incidence of diphtheritic tracheitis to unimmunized children only. Reports of this are largely limited in modern literature, compared to the beginning of the century when tracheostomy was a routine practice to circumvent acute airway obstruction due to formation of pseudomembranes [16].

Fayon et al. [17] studied independent risk factors for development of bacterial tracheitis in a large series of children admitted to the PICU (n = 955), and found that the incidence of bacterial nosocomial tracheitis in that population was about 1.8 %. The pathogens isolated in this series were in agreement with other studies of bacterial tracheitis, comprising *Staphylococcus aureus* and gram-negative bacteria, and sometimes, mixed flora. In this population, tracheitis was attributed to young age, with small-sized airways in which thick secretions and mucosal inflammation being blamed for impairment of air flow and increased stasis. Head trauma, neuromuscular blockade and mechanical ventilation were independent variables that increased the risk of infection, but the last two risk factors may be physiologically collinear, given that most patients who were administered neuromuscular blockade were intubated, and vice versa.

Given the evolution of design features of modern day endotracheal tubes as well as enhanced monitoring of cuff pressures, reports of laryngotracheitis induced by indwelling endotracheal tubes have largely been limited to historic data [18]. Modern endotracheal tubes use materials that intrinsically inhibit or are coated with substances such as micronized silver to reduce bacterial growth by providing less scaffolding for colonization [19, 20].

Infectious agents such as *Mycobacterium tuberculosis* and fungi have been previously reported to have caused isolated instances of tracheal infection with a picture of long-term respiratory failure requiring a tracheostomy during the course of treatment that may be prolonged [21]. Chronic aspiration as well as gastroesophageal reflux (GERD) may accelerate laryngotracheal injury facilitating the development of tracheitis in those children.

Clinical Presentation

Despite the narrow spectrum of pathogens isolated from the plethora of tracheal infections described, these can have varied presentations, and typically differ in the outpatient vis-à-vis inpatient setting.

Acute viral croup manifests in the form of a viral prodrome characterized by clear rhinorrhea, low-grade fever, sore throat (in older children) and cough [22]. This usually lasts about 12–72 h, and typically progresses to hoarseness and the pathognomonic *croupy* cough that has a bark-like character. Rarely, febrile convulsions can occur. Nighttime symptoms are usually worse which frequently prompts the parents to seek care in the emergency room.

The typical course of progression goes through stridor that is inspiratory in nature but may also be associated with an expiratory component that results from unique features of the larynx in young children [23]. The infant larynx is narrowest in the subglottic segment, and inflammation of this area results in a fixed obstruction that leads to expiratory stridor. Children presenting multiple times with acute viral croup may have a masked presentation of subglottic stenosis wherein the already narrowed subglottic larynx is further reduced in diameter due to croup-related inflammation [24]. Hoarseness results from edema of the true vocal cords, often reducing their mobility. Wheezing is infrequently present. With increased severity, suprasternal and intercostal retractions may be present, and tachycardia and tachypnea are relatively common. It is important to note that reduction in the intensity of stridor in a sick-appearing child may be sign of impending respiratory failure as airflow may be reduced to the point where stridor may not be present.

When an infectious cause is not present in croup, the clinical course is abbreviated, with the noticeable absence of the viral prodrome. This condition is frequently referred as “spasmodic croup”, although episodic croup is a more appropriate term as it is typically triggered by an allergic etiology and often recurs [25]. Pediatric angioedema shares features with croup, but is often associated with facial or neck swelling that is acute in onset [26]. Rarely, an undetected foreign body may masquerade as acute croup. Although a viral prodrome may be absent, an unsuspecting physician may be drawn into an acute airway emergency due to commonality of symptoms [27].

The severity of viral croup may be assessed using one of the many scoring systems available. The most well-known of these, the Westley Croup Score [28], utilizes key clinical signs including chest retractions, stridor, cyanosis, level of consciousness and air entry to obtain a composite score that is predictive of the need for intubation. As croup is primarily a clinical diagnosis, the utility of the Westley Score, as with other stratification systems, such as the Alberta Clinical Practice Guideline Working Group [29], may be limited to use in a research scenario. For example, using the Westley Score, Johnson et al. [30] showed that $\geq 85\ \%$ of children present with symptoms of generally mild croup, and less than 1 % were diagnosed with severe croup.

Peltola et al. [31] studied the clinical courses of croup caused by parainfluenza and influenza viruses to highlight the differences in morbidity caused by the different viral strains in hospitalized children. In general, there were no significant differences in the patterns of clinical features due to infections with the three parainfluenza subtypes, except that parainfluenza 3 was associated with wheezing. However, children with croup due to microbiologically-confirmed influenza virus tended to be hospitalized for longer (4 days *vs.* 2 days for parainfluenza). In addition, the rates of readmission were higher for influenza due to the relapsing course of respiratory distress during the few days following discharge. The requirements for corticosteroids as well as supplemental oxygen also tended to be higher for those caused by influenza virus, emphasizing its enhanced virulence.

Notwithstanding the generally predictable course of viral croup, it is important to differentiate it from other acute disorders of the pediatric airway. Rapidity in progression to high fever, odynophagia, anxiety and relative aphonia should always alert the practitioner to supraglottitis (epiglottitis), which is a rare occurrence following introduction of universal immunization against *Hemophilus influenzae* type b. Posturing in the upright position and extension of the neck with drooling in an anxious-appearing child mandates the need to secure the airway in a controlled setting such as the operating room. Care should be taken to not agitate the child for that may precipitate respiratory collapse. If there is history to suggest incomplete immunization, laryngeal diphtheria should be considered. This condition tends to have a slower progression, and has historically been associated with the presence of exudative membranes in the oropharynx.

Bacterial tracheitis typically is a secondary infection following a primary viral respiratory infection due to a cascade of events resulting from tracheal mucosal injury, impaired phagocytic function and cytopathic effects of the viral infection. This condition usually is recognized after reasonable efforts to treat viral croup have failed. Children with bacterial tracheitis are acutely ill, with symptoms to suggest dehydration and organ failure in the presence of other host factors such as immunodeficiency. Often seen in an inpatient setting in children admitted to the ICU with respiratory failure, bacterial tracheitis can have a variable presentation in the absence of pathognomonic clinical signs [32].

The cardinal initial signs of bacterial tracheitis include cough, stridor and a rapidly changing course of illness that progresses to respiratory failure quickly. Children affected are usually older (>5 years). Other symptoms on admission may include choking episodes, dyspnea, dysphagia, neck pain, dysphonia and agitation. In one study by Bernstein et al. [33], children younger than 5 years of age were twice as likely to be intubated, compared to older children. The same study compared changing figures for mortality—prior to the 1940s, the mortality rate for bacterial tracheitis approached 40 %, but with advances in mechanical ventilation and airway management, that figure has dropped to 0–20 % in more recent series.

Diagnostic Tests

From the majority of studies, it is clear that the diagnosis of acute viral croup is chiefly based on clinical examination and does not necessitate laboratory testing. That said, if there is suspicion for a concurrent lower respiratory tract infection, white blood cell count with differential, as well as routine postero-anterior/lateral chest and neck radiographs may be indicated. In viral croup, the white count is often at the high end of normal, and may be higher in approximately 50 % of hospitalized children [34]. Administration of corticosteroids may cause leukocyte demargination, which can lead to spuriously elevated counts during the course of treatment.

Plain film radiography often is utilized to evaluate laryngotracheal edema in croup, but has inconsistent results. The typical picture is that of narrowing of laryngeal air column in the subglottic segment, approximately for ~5–10 mm below the level of the vocal cords, resulting from mucosal edema [35]. This has been historically referred to as the *steeple* sign (Fig. 12.1), but is observed only in ~50 % of instances [23]. This, coupled with reduced sensitivity for differentiating between viral croup, epiglottitis and bacterial tracheitis undermines the usefulness of routine radiographs for diagnosis. However, some investigators such as Mills et al. [36], have reported sensitivity and specificity of >90 % respectively. The best practice in these circumstances is to consider radiographs in those children in whom the clinical presentation is atypical and whose respiratory status is stable enough to undergo positioning prior to obtaining the films [23].

Alveolar gas exchange is usually not affected by viral croup, unless there is concurrent presence of laryngotracheobronchitis, asthma or pulmonary insufficiency [23]. Thus, pulse oximetry and respiratory rate have been shown to have poor correlation with clinical status or hypoxia due to artifacts [37]. Evidently, the uncompromised standard is clinical observation with pulse oximetry as a useful adjunct in instances wherein the lower airway is also affected.

In cases where operative control of the airway is required, telescopic tracheobronchoscopy, aided by the ventilating bronchoscope provides the gold standard for assessment of the airway in severe croup, or when alternate pathology, such as supraglottitis, is suspected. In the ambulatory setting, children who present with recurrent croup should be examined for concurrent abnormalities. Chun et al. [38] evaluated 30 children who were previously diagnosed with recurrent episodes of croup. A third of these children were found to have synchronous lesions such as subglottic stenosis, edema and

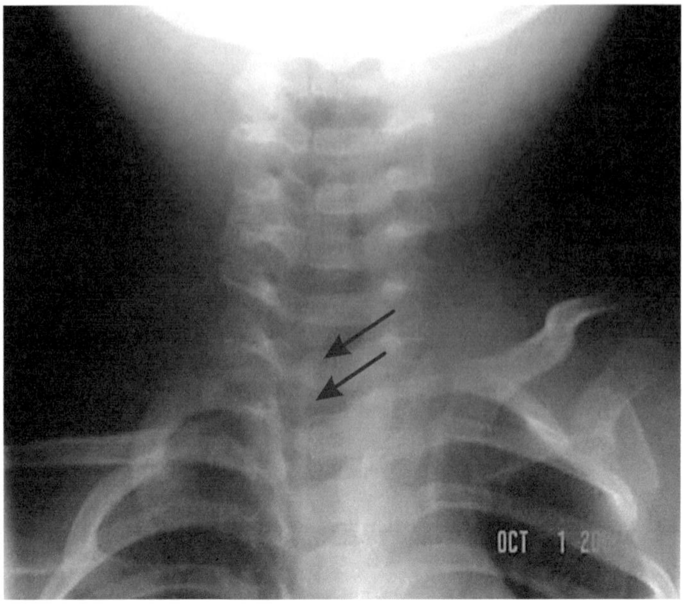

Fig. 12.1 Antero-posterior view of a plain film radiograph showing a long segment of subglottic and tracheal inflammation in a child with croup

cysts. In the same study, abnormal rigid endoscopic findings were more likely to be seen in children under the age of 3 years, highlighting the need for a higher index of suspicion and lower threshold for performing airway endoscopy in this age group.

Microbiologic investigations to determine etiology are increasingly being performed due to the availability of molecular and standard virologic methods. These tests are usually not recommended for diagnosis in mild cases of croup, but may be warranted in children hospitalized and/or requiring mechanical ventilation. Real-time polymerase chain reaction (RT-PCR) and viral cultures are also indicated with atypical courses of the infection, as described by reports of novel pathogenic strains for viral croup, e.g. coronavirus NL63 detected in samples isolated from Europe [39]. An improved panel based on an RT-PCR assay has been developed for influenza A and B viruses, RSV and parainfluenza 1, 2, 3 and 4. According to one study, the application of PCR increases the sensitivity of respiratory viral diagnosis, with results being made available within 6 h, thus increasing clinical relevance [40]. With claimed sensitivity of ~80 % and specificity approaching 100 %, several authors have increasingly validated their cost-effectiveness [41]. As mentioned earlier, the routine use of these tests in mild croup is unsubstantiated.

In children undergoing rigid endoscopy or endotracheal intubation for bacterial tracheitis and other serious airway infections, routine contact bacterial cultures and broncho-alveolar lavage with cultures may be obtained to facilitate culture-directed therapy. Jones et al. [42] first described laryngoscopically-directed cultures in bacterial tracheitis from copious mucopurulent material obtained from the subglottis, which grew *S. aureus* in most instances (Fig. 12.2). Plain film radiographs in these instances are consistent with progression of an inflammatory response (Fig. 12.3). These results have been replicated from a number of other centers [32, 43, 44].

Treatment

The treatment of tracheal infections has evolved over the course of the twentieth century, from initial descriptions of primitive endotracheal intubation to tracheostomy performed for acute airway distress secondary to laryngeal diphtheria [1–3]. The first recognized form of treatment was the use of mist

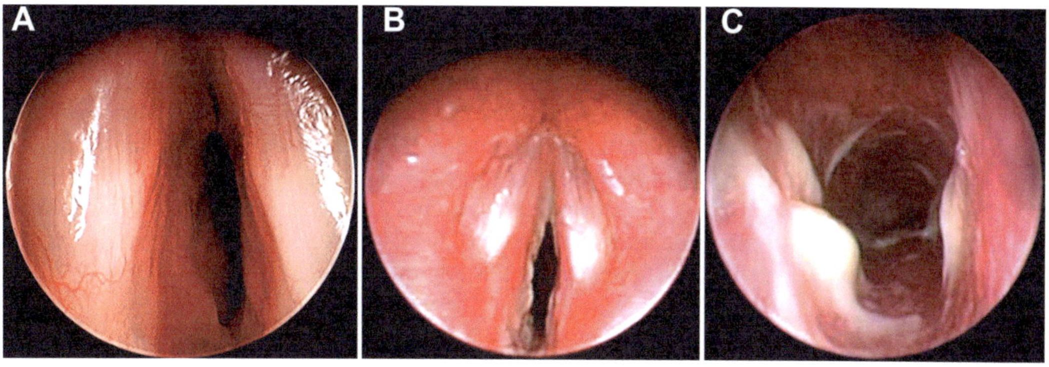

Fig. 12.2 Endoscopic photographs of (**a**) early bacterial tracheitis, with increase in exudates seen in the subglottis without overt purulence, (**b**) crusting and purulence seen that progressed to (**c**) erythema, pseudomembranes and overall inflamed-appearing tracheal mucosa

Fig. 12.3 Lateral plain firm radiograph showing marked haziness in the air column within the trachea, signifying ongoing inflammation. Arrows point to anatomical changes that can be due to ongoing tracheal inflammation

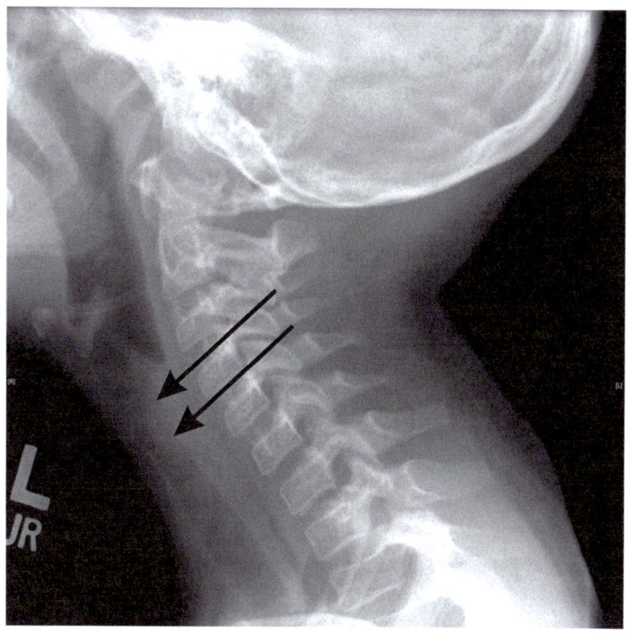

(humidified aerosol) produced by hot water, historically reported by keeping children close to a running tub with the door closed, leading to accumulation of mist. Discovery of therapeutic benefits from the use of corticosteroids and racemic epinephrine have revolutionized the manner in which croup is treated, and advanced in mechanical ventilation as well as development of rigid telescopes have improved treatment of tracheal infections of bacterial origin as well. These therapeutic strategies are summarized below.

Use of Humidified Air

Croup kettles were first introduced in the late nineteenth century to provide aerosolized mist to alleviate the symptoms of viral croup [45]. Later, cool mist was observed to have the same degree of therapeutic benefit as warm mist, and this avoids the risk of burns. There are at least three postulated mechanisms, which include (i) a soothing effect on inflamed mucosa, (ii) reduced viscosity of tracheal secretions and (iii) activation of laryngeal mechanoreceptors leading to reduction of turbulence [23]. However, humidity may also trigger bronchospasm, thus the duration of therapy should be carefully monitored. Recent studies have, however, shown that the benefits offered by mist treatment may be overemphasized. Three separate studies, that did not include untreated controls, determined that the efficacy of aerosolized mist may not be proportional to the degree of mist saturation, for e.g. the effects of humidity at three different levels (100 %, 40 % and 33 %) remained the same [46]. In yet another study, the effect of nebulized saline was identical to mist. Lastly, a recent Cochrane review of data concluded that the benefit of mist therapy remains unproven [47].

Use of Corticosteroids

Despite the various recommendations for dosages, routes and drugs for use of corticosteroids, a number of large-scale studies have exemplified their therapeutic efficacy. Their mechanism of action is related to the reduction of vascular permeability, resulting in a reduction of laryngeal and tracheal mucosal inflammation. Russell et al. [48] in a Cochrane Collaboration reviewed 38 studies and showed that corticosteroids resulted in a rapid improvement of Westley score, fewer return visits and/or readmissions, reduction of stay in the emergency room as well as the overall need for concurrent use of epinephrine. The benefits are not readily apparent in children with mild croup as the symptoms begin to resolve in about the same time taken for steroids to show treatment benefit.

Following adoption of corticosteroids as a standard first line of therapy in acute viral croup, overall hospitalization and the burden of the disease on healthcare systems worldwide began to fall. This was acknowledged following the guidelines formulated by the Canadian Pediatric Society that encouraged the use of intravenous dexamethasone as initial treatment of croup [9]. Among steroids, dexamethasone is used in a dose of 0.6 $mg \cdot Kg^{-1}$ body weight given either orally or by the intramuscular route. As dexamethasone is a potent steroid with a prolonged half-life, repeat doses are often unnecessary.

Other investigators have shown that orally administered dexamethasone is as efficacious as parenteral formulations. The choice of route should hence be determined based on cost and availability. Yet another study failed to show differences in therapeutic benefit between three different doses (0.15, 0.3 and 0.6 $mg \cdot Kg^{-1}$) of dexamethasone, so a single dose (0.6 $mg \cdot Kg^{-1}$; maximum of 8 mg) may be sufficient in the outpatient setting [49]. A double-blind, randomized control trial compared three different treatment strategies that included placebo, nebulized budesonide and oral dexamethasone [50]. In this study, the overall rates of hospitalization were much less in the group treated with dexamethasone (23 %), compared with budesonide (38 %) and far less compared with placebo (77 %). Other studies have also advocated for the use of aerosolized budesonide given the rapidity of its action and effectiveness comparable to that of nebulized epinephrine [51, 52].

Use of Epinephrine

The primary benefit offered by the use of aerosolized/nebulized epinephrine is the reduced need for intubation. Early studies showed immediate clinical benefit with use of 2.25 % racemic epinephrine, and the more recent studies demonstrated the same amount of benefit for L-epinephrine at a ratio of 1:1000 used with 5 mL saline [53]. Initial studies represented a major paradigm shift in management of children with severe croup, obviating the need for endotracheal intubation or tracheostomy [54]. The therapeutic effects of epinephrine are mediated via α-adrenergic receptors that results in constriction of capillary arterioles and reduced inflammation. Unfortunately, although the effects are almost immediate, they only last approximately 2 h, and hence the child should be watched for a reasonable period of time prior to discharge. This therapy may be suitable even in the outpatient setting if the observation period is adequate, although lack of improvement at about an hour following treatment may convert an outpatient encounter to hospitalization [55]. When conditions such as tetralogy of Fallot, tachycardia or ventricular outlet obstruction co-exist, epinephrine should be used cautiously [23]. With the peak effect occurring between 30 and 60 min, the child should be carefully monitored for the rebound effect—which usually occurs 3 h after treatment. The recommended dose is thus 2.25 % (0.25 mL in 3.75 mL of saline) for children <6 months of age and 0.5 mL for infants and children >6 months. Substituting isotonic with hypertonic saline (3 %) may enhance the effect by absorbing water from the submucosa.

Other Therapies

When respiratory failure is impending (cyanosis, severe retractions with lack of airflow, and persistent desaturations), endotracheal intubation is indicated until laryngeal edema resolves. This is usually transient and rarely evolves into a need for long-term mechanical ventilation, In children treated with steroids during the course of intubation, the time to extubation is shortened and the need for reintubation also is reduced [56]. Use of the physiologic leak test, by either vocalization around the cuff, or sustained difference in inspiratory and expiratory tidal volumes serves as a guide for extubation in these children.

Since its description in 1979, use of helium as a carrier for oxygen (heliox) has beneficial effects in reducing eddy currents that interact with each other and thereby reduce turbulent flow. Heliox is routinely used in children with post-extubation stridor to reduce the risk of re-intubation. As an appreciable number of children with severe croup progress to respiratory failure needing an artificial airway, using heliox can reduce the work of breathing by easing the delivery of oxygen to the lower airway past the site of obstruction. Assessments with Croup Scores and blood gas analyses reaffirm the beneficial role of heliox as a useful adjunct to potentially circumvent the need for endotracheal intubation [57]. A randomized trial showed benefit comparable to racemic epinephrine in moderate to severe croup [58].

As the etiology of croup is not bacterial, there is no role for routine use of antibiotics. In the past, inappropriately prescribed antibiotics have been reported to cause superinfections, prolongation of hospital stay as well as general increase in costs [29]. However, when the diagnosis of bacterial tracheitis is strongly suspected, the management changes wherein culture-directed antibiotic therapy is the gold standard of treatment. Empiric therapy with coverage that includes *S. aureus*, *S. pyogenes*, *S. pneumoniae and H. influenzae* is indicated. In an era when both hospital-acquired and community-acquired methicillin-resistant *S. aureus* (MRSA) are prevalent, the combination of vancomycin and a third generation cephalosporin (such as cefotaxime or ceftriaxone) is a reasonable choice until identification and susceptibility of the causative organism is established. In an intubated patient, tracheal aspirates should be obtained. A very useful adjunct to anti-microbial therapy is the use of frequent pulmonary toilet and debridement of tracheal pseudomembranes under bronchoscopic guidance [59]. In the presence of other co-morbidities such as immunosuppression, mortality increases. Reported complications of bacterial tracheitis include pneumomediastinum, sepsis and multi-organ failure, bronchospasm and impaired gas-exchange due to the burden of pseudomembranes with toxic shock syndrome [60]. Severe croup caused by influenza viruses as a part of epidemics may require treatment with neuraminidase inhibitors [61].

With the increasing number of options to treat croup, an algorithm is useful to stratify the burden of the disease and dictate an appropriate protocol. This is shown in Fig. 12.4.

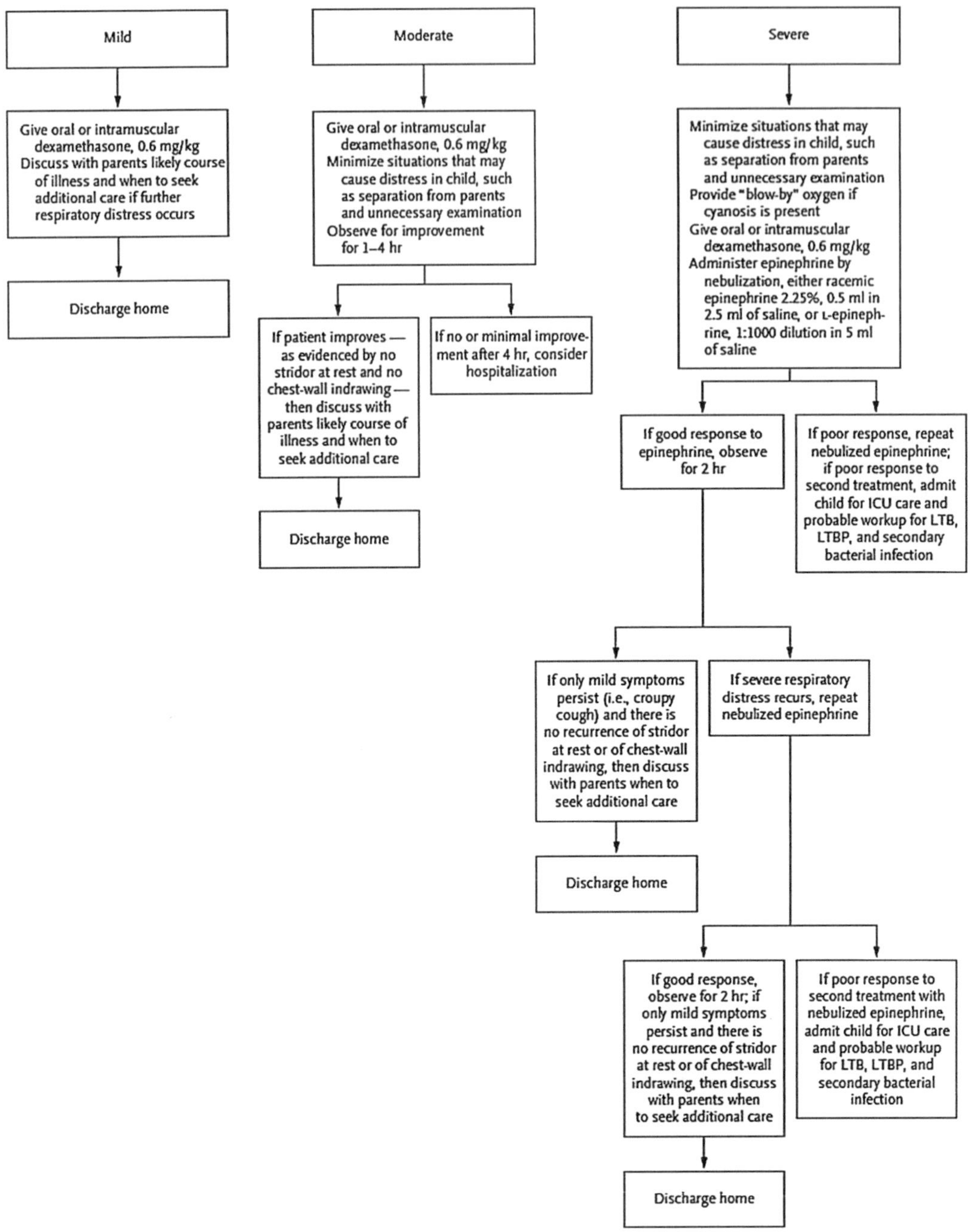

Fig. 12.4 Algorithm to treat croup in the outpatient setting. (From The New England Journal of Medicine. Cherry JD, Clinical practice. Croup. Vol. 358, pp. 384–91 [62]. © 2008 Massachusetts Medical Society. Reprinted with permission from the Massachusetts Medical Society.)

Conclusions

Despite the relative commonality of laryngotracheal infections, there are no clearly defined guidelines by national organizations for their treatment. The clinical picture can be often frightening to the parents who bring the child to the emergency room. Fortunately, the vast majority of children show signs of rapid improvement after initiation of treatment using steroids and racemic epinephrine. Only a very small proportion of children require hospitalization and an even smaller proportion require intubation and mechanical ventilation. Complications are rare exceedingly rare. In contrast, bacterial tracheitis may have varied presentations and often requires endotracheal intubation and debridement in the operating room. Mortality is higher but early institution of culture-directed therapy is known to reduce the severity of disease and the incidence of complications. It is important for the astute clinician to recognize the symptoms of croup and maintain a high index of suspicion for conditions that masquerade as croup, such as a foreign body, supraglottitis (epiglottitis), subglottic stenosis and other anatomic abnormalities.

References

1. Green H. Remarks on croup and its treatment. New York: Baker, Godwin & Company, printers; 1854.
2. O'Dwyer J. Fifty cases of croup in private practice treated by intubation of the larynx, with a description of the method and of the dangers incident thereto. Med Rec. 1887;32:557–61.
3. Talbot I. Tracheotomy in croup. N Engl Med Gazette. 1866;1:18.
4. Hopkins A, Lahiri T, Salerno R, Heath B. Changing epidemiology of life-threatening upper airway infections: the reemergence of bacterial tracheitis. Pediatrics. 2006;118(4):1418–21.
5. Gill JR, Sheng ZM, Ely SF, Guinee DG, Beasley MB, Suh J, et al. Pulmonary pathologic findings of fatal 2009 pandemic influenza A/H1N1 viral infections. Arch Pathol Lab Med. 2010;134(2):235–43.
6. Fisher RG, Boyce TG, Moffet HL. Moffet's pediatric infectious diseases: a problem-oriented approach. Philadelphia: Lippincott Williams & Wilkins; 2005.
7. Denny FW, Murphy TF, Clyde Jr WA, Collier AM, Henderson FW. Croup: an 11-year study in a pediatric practice. Pediatrics. 1983;71(6):871–6.
8. McConnochie KM, Hall CB, Barker WH. Lower respiratory tract illness in the first two years of life: epidemiologic patterns and costs in a suburban pediatric practice. Am J Public Health. 1988;78(1):34–9.
9. Segal AO, Crighton EJ, Moineddin R, Mamdani M, Upshur RE. Croup hospitalizations in Ontario: a 14-year time-series analysis. Pediatrics. 2005;116(1):51–5.
10. Marx A, Torok TJ, Holman RC, Clarke MJ, Anderson LJ. Pediatric hospitalizations for croup (laryngotracheobronchitis): biennial increases associated with human parainfluenza virus 1 epidemics. J Infect Dis. 1997;176(6):1423–7.
11. Tebruegge M, Pantazidou A, Thorburn K, Riordan A, Round J, De Munter C, et al. Bacterial tracheitis: a multi-centre perspective. Scand J Infect Dis. 2009;41(8):548–57.
12. Vargosko AJ, Chanock RM, Huebner RJ, Luckey AH, Kim HW, Cumming C, et al. Association of type 2 hemadsorption (parainfluenza 1) virus and Asian influenza a virus with infections croup. N Engl J Med. 1959; 261(1):1–9.
13. Nicholson KG. Impact of influenza and respiratory syncytial virus on mortality in England and Wales from January 1975 to December 1990. Epidemiol Infect. 1996;116(1):51–63.
14. Joffe S, Escobar GJ, Black SB, Armstrong MA, Lieu TA. Rehospitalization for respiratory syncytial virus among premature infants. Pediatrics. 1999;104(4 Pt 1):894–9.
15. Conley SF, Beste DJ, Hoffmann RG. Measles-associated bacterial tracheitis. Pediatr Infect Dis J. 1993;12(5):414–5.
16. Berner R, Leititis JU, Furste HO, Brandis M. Bacterial tracheitis caused by Corynebacterium diphtheriae. Eur J Pediatr. 1997;156(3):207–8.
17. Fayon MJ, Tucci M, Lacroix J, Farrell CA, Gauthier M, Lafleur L, et al. Nosocomial pneumonia and tracheitis in a pediatric intensive care unit: a prospective study. Am J Respir Crit Care Med. 1997;155(1):162–9.
18. Jordan WS, Graves CL, Elwyn RA. New therapy for postintubation laryngeal edema and tracheitis in children. JAMA. 1970;212(4):585–8.

19. Rello J, Kollef M, Diaz E, Sandiumenge A, del Castillo Y, Corbella X, et al. Reduced burden of bacterial airway colonization with a novel silver-coated endotracheal tube in a randomized multiple-center feasibility study. Crit Care Med. 2006;34(11):2766–72.
20. Bauer TT, Torres A, Ferrer R, Heyer CM, Schultze-Werninghaus G, Rasche K. Biofilm formation in endotracheal tubes. Association between pneumonia and the persistence of pathogens. Monaldi Arch Chest Dis. 2002; 57(1):84–7.
21. Graf J, Stein F. Tracheitis in pediatric patients. Semin Pediatr Infect Dis. 2006;17(1):11–3.
22. Knutson D, Aring A. Viral croup. Am Fam Physician. 2004;69(3):535–40.
23. Malhotra A, Krilov LR. Viral croup. Pediatr Rev. 2001;22(1):5–12.
24. Holinger P, Kutnick S, Schild J, Holinger L. Subglottic stenosis in infants and children. Ann Otol Rhinol Laryngol. 1975;85(5 Pt. 1):591–9.
25. Koren G, Frand M, Barzilay Z, MacLeod SM. Corticosteroid treatment of laryngotracheitis v spasmodic croup in children. Am J Dis Child. 1983;137(10):941–4.
26. Shah UK, Jacobs IN. Pediatric angioedema: ten years' experience. Arch Otolaryngol Head Neck Surg. 1999;125(7):791–5.
27. Gay Jr BB, Atkinson GO, Vanderzalm T, Harmon JD, Porubsky ES. Subglottic foreign bodies in pediatric patients. Am J Dis Child. 1986;140(2):165–8.
28. Westley CR, Cotton EK, Brooks JG. Nebulized racemic epinephrine by IPPB for the treatment of croup: a double-blind study. Am J Dis Child. 1978;132(5):484–7.
29. Wang EE, Einarson TR, Kellner JD, Conly JM. Antibiotic prescribing for Canadian preschool children: evidence of overprescribing for viral respiratory infections. Clin Infect Dis. 1999;29(1):155–60.
30. Johnson DW. Croup. BMJ Clin Evid. 2009;2009:0321.
31. Peltola V, Heikkinen T, Ruuskanen O. Clinical courses of croup caused by influenza and parainfluenza viruses. Pediatr Infect Dis J. 2002;21(1):76–8.
32. Miranda AD, Valdez TA, Pereira KD. Bacterial tracheitis: a varied entity. Pediatr Emerg Care. 2011;27(10):950–3.
33. Bernstein T, Brilli R, Jacobs B. Is bacterial tracheitis changing? A 14-month experience in a pediatric intensive care unit. Clin Infect Dis. 1998;27(3):458–62.
34. Postma DS, Jones RO, Pillsbury 3rd HC. Severe hospitalized croup: treatment trends and prognosis. Laryngoscope. 1984;94(9):1170–5.
35. Kaditis AG, Wald ER. Viral croup: current diagnosis and treatment. Pediatr Infect Dis J. 1998;17(9):827–34.
36. Mills JL, Spackman TJ, Borns P, Mandell GA, Schwartz MW. The usefulness of lateral neck roentgenograms in laryngotracheobronchitis. Am J Dis Child. 1979;133(11):1140–2.
37. Stoney PJ, Chakrabarti MK. Experience of pulse oximetry in children with croup. J Laryngol Otol. 1991;105(4):295–8.
38. Chun R, Preciado DA, Zalzal GH, Shah RK. Utility of bronchoscopy for recurrent croup. Ann Otol Rhinol Laryngol. 2009;118(7):495–9.
39. van der Hoek L, Sure K, Ihorst G, Stang A, Pyrc K, Jebbink MF, et al. Croup is associated with the novel coronavirus NL63. PLoS Med. 2005;2(8), e240.
40. Templeton KE, Scheltinga SA, Beersma MF, Kroes AC, Claas EC. Rapid and sensitive method using multiplex real-time PCR for diagnosis of infections by influenza a and influenza B viruses, respiratory syncytial virus, and parainfluenza viruses 1, 2, 3, and 4. J Clin Microbiol. 2004;42(4):1564–9.
41. Syrmis MW, Whiley DM, Thomas M, Mackay IM, Williamson J, Siebert DJ, et al. A sensitive, specific, and cost-effective multiplex reverse transcriptase-PCR assay for the detection of seven common respiratory viruses in respiratory samples. J Mol Diagn. 2004;6(2):125–31.
42. Jones R, Santos JI, Overall Jr JC. Bacterial tracheitis. JAMA. 1979;242(8):721–6.
43. Salamone FN, Bobbitt DB, Myer CM, Rutter MJ, Greinwald Jr JH. Bacterial tracheitis reexamined: is there a less severe manifestation? Otolaryngol Head Neck Surg. 2004;131(6):871–6.
44. Liston SL, Gehrz RC, Jarvis CW. Bacterial tracheitis. Arch Otolaryngol. 1981;107(9):561–4. Chicago, Ill: 1960.
45. Porter L. Management of the sick infant. South Med J. 1927;20(7):576.
46. Scolnik D, Coates AL, Stephens D, Da Silva Z, Lavine E, Schuh S. Controlled delivery of high vs low humidity vs mist therapy for croup in emergency departments: a randomized controlled trial. JAMA. 2006;295(11):1274–80.
47. Moore M, Little P. Humidified air inhalation for treating croup. Cochrane Database Syst Rev. 2006;3, CD002870.
48. Russell KF, Liang Y, O'Gorman K, Johnson DW, Klassen TP. Glucocorticoids for croup. Cochrane Database Syst Rev. 2011;1, CD001955.
49. Rittichier KK, Ledwith CA. Outpatient treatment of moderate croup with dexamethasone: intramuscular versus oral dosing. Pediatrics. 2000;106(6):1344–8.
50. Johnson DW, Jacobson S, Edney PC, Hadfield P, Mundy ME, Schuh S. A comparison of nebulized budesonide, intramuscular dexamethasone, and placebo for moderately severe croup. N Engl J Med. 1998;339(8):498–503.
51. Fitzgerald D, Mellis C, Johnson M, Allen H, Cooper P, Van Asperen P. Nebulized budesonide is as effective as nebulized adrenaline in moderately severe croup. Pediatrics. 1996;97(5):722–5.

52. Klassen TP, Feldman ME, Watters LK, Sutcliffe T, Rowe PC. Nebulized budesonide for children with mild-to-moderate croup. N Engl J Med. 1994;331(5):285–9.
53. Cherry JD. State of the evidence for standard-of-care treatments for croup: are we where we need to be? Pediatr Infect Dis J. 2005;24(11 Suppl):S198–202; discussion S1.
54. Adair JC, Ring WH, Jordan WS, Elwyn RA. Ten-year experience with IPPB in the treatment of acute laryngotracheobronchitis. Anesth Analg. 1971;50(4):649–55.
55. Prendergast M, Jones JS, Hartman D. Racemic epinephrine in the treatment of laryngotracheitis: can we identify children for outpatient therapy? Am J Emerg Med. 1994;12(6):613–6.
56. Tibballs J, Shann FA, Landau LI. Placebo-controlled trial of prednisolone in children intubated for croup. Lancet. 1992;340(8822):745–8.
57. Duncan PG. Efficacy of helium—oxygen mixtures in the management of severe viral and post-intubation croup. Can Anaesth Soc J. 1979;26(3):206–12.
58. Weber JE, Chudnofsky CR, Younger JG, Larkin GL, Boczar M, Wilkerson MD, et al. A randomized comparison of helium-oxygen mixture (Heliox) and racemic epinephrine for the treatment of moderate to severe croup. Pediatrics. 2001;107(6), E96.
59. Sofer S, Duncan P, Chernick V. Bacterial tracheitis—an old disease rediscovered. Clin Pediatr. 1983;22(6):407–11.
60. Kasian GF, Bingham WT, Steinberg J, Ninan A, Sankaran K, Oman-Ganes L, et al. Bacterial tracheitis in children. CMAJ. 1989;140(1):46–50.
61. Bridges CB, Harper SA, Fukuda K, Uyeki TM, Cox NJ, Singleton JA. Prevention and control of influenza. Recommendations of the Advisory Committee on Immunization Practices (ACIP). MMWR Recomm Rep. 2003;52(RR-8):1–34; quiz CE1–4.
62. Cherry JD. Clinical practice. Croup. N Engl J Med. 2008;358(4):384–91.

Part IV
Neck

Chapter 13
Infectious Lymphadenopathy

Andrea T. Cruz and Daniel C. Chelius

Introduction

Lymphadenopathy is defined as swelling of the lymph nodes, whereas lymphadenitis is defined as tender inflammation of lymph nodes. Lymphadenopathy is common in young children, as lymphatic tissue is most prominent in children 2–7 years of age. The differential diagnosis of lymphadenopathy is broad, but can be conceptualized by distribution (regional versus generalized) and by chronicity (acute versus chronic) (Table 13.1), in addition to by etiology. Obtaining a thorough travel, vaccination, and exposure history is critical for identification of imported infections or of vaccine-preventable diseases more common in other countries. A list of infections causing lymphadenopathy more common in returned travelers is provided in Table 13.2.

Localized Adenopathy

Knowledge of lymphatic drainage patterns can help the clinician determine possible causes of adenopathy. The most common causes of anterior cervical adenopathy will be viral respiratory infections, as these nodes drain the upper airway. Posterior cervical or occipital adenopathy can be seen with scalp infections, including kerions associated with tinea capitis, as these nodes drain the posterior neck and scalp. Preauricular nodes are more commonly associated with conjunctivitis (classically, adenovirus) or other superficial ocular infections. Parinaud's oculoglandular syndrome is the combination of unilateral conjunctivitis with an ipsilateral preauricular node. Parinaud's has been associated with tularemia [1], cat scratch disease [2], Epstein-Barr virus (EBV) [3], and *Yersinia enterocolitica* [4].

A.T. Cruz, M.D., M.P.H. (✉)
Department of Pediatrics, Baylor College of Medicine, 6621 Fannin Street, Suite A2210, Houston, TX 77030, USA
e-mail: acruz@bcm.edu

D.C. Chelius, M.D., F.A.A.P.
Department of Otolaryngology – Head and Neck Surgery, Baylor College of Medicine, Houston, TX, USA

Texas Children's Hospital, Houston, TX, USA
e-mail: dannychelius@gmail.com

T.A. Valdez, J.G. Vallejo (eds.), *Infectious Diseases in Pediatric Otolaryngology*,
DOI 10.1007/978-3-319-21744-4_13

Table 13.1 Most common causes of regional cervical infectious lymphadenopathy and lymphadenitis

Site	Region(s) drained by that node	Etiologies
Cervical	Head/neck	Viral upper respiratory tract infections
		Pyogenic infections of head/neck
		Actinomycosis
		Cat scratch[a]
		CMV, EBV
		Kawasaki disease
		Nocardia
		Non-tuberculous mycobacteria[a]
		Toxoplasmosis
		Tuberculosis[a]
		Tularemia
Occipital	Posterior neck and scalp	Rubella
		Seborrheic dermatitis
		Tinea capitis
Preauricular	Conjunctivae, eyelids	Viral conjunctivitis (including adenovirus)
		Parinaud's oculoglandular syndrome
		Cat scratch disease[a]
		Chlamydia trachomatis
		Tularemia
Submaxillary, submental	Oral cavity, lips	Dental caries or abscesses
		Herpangina
		Herpetic gingivostomatitis
Supraclavicular	Intrathoracic, abdomen, arms, thyroid	Tuberculosis[a]
		Nontuberculous mycobacteria[a]
Generalized lymphadenopathy		Large DNA viruses: CMV, EBV, HSV, VZV
		Brucella
		HIV infection (acute or chronic[a])
		Leishmaniasis
		Leptospirosis
		Lyme disease
		Measles
		Mumps
		Syphilis[a]
		Toxoplasmosis[a]
		Tuberculosis[a]
		Tularemia

[a]More chronic infections

CMV cytomegalovirus; *EBV* Epstein-Barr virus; *HIV* human immunodeficiency virus, *HSV* herpes simplex virus, *VZV* varicella zoster virus

Signs of inflammation also can help differentiate among the causes of localized infectious lymphadenopathy. Nontender adenopathy should lead the clinician away from most pyogenic causes, and should increase the index of suspicion for viral upper respiratory infections (URIs) or mycobacterial disease, depending upon the duration of illness. More indolent infections (actinomycosis, nocardiosis) may present without pyrexia. The epidemiology, clinical manifestations, diagnosis, and treatment of the most common causes of pediatric lymphadenopathy are summarized in Table 13.3.

Table 13.2 Infections causing lymphadenopathy more common in returned travelers

Class	Organisms	Region(s)	Epidemiology	Signs/symptoms
Bacteria	Brucellosis (*Brucella* species)	Worldwide, but more common in Central and South America, Russia, Middle East	Contact with tissues of infected farm animals or unpasteurized dairy products	Fever, chills, weight loss, hepatosplenomegaly, generalized adenopathy
	Leptospirosis	Worldwide, but more common in tropical climates (and after flooding)	Contact with contaminated water or urine of rodents, opossums, raccoons, or farm animals	Generalized adenopathy, fever, myalgias, conjunctival suffusion, retro-orbital pain, jaundice
	Melioidosis (*Burkholderia pseudomallei*)	Northern South America, Indian sub-continent, southeast Asia, northern Australia	More common during the monsoonal wet season	Suppurative parotitis, generalized adenopathy, septic arthritis, pericarditis, necrotizing fasciitis, hepatosplenic abscesses, pneumonia
	Plague (*Yersinia pestis*)	The Americas (rural regions), Africa, Asia; in the United States, is endemic in western states	Bite from rodent fleas; pneumonic form can be transmitted person-to-person	Regional adenopathy (buboes) most common in inguinal region, but can be seen in cervical or axillary regions, fever, purpura
	Tularemia (*Francisella tularensis*)	Most U.S. cases occur in the summer.	Rabbits, rodents, beavers, ticks, handling of dead animals	Parinaud's, fever, ulceroglandular syndrome
Viruses	HIV	Highest rates in sub-Saharan Africa	Sexual, blood products, mother-to-child transmission, injecting drug use	See text and Table 13.3
	Measles (rubeola)	Most cases imported from Asia and Africa	Airborne transmission; incredibly infectious	Fever, conjunctivitis, blanchable erythematous rash starting on head and progressing to feet
	Mumps	Most cases imported from Asia, Eastern Europe	Droplet precautions until 5 days after onset of parotitis	Parotitis, aseptic meningitis, orchitis, arthritis
Parasitic or protozoal	Filariasis (*Wucheria bancrofti*, *Brugia* species)	Caribbean, Africa, Asia, Pacific Islands	Transmitted by bite of infected mosquitoes	Localized adenopathy associated with adult worms; lymphedema and hydroceles rare in children
	Leishmaniasis	Africa, Indian sub-continent	Transmitted by the phlebotomine sand fly	Cutaneous from with papule progressing to a destructive erosive lesion, most common on face; regional adenopathy. Visceral form (kala-azar) with fever, organomegaly, generalized adenopathy
	Malaria (*Plasmodium* species)	Worldwide, except North America, Western Europe, Scandinavia, Australia/New Zealand	Bite of infected mosquito, which often feed at night. Most common in children returning to parents' native countries who do not obtain antimalarial prophylaxis	Fever, chills, malaise, hepatosplenomegaly, generalized adenopathy; can see CNS, renal involvement or respiratory failure
Fungal	Blastomycosis (*B. dermatitidis*)	Africa, India, Central/South America (as well as southern and central United States)	Inhalation of organisms from soil; no person-to-person transmission	Cutaneous lesions can be polymorphic: ulcers, pustules, verrucous, nodular; disseminated disease also can occur

CNS central nervous system, *HIV* human immunodeficiency virus, *U.S.* United States

Table 13.3 Epidemiology, clinical manifestations, diagnosis, and treatment of common causes of lymphadenopathy in children

Class	Organism(s)	Epidemiology/infection control	Symptoms	Diagnosis	Treatment
Bacteria	Acute pyogenic (*Staphylococcus aureus*, *Streptococcus pyogenes*)	Can be part of endogenous flora	Pharyngitis, abscess, cellulitis (need to evaluate for deep neck infection)	Culture Rapid assays	*S. pyogenes*: penicillin or amoxicillin
				for *S. pyogenes*	*S. aureus*: TMP-SMX, clindamycin, or cephalexin depending on MRSA rates in the area
	Actinomycosis (*A. israelii*)	Endogenous human flora causing disease after breakdown in mucocutaneous barriers (including after human bites) or in HIV-infected or CGD patients	Cervicofacial most common: hard nodular lesions on mandible, draining sinus tracts, submandibular adenopathy	Anaerobic culture of normally sterile sites	Penicillin or ampicillin IV× 4–6 weeks followed by months of oral suppressive therapy
				Yellow 'sulfur' granules visualized on microscopy	
	Brucellosis (*B. melitensis* and other species)	Zoonotic infection; associated with handling aborted non-human animal fetuses, consumption of unpasteurized milk or undercooked food	Fever, night sweats, malaise, generalized adenopathy, hepatosplenomegaly, arthritis	Culture (need to be held for weeks)	Combination therapy to prevent relapse: rifampin plus either doxycycline or TMP-SMX. For serious infections, gentamicin as part of initial regimen is indicated
				Serology	
	Cat-scratch (*Bartonella henselae*)	Scratch from cat or bite from infected flea	Localized adenopathy; poorly healing papule; 30 % with fever; hepatosplenic lesions	Serology	Optimal therapy unclear. While usually resolves in 4–6 weeks, symptoms may abate more quickly if children receive antibiotics (azithromycin, fluoroquinolones, TMP-SMX)
				Histopathology	
	Chlamydia trachomatis	Trachoma exceedingly rare in the US, but a common cause of childhood visual loss in developing nations	Isolated conjunctivitis (develops several days-weeks after birth), not associated with scarring; should be evaluated for chlamydial pneumonia	Nucleic acid amplification tests	Conjunctivitis/pneumonia: oral erythromycin × 14 days
			Trachoma: corneal neovascularization	Culture for documentation of suspected sexual abuse	Trachoma: azithromycin 20 mg/kg as single dose recommended by WHO
	Leptospirosis	Urine or placental tissue of infected animals	Biphasic illness with initial fever, conjunctival suffusion, myalgias. Immune-mediated phase with adenopathy, aseptic meningitis, purpuric rash	Serology	Penicillin
					Can see Jarisch-Herxheimer reaction after starting penicillin

	Lyme disease (*B. burgdorferi*)	Bit of deer ticks (*Ixodes*)	Early localized: erythema migrans with fever, malaise, painless adenopathy. Other: carditis, arthritis, meningo-encephalitis	Early in illness, clinical diagnosis, as serologies take up to a month to become positive	Early localized: amoxicillin or doxycycline
					Early disseminated, late disease: amoxicillin or doxycycline; ceftriaxone or IV penicillin for carditis, meningitis, encephalitis, or persistent/recurring arthritis
	Nocardiosis (*Nocardia nova, brasiliensis, farcinica*)	Direct inoculation into skin from vegetative material	Tender shallow ulcers, spread in lymphatic pattern; disseminated disease in immunocompromised children	Culture (indolent organism; need to hold cultures for weeks)	TMP-SMX× 6–12 weeks
					Abscess drainage decreases frequency of satellite lesions
				Weakly acid-fast	Add amikacin or ceftriaxone for deeper infections in immunocompromised hosts
	Non-tuberculous mycobacteria	Most common in preschool-aged children	Nontender chronic lymphadenopathy; overlying violaceous discoloration of skin; formation of sinus tracts	Culture (yield will be low if swabs are sent; instead, caseous material should be drawn up in a syringe and sent directly to the laboratory; characteristic exam and history may favor surgical treatment prior to biopsy)	Combination therapy with azithromycin and either rifampin or ethambutol for the most common isolate, *Mycobacterium avium* complex (MAC)
					Complete excision is superior to medical therapy for otherwise healthy children with isolated adenopathy
	Tuberculosis (scrofula)	Airborne transmission; N95 mask and negative-pressure room should be utilized	Nontender cervical or supraclavicular nodes; fever. Skin discoloration rare	Culture (often negative, in which case use triad of positive TST, history of contact with an adult with contagious TB, and compatible clinical or radiographic findings)	Isoniazid, rifampin, ethambutol, and pyrazinamide unless drug resistance is suspected or confirmed
				PCR	
	Tularemia	Contact with rodents, lagomorphs (rabbits, hares), ticks, beavers, deer flies; aerosolization during yard work	Fever, chills, headache, Parinaud's oculoglandular syndrome; ulceroglandular syndrome (skin ulcers with tender adenopathy)	Serology	Streptomycin or gentamicin × 10 days
				Culture is hazardous to laboratory personnel	Alternative: fluoroquinolones, doxycycline

(continued)

Table 13.3 (continued)

Class	Organism(s)	Epidemiology/infection control	Symptoms	Diagnosis	Treatment
Viral	Adenovirus	Cause of epidemic keratoconjunctivitis	Fever, conjunctivitis, preauricular adenopathy, pharyngitis, hepatitis, hemorrhagic cystitis	Culture	Supportive care unless child is immunosuppressed or has life-threatening disease
				PCR	
				Rapid assays	
	CMV	Most common congenital infection in the U.S. (only 10 % symptomatic at birth)	Fever, fatigue, hepatitis, pharyngitis;	Titers	Supportive care unless child is immunosuppressed or has life-threatening disease
				PCR	
			splenomegaly less common than in EBV	Culture	
	EBV	90 % of U.S. adults have been infected with EBV	Pharyngitis, splenomegaly, fatigue, periorbital edema	Titers	Supportive
				PCR	
	HHV-8 (Castleman's disease; Kaposi sarcoma)	Seroprevalence highest in the Mediterranean, Africa, the Middle East, and the Amazon basin	Fever, disseminated adenopathy, masses in mediastinum, head, and neck	PCR	
		Castleman's most common in adolescents		Serology	Supportive unless develop HHV-8-associated malignancies (e.g., lymphoma, Kaposi sarcoma)
	HIV	Vertically-acquired infection now rare in U.S. Unusual mode of transmission: premastication of food for infants	Acute HIV infection: fever, malaise, pharyngitis, generalized adenopathy	PCR	Antiretroviral therapy
				Serology (may be negative in acute HIV infection)	
		Should be part of screening for adopted and immigrant children	Chronic HIV infection: failure to thrive, hepatosplenomegaly, dermatitis, opportunistic infections	Viral load	Prophylaxis against opportunistic infections
	Measles	Airborne transmission; one of the most contagious infectious agents; N95 mask and negative-pressure room should be utilized	Cephalocaudad erythematous maculopapular rash that becomes confluent; conjunctivitis; Koplik spots rare, transient	Serology	Supportive care. Vitamin A has been shown to decrease measles mortality in developing nations
	Mumps	The only cause of epidemic parotitis	Parotitis, aseptic meningitis, orchitis, arthritis	PCR	Supportive care
				Serology of limited utility, as IgM response is very transient	

Fungal	Tinea capitis (*Trichophyton*, *Microsporum* species)	Fungi can remain viable on fomites for days-weeks	Focal alopecia, brittle hair, kerion formation	Potassium hydroxide wet mounts show arthroconidia within hair shaft	Griseofulvin
	Blastomycosis (*B. dermatitidis*)	Endemic in soil in south/central United States and other regions [Table 13.2]	Multiple cutaneous findings [see Table 13.2] with nontender adenopathy	Culture on Sabouraud media Visualization of thick-walled, broad-based budding yeast in tissue	Amphotericin (use of oral agents has not been well-studied in children)
	Coccidioidomycosis (*C. immitis*)	Endemic in soil in southwestern United States	Pneumonia (mimics TB); fever, malaise, erythema nodosum, skin/soft tissue infections in areas of penetrating trauma with regional adenopathy	Serology (acute, convalescent) Visualization of spherules in infected body fluid	Fluconazole or itraconazole for 6–12 months if have severe clinical manifestations or are immunocompromised hosts
				Culture is hazardous to laboratory personnel	(treatment of uncomplicated primary infection in normal hosts is controversial)
Other	Kawasaki	Over 80 % of cases occur in preschool-aged children	Fever ≥5 days plus ≥4/5: rash; cervical adenopathy (≥1.5 cm in diameter), hand/pedal edema, mucosal changes, conjunctivitis	Clinical diagnosis with supporting laboratory data: anemia, thrombocytosis, leukocytosis, elevated ALT, sterile pyuria, hypoalbuminemia	IVIG, high-dose aspirin
	Kikuchi	Rare finding; most common in Asian adolescents	Fever, disseminated adenopathy, fatigue	Necrotizing lymphadenitis seen on pathology of excisional biopsy Diagnosis of exclusion	Supportive care. Corticosteroids and nonsteroidal anti-inflammatories used for severe symptoms or long duration of illness

ALT alanine aminotransferase, *CGD* chronic granulomatous disease, *CMV* cytomegalovirus, *EBV* Epstein-Barr virus, *HIV* human immunodeficiency virus, *IV* intravenous, *IVIG* intravenous immunoglobulin, *MRSA* methicillin-resistant *S. aureus*, *PCR* polymerase chain reaction, *TB* tuberculosis, *TMP-SMX* trimethoprim-sulfamethoxazole *TST* tuberculin skin test, *WHO* World Health Organization

Acute Localized Lymphadenopathy

The most common causes of acute localized cervical lymphadenopathy are viral upper respiratory tract infections (URIs). These nodes usually are subcentimeter, bilateral, mobile, minimally tender, and nonfluctuant. The natural history is that these nodes typically return to their normal size within 1 month. Other viral infections, such as cytomegalovirus (CMV) and Epstein-Barr virus (EBV) can cause both localized and generalized lymphadenopathy and are described in the latter section.

Acute pyogenic bacteria are the second most common cause of acute localized cervical adenopathy. The two most common pathogens are *Streptococcus pyogenes* (group A streptococcus, GAS) and *Staphylococcus aureus*. GAS accounts for 15–36 % of exudative pharyngitis cases in children and adolescents [5]. The Centor criteria have been used to help clinically differentiate viral from GAS pharyngitis. Children receive one point for each of the following: fever; absence of cough; exudative tonsillitis; and tender anterior cervical nodes. Children with scores of <2 should not be tested by rapid streptococcal assays, as positive results in this group are more likely to reflect false positives from GAS carriage in the posterior pharynx [6].

When evaluating a child for pyogenic adenitis, it is imperative that clinicians evaluate for deeper neck infections, including peritonsillar abscesses, retropharyngeal abscesses, and Lemierre's syndrome [7]. Peritonsillar abscesses are most common in adolescents, and are characterized by unilateral swelling of the tonsils, change in caliber of the voice, trismus, unilateral odynophagia, displacement of the uvula toward the unaffected side, and fever. Lymphadenopathy of the jugulo-digastric nodes is most common. The diagnosis is clinical, though in some cases computed tomography (CT) is useful to evaluate for deeper extension of the abscess prior to bedside drainage. In contrast, retropharyngeal abscesses (RTAs) are most common in preschool-aged children, and are associated with nuchal rigidity or torticollis, difficulty swallowing, drooling, stridor, and fever. While a soft-tissue lateral neck radiograph can suggest an RTA if there is increased prevertebral space, CT of the neck is useful to better delineate the anatomy prior to operative intervention. Lemierre's syndrome is comprised of a deep neck abscess associated with septic thrombophlebitis of the internal jugular vein, and septic pulmonary emboli. A palpable cord in the lateral neck in a toxic-appearing child can be the first indication of Lemierre's. While now the most common etiology is *S. aureus* [7], anaerobes (especially *Fusobacterium necrophorum*) were the initial organisms described for Lemierre's.

The treatment of choice for GAS is penicillin or amoxicillin, as there has never been a GAS isolate resistant to beta-lactams. As such, use of broader spectrum antibiotics, such as cephalosporins or amoxicillin-clavulanate, offers no benefit for initial treatment or to prevent relapse in children [8]. Macrolide resistance is approximately 5 % in the United States [9] and clindamycin resistance is approximately 20–25 % [10]. Empiric use of clindamycin for peritonsillar abscesses or RTAs depends on the level of clindamycin-resistance among *S. aureus* isolates in an area. Children with suspected Lemierre's should receive broad-spectrum antibiotics covering both methicillin-resistant *S. aureus* and also anaerobes (e.g., vancomycin plus metronidazole).

Facial cellulitis in children often is of odontogenic origin. Other causes include: GAS cellulitis, impetigo, or erysipelas; *S. aureus*; group B streptococcus (*S. agalactiae*) in infants, and *Haemophilus influenza* type B in unimmunized children. Fat necrosis of the cheeks ("popsicle panniculitis") is characterized by tender, red, indurated marks on the medial cheeks in preschool-aged children and can mimic facial cellulitis; fever and adenopathy are absent in this condition.

A special consideration in children with cervical adenopathy is Kawasaki disease. This condition, the etiology of which is unknown, can cause coronary artery aneurysms. Kawasaki's is characterized by at least 5 days of fever in association with four of the five clinical features: bilateral nonpurulent bulbar conjunctival injection; swelling of the hands or feet (or periungual desquamation); strawberry tongue or cracked red lips; polymorphous rash (of any type except bullous or vesicular); and cervical adenopathy at least 1.5 cm in diameter. While there is no single test for Kawasaki, supporting laboratory features include hypoalbuminemia, anemia, transaminitis, thrombocytosis, leukocytosis, and sterile pyuria [11]. As treatment of Kawasaki with high-dose aspirin and intravenous immunoglobulin within the first 10 days of illness can reduce the rate of coronary aneurysms, it is an important that the otolaryngologist be cognizant of Kawasaki disease.

Cat-scratch disease, caused by *Bartonella henselae*, is characterized by localized adenopathy. While cat-scratch disease is most common in the axillary region after a cat scratch to the upper extremity, scratches to the face can result in cervical adenopathy. There is often an indolent, slowly-healing papule at the site of the cat scratch. The infected lymph nodes are tender, erythematous, fluctuant, and will occasionally spontaneously drain. In some pediatric case series, hepatosplenic cat-scratch is among the most common causes of fever of unknown origin [12]. Most lesions will resolve spontaneously in 4–6 weeks; antibiotics may decrease symptom duration, but while multiple antibiotics have been used successfully (including macrolides, rifampin, fluoroquinolones, and trimethoprim-sulfamethoxazole), the optimal regimen and duration are unknown.

Subacute or Chronic Localized Lymphadenopathy

Several more indolent pathogens can cause chronic localized lymphadenopathy in immunocompetent hosts. These include tuberculosis, nontuberculous mycobacteria (NTM), actinomycosis, and nocardiosis. Lymphadenopathy caused by these pathogens usually is non-tender or minimally tender, except for *Nocardia*. Clinical findings and diagnostic and therapeutic options are listed in Table 13.3.

Pediatric tuberculosis (TB) lymphadenopathy (scrofula) is characterized by painless cervical or supraclavicular adenopathy. The nodes may seem rubbery and rarely appear matted. Similar to NTM nodes, they can become adherent to the overlying skin and subsequently a sinus tract can develop. Disseminated tuberculous lymphadenopathy can be seen as an early finding in lympho-hematogenous spread of the bacteria. Fine-needle aspirate has been shown to be a safe, effective way to obtain cultures in children [13]. In addition to acid-fast culture, evaluation of a child with suspected tuberculous lymphadenopathy should include a chest radiograph to evaluate for intrathoracic involvement. As many children with tuberculosis have negative cultures, the diagnosis often is made on the basis of a positive tuberculin skin test (TST) (or interferon gamma release assay, a more specific blood-based assay than the TST), contact with a person known to have TB, and compatible clinical or radiographic findings [14]. In areas with high incidence rates for TB, symptom-based algorithms can accurately differentiate tuberculous lymphadenopathy from other causes. One model found that with lymphadenopathy for at least 4 weeks refractory to oral antibiotics, without an obvious superficial lesion in the region drained by that node, and with a node at least 2 × 2 cm in diameter, the sensitivity for tuberculosis was 89 % and the specificity was 98 % [15]. However, in most industrialized nations, where TB rates are low, this algorithm would result in many false positive evaluations. Multidrug therapy (e.g., isoniazid, rifampin, ethambutol, and pyrazinamide for drug-susceptible isolates) administered as directly observed therapy for at least 6 months is the standard of care [16].

NTM lymphadenitis can be caused by a number of environmentally ubiquitous species. Immunocompetent, preschool-aged children are the most common group in which NTM adenopathy is seen. In the United States, *Mycobacterium avium* complex (MAC) and *M. kansasii* are the most common isolates, but there is substantial regional variation in NTM species distribution, and species also display wide heterogeneity in antibiotic susceptibilities. NTM adenopathy is most common in the submandibular region, followed by preauricular and submental nodes. The nodes typically are non-tender, unilateral, and slowly growing (maximum size is usually <4 cm). With time, the nodes will become fluctuant and the overlying skin will become erythematous and then violaceous. This appearance is very specific to atypical mycobacterial lymphadenopathy (Fig. 13.1). Similar to with tuberculous adenopathy, sinus tract formation is also a complication; this risk is increased if NTM is not suspected and

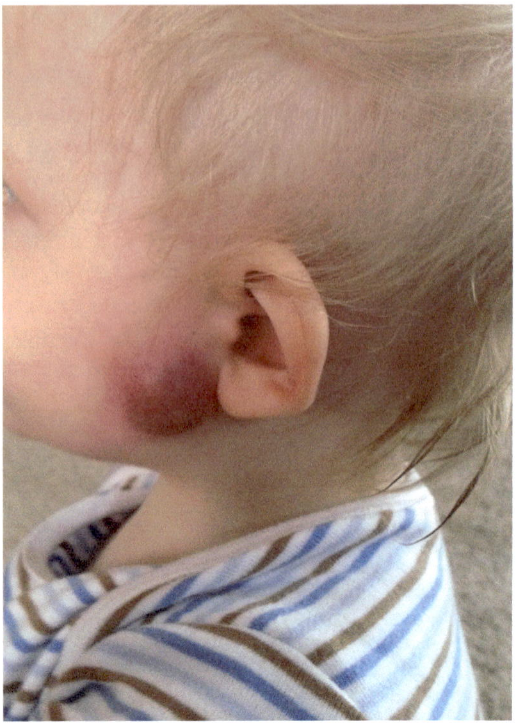

Fig. 13.1 Typical violaceous appearance of atypical mycobacterial lymphadenitis

a node is incised, as would be done for routine pyogenic pathogens. Despite being environmentally ubiquitous, NTM species can be quite hydrophobic. As a consequence, culture yield will be diminished if specimens are simply swabbed and sent to the laboratory. Instead, curettage material should be drawn into a syringe and sent to the laboratory in that fashion. Diagnosis and definitive treatment is surgical excision. If a node can be excised *en toto*, there is excellent evidence in the otolaryngology literature that surgical management is superior to medical management [17]. However, the location of the nodes poses barriers to excision, as the facial nerve courses along the path of submental nodes and preauricular nodes can frequently involve the first divisions of the nerve. In cases where there are significant skin changes the surgeon must be aware that there may not be an adequate surgical resection plane, which can pose a greater risk to the facial nerve. When there is high risk to the facial nerve due to depth of involvement in the preauricular area or location along the path of the peripheral nerve branches, some authors have advocated curettage as an alternative to excision. A recent meta-analysis found at least temporary facial weakness complicated 10 % of complete excisions versus 0 % of curettage procedures [18]. In this meta-analysis, the pooled cure rate with complete excision was 88.5 %, whereas complete resolution with curettage alone was only 61 % and with antibiotics alone was 67 %.

As a consequence of facial nerve risk, medical management often is necessary, with surgical intervention being reserved for those children who fail antibiotic therapy. To decrease the risk of selecting for drug resistance when antibiotic therapy is elected, children with suspected NTM adenopathy should be treated with combination therapy. Monotherapy with a single antibiotic should never be used for suspected mycobacterial disease. The backbone of therapy for MAC is macrolides; while both clarithromycin and azithromycin can be used, the latter is preferable because the suspension form tastes better and the single-daily dosing of azithromycin will facilitate adherence by the family. The second drug used typically is either ethambutol or rifampin [19]. It is important that families are notified about the orange discoloration to the urine and inactivation of oral contraceptives caused by rifampin.

Table 13.4 Treatment recommendations for non-tuberculous mycobacterial lymphadenitis by clinical stage

Clinical stage	Clinical characteristics	Treatment recommendation
I	Painless, firm	Antibiotics[a]
	Adherent to overlying skin	
	Increased vascularity	
II	Fluctuance	Antibiotics
		Fine needle aspiration(FNA) +/−
		Curettage +/− staged excision
		Complete excision
III	Skin changes—violaceous coloration	Antibiotics
	Thinning of skin, parchment-like changes, shiny appearance	FNA +/−[b]
		Curettage +/− staged excision
IV	Fistulization	Antibiotics
		Complete excision +/− staged wound closure

Source: Adapted from Penn et al. [21] with permission from Elsevier
[a]Though not proposed in this paper, some authors would still consider complete excision if the diagnosis is strongly suspected
[b]Some authors would defer FNA given the characteristic violaceous color and would proceed with curettage versus excision

The choice of medical versus surgical intervention versus watchful waiting and the type of surgical intervention should be discussed at length with the patient (if practical) and their family. In most cases, NTM lymphadenitis will resolve without intervention in 6–12 months [20]. However, at least 60 % of children will develop draining fistulas and cosmetically significant scarring when observation alone is employed [18]. Therefore, the selection of treatment modality must include consideration of the risk to the facial nerve, likely cosmetic outcomes, antibiotic side effects, and the family's tolerance of fistulization and drainage for up to a year in the event of non-treatment. While most authors agree that when complete excision is feasible without significant risk to the facial nerve, it should be the first treatment option, the plan should be tailored to the individual. Though there is no consensus on a complete treatment algorithm for NTM lymphadenopathy, Penn et al. [21] proposed a useful set of guidelines regarding antibiotics, excision, curettage and staged excision, and FNA (Table 13.4).

Differentiating TB from NTM can be challenging. Several features can be more suggestive of NTM versus TB. These include younger age (preschool versus adolescent), lack of TB risk factors (including birth in a low TB-incidence nation); normal chest radiograph; negative TSTs or interferon gamma release assays in family members; presence of microabscesses; lack of caseation; ill-defined granulomas, and characteristic purple discoloration of the skin [22, 23]. If empiric treatment is needed before culture results become available and it is epidemiologically difficult to differentiate NTM from TB in a child, there is a regimen that can offer three antibiotics to treat each condition: isoniazid, rifampin, ethambutol, and azithromycin. Here, the first three antibiotics treat TB and the latter three offer empiric coverage for the most common NTM species. The downside to this regimen is that by excluding pyrazinamide from the empiric regimen, then the TB treatment course may be longer.

Actinomycosis can cause disease in three sites: cervicofacial (the most common), thoracic (following aspiration), and abdominal (following penetrating trauma). The two most common predisposing comorbidities for disseminated actinomycosis are HIV infection and chronic granulomatous disease (CGD). The inciting event for cervicofacial actinomycosis is odontogenic (extraction, infection, trauma). Children develop localized nodular mandibular lesions ("lumpy jaw") which may progress to fistulous sinus tracts. Submental adenopathy is most common. Anaerobic cultures should be sent for *Actinomyces*, and demonstration of beaded Gram-positive rods with yellow 'sulfur' granules on microscopy help solidify the diagnosis. Initial therapy is parenteral penicillin or ampicillin for at least 1 month, followed by months of oral suppressive therapy [24].

Nocardiosis is caused by any of several environmentally ubiquitous bacteria. In immunocompetent children, the most common manifestation is cutaneous disease after direct inoculation from vegetative material [25]. Painful shallow ulcers surrounded by smaller satellite lesions, with spread along lymphatic channels, are seen along with tender regional adenopathy. While some examination findings mimic those of pyogenic bacteria, the course is more indolent than with GAS or *S. aureus*. In immunocompromised patients, including those with CGD, pulmonary, central nervous system, and disseminated disease may be seen. As these are indolent pathogens, cultures need to be kept for several weeks to optimize microbiologic diagnosis; weakly acid-fast staining of organisms may be the first clue to *Nocardia*. Trimethoprim-sulfamethoxazole is the backbone of therapy.

Generalized Adenopathy

Supraclavicular, cervical, occipital, and preauricular nodes may also be enlarged as part of generalized lymphadenopathy in childhood. Certain examination and radiographic findings have been more associated with malignancy: supraclavicular location, fixed nodes, and abnormal chest radiography [26]. Duration of adenopathy, tenderness, fever, splenomegaly, and unilateral versus bilateral do not reliably differentiate between infectious and oncologic etiologies.

Acute Generalized Adenopathy

CMV, EBV, herpes simplex virus (HSV), and human herpesvirus-8 (HHV-8) are all large DNA viruses capable of causing generalized adenopathy. In young children, the manifestations of these viruses cannot be differentiated from viral URIs, except that the duration of fever may be longer. The clinical presentation in older and immunocompromised children has more variation (Table 13.3). As a general rule, treatment is supportive for the previously healthy child.

Acute HIV infection is caused by widespread dissemination of the virus immediately after a child is infected. Symptoms include fever, weight loss, disseminated non-tender lymphadenopathy, headaches, pharyngitis, and headaches; thus, it is difficult to distinguish acute HIV infection from the symptoms of the large DNA viruses [27]. As the symptoms occur days to weeks after infection, serologies are negative. Diagnosis is based on quantitative or qualitative PCR or on viral load. Children with acute HIV infection should be screened for other sexually transmitted infections.

Tularemia is a zoonotic infection of lagomorphs (rabbits, hares), rodents, and cats, and can be transmitted by contact with one of these animals or by the bite of an infected tick or deer fly. Tularemia can cause several syndromes, the most common of which is ulceroglandular tularemia. These patients have generalized or localized adenopathy (ranging up to 7 cm in diameter) in association with a papular inoculation site that later becomes ulcerative. Glandular syndrome, without an inoculation site, is the next most common presentation. In order of descending frequency, cervical, occipital, axillary, and inguinal adenopathy can be seen [28]. Parinaud's oculoglandular syndrome is the third most common manifestation, with conjunctivitis and preauricular adenopathy [1]. The diagnosis is based on serologies, as it is dangerous to grow the organism in the laboratory, and aminoglycosides are the treatment of choice.

Brucellosis is a zoonotic disease transmitted to humans through consumption of unpasteurized milk, raw or undercooked foods, or handling tissue of infected animals. Disease is more common in Hispanic children, and the two U.S. states with the most cases are Texas and California [29]. Symptoms include fever and influenza-like symptoms; examination is notable for generalized adenopathy (tender or non-tender) and hepatosplenomegaly. *Brucella* can cause osteomyelitis as well, and has a predilection for the sacro-iliac joint. Diagnosis is by blood culture; however, since the bacterium is very slow-growing, cultures need to be held for a minimum of 4 weeks. Combination antibiotic therapy is needed to affect cure and decrease relapse rate. Rifampin with either doxycycline (for children ≥8-years-old) or trimethoprim-sulfamethoxazole for approximately 6 weeks is recommended. Monotherapy is not recommended. For more severe disease, an aminoglycoside should be added to the initial regimen.

It is estimated that there were approximately 23,000 cases of syphilis in persons 15–24 years of age in the US in 2008 [30]. The rate of congenital syphilis is now approximately 12/100,000, with most cases occurring in the South; 50 % are born to African-American mothers, 31 % to Hispanic mothers [31]. Congenital syphilis can present as generalized lymphadenopathy in children with snuffles (copious nasal discharge), organomegaly, and rashes. In addition for adolescents or sexually abused children, diffuse lymphadenopathy, along with a maculopapular rash of the palms and soles, can be the presenting findings of secondary syphilis. The diagnosis of congenital syphilis is complex. In addition to obtaining results of maternal treponemal tests and treatment history, infants should be evaluated by physical examination, RPR, and VDRL. The treatment of choice (and the only acceptable treatment for pregnant women) is parenteral penicillin G.

Leptospirosis is caused by a spirochete excreted in the urine of infected animals and is more common after areas have been flooded [32]. The most common manifestations are fever, non-purulent conjunctival suffusion, and leg/lumbar myalgias. In the second (immune-mediated) phase, tender adenopathy, rash, and aseptic meningitis may be seen. Complications can include renal failure, hepatorenal syndrome, shock, and hemorrhagic pneumonitis. The diagnosis is based on serologies, as cultures require special media and handling. The treatment of choice is parenteral penicillin.

Lyme disease is caused by a spirochete and transmitted for deer ticks (*Ixodes*); most U.S. cases occur in the northeast and Great Lakes region. Early localized disease is characterized by erythema migrans (bull's eye lesions) at the site of the tick bite. Secondary spirochetemia results in fever and an influenza-like illness. Later complications can involve joints, the central nervous system, and the conduction system [33]. Diagnosis is clinical in early localized disease, as serologies may take up to 4 weeks to become positive. The treatment of choice for most forms is amoxicillin for young children and doxycycline for children ≥8 years of age.

Chronic Generalized Adenopathy

The differential diagnosis of infectious causing chronic generalized adenopathy is narrow, but includes some life-threatening infections. The otolaryngologist may be asked to see these children for enlarged cervical nodes prior to other adenopathy being recognized. The differential diagnosis includes chronic HIV infection, fungal disease, toxoplasmosis, and leishmaniasis.

Children with long-standing untreated HIV infection commonly have generalized adenopathy. In most cases, this is due to viral infiltration of lymphatic tissue, but adenopathy may also reflect opportunistic infections to which HIV-infected children are susceptible: EBV-associated lymphomas or HHV-associated Kaposi sarcoma. The CDC classification for HIV infection in children lists having adenopathy (≥0.5 cm at more than two sites or bilateral adenopathy at one site) as meeting clinical category A (mildly symptomatic) criteria [34]. Biopsy for aerobic, anaerobic, fungal, and acid-fast cultures and for flow cytometry may be needed to exclude other causes of adenopathy. Adenopathy improves and may resolve after initiation of antiretroviral therapy. Certain fungal infections can be associated with generalized adenopathy; the two most common seen in the United States are blastomycosis and coccidioidomycosis. Blastomycosis is endemic in the south/central United States as well as in Central/South America, India, and Africa (Table 13.3). While pulmonary, skeletal, and disseminated infections can occur (and may mimic TB), the most common site causing adenopathy is cutaneous blastomycosis [35]. Manifestations are polymorphous and include ulcers, pustules, and verrucous lesions. The diagnosis is by culture or by staining of tissue, which may demonstrate thick-walled, broad-based budding yeast. Amphotericin remains the treatment of choice in children.

Coccidioidomycosis is endemic to the southwestern United States. While pulmonary disease is self-limited and disseminated infection rare in immunocompetent children, cutaneous and skin/soft tissue disease can occur and are associated with nontender adenopathy [36]. The skin findings, similar to with blastomycosis, are protean and include erythema nodosum, erythema multiforme, and maculopapular rashes. The diagnosis is made by serology or visualization of spherules in tissue; this fungus can be transmitted in the laboratory setting, and laboratory personnel must be warned when handling specimens if coccidioidomycosis is suspected. The treatment is fluconazole or itraconazole.

Toxoplasma gondii is a protozoan transmitted from infected cat feces. Congenital toxoplasmosis may present with generalized lymphadenopathy in addition to other clinical (jaundice, diarrhea), laboratory (pancytopenias), examination (chorioretinitis, hepatosplenomegaly, rash, pneumonitis), and radiographic findings (microcephaly, intracranial calcifications, hydrocephaly). Post-natally acquired toxoplasmosis usually is asymptomatic except for in immunocompromised hosts. In these persons, fever, malaise, sore throat, and isolated cervical or generalized adenopathy can be seen. The diagnosis is based on serologies (however, IgM can remain elevated for years) or PCR. Treatment with pyrimethamine and sulfadiazine usually is limited to infants with significant complications with vertically-acquired toxoplasmosis or to immunocompromised hosts [37].

Leishmania species are spread by the phlebotomine sand fly and can cause three clinical syndromes: cutaneous; mucosal; and visceral (kala-azar). Cutaneous leishmaniasis begins as an erythematous papule that evolves into a shallow painless ulcer with satellite lesions and non-tender localized adenopathy. Spread occurs along lymphatic channels, similar to cutaneous blastomycosis, but resolves spontaneously after weeks to years with a residual atrophic scar. In contrast, mucosal leishmaniasis lesions are more aggressive and can cause local tissue destruction around the face; localized adenopathy is a less prominent finding with this form. Visceral leishmaniasis involves spread to the reticuloendothelial system with splenic and marrow involvement. Disseminated adenopathy is common in east Africa. Kala-azar is almost uniformly fatal if untreated [38]. Visualization of the parasite (amastigotes) in infected tissue is diagnostic. Serologies are not routinely available in endemic settings. Treatment should be managed in conjunction with experts at the Centers for Disease Control and Prevention. Amphotericin often is used for visceral leishmaniasis.

Surgical Evaluation of Lymphadenopathy

The most common role of the Head and Neck surgeon in cases of cervical lymphadenopathy other than NTM adenopathy or suppurative adenopathy with skin involvement is to assist in establishing the diagnosis (Table 13.4) [21]. Fine needle aspiration is helpful in the diagnosis in patients with persistent cervical lymphadenopathy. This technique is minimally invasive, reliable and with few reported complications. Van de Schoot et al. [39] showed fine needle aspiration results of 86 % sensitivity and 96 % specificity in 39 patients with lymphadenopathy. In this study 61 % of patients only required fine needle aspiration without any need for open excisional biopsy. However, a systematic review of the literature in 2014 reported a sensitivity range as low as 67 % and emphasized that FNA should not be relied upon to exclude malignancy [40]. Another limitation of fine needle aspiration is that it requires an experienced pediatric cytopathologist, which may not be available at many institutions [41].

Open Biopsy is still the gold standard for histologic diagnosis of cervical lymphadenopathy in pediatric patients. Unfortunately, there are no clear guidelines on when a lymph node should be biopsied as emphasized in Locke's systematic literature review. Some clinical features that should suggest open biopsy are listed (Table 13.5) [42]. While the need for open biopsy in the general population seen by primary care providers is likely small, biopsy should be considered in cases of progressively enlarging lymphadenopathy, systemic signs and symptoms suggesting malignancy, and lymphadenopathy larger than 2 cm that persists for over 4–6 weeks and fails to respond to antibiotics or other diagnostic

Table 13.5 Recommendations for surgical excision or biopsy for cervical lymphadenopathy

Therapeutic
Atypical mycobacterial lymphadenopathy
To establish diagnosis
Rapidly enlarging lymph node over 2 weeks
High suspicion of malignancy (supraclavicular nodes, systemic signs of weight loss, fever, hepatosplenomegaly, arthralgias)
Lymphadenopathy larger than 2 cm that persists for over 4–6 weeks without responding to antibiotic treatment
Presence of abnormal chest radiograph with cervical lymphadenopathy

Source: Adapted from Rosenberg et al. [42] with permission from Elsevier

measures, a. Ultrasound features have shown promise in predicting benign or malignant nature of enlarged lymph nodes, but further study is required [40]. Benign reactive lymphoid hyperplasia is still the most common finding in open biopsy as well as in fine needle aspiration.

Conclusion

In summary, cervical lymphadenopathy is common in the pediatric population. A large number of lymphadenopathies are associated with infectious organisms. Therefore, the differential diagnosis is broad and a thorough clinical history and physical examination are important to establish the correct diagnosis. Antimicrobial therapy is the treatment of choice for the vast majority of these cases. Surgical management, with a few exceptions, is often limited to help establish a diagnosis and rule out other causes of lymphadenopathy such as malignancy.

References

1. Thompson S, Omphroy L, Oetting T. Parinaud's oculoglandular syndrome attributable to an encounter with a wild rabbit. Am J Ophthalmol. 2001;131(2):283–4.
2. Grando D, Sullivan LJ, Flexman JP, Watson MW, Andrew JH. *Bartonella henselae* associated with Parinaud's oculoglandular syndrome. Clin Infect Dis. 1999;28(5):1156–8.
3. Meisler DM, Bosworth DE, Krachmer JH. Ocular infectious mononucleosis manifested as Parinaud's oculoglandular syndrome. Am J Ophthalmol. 1981;92(5):722–6.
4. Chin GN, Noble RC. Ocular involvement in *Yersinia enterocolitica* infection presenting as Parinaud's oculoglandular syndrome. Am J Ophthalmol. 1977;83(1):19–23.
5. Linder JA, Bates DW, Lee GM, Finkelstein JA. Antibiotic treatment of children with sore throat. JAMA. 2005;294(18):2315–22.
6. Fine AM, Nizet V, Mandl KD. Large-scale validation of the Centor and McIsaac scores to predict group A streptococcal pharyngitis. Arch Intern Med. 2012;172(11):847–52.
7. Kizhner V, Samara G, Panesar R, Krespi YP. Methicillin-resistant *Staphylococcus aureus* bacteremia associated with Lemierre's syndrome: case report and literature review. J Laryngol Otol. 2013;127(7):721–3.
8. Van Driel ML, De Sutter AI, Keber N, Habraken H, Christiaens T. Different antibiotic treatments for group A streptococcal pharyngitis. Cochrane Database Syst Rev. 2013;10, CD004406.
9. Villaseñor-Sierra A, Katahira E, Jaramillo-Valdivia AN, et al. Phenotypes and genotypes of erythromycin-resistant *Streptococcus pyogenes* strains isolated from invasive and non-invasive infections from Mexico and the United States during 1999–2010. Int J Infect Dis. 2012;16(3):e178–81.
10. Chen I, Kaufisi P, Erden G. Emergence of erythromycin- and clindamycin-resistant *Streptococcus pyogenes* emm 90 strains in Hawaii. J Clin Microbiol. 2010;49(1):439–41.
11. Newburger JW, Takahashi M, Gerber MA, et al. Diagnosis, treatment, and long-term management of Kawasaki disease: a statement for health professionals from the Committee on Rheumatic Fever, Endocarditis, and Kawasaki Disease, Council on Cardiovascular Disease in the Young, American Heart Association. Pediatrics. 2004;114(6):1708–33.
12. Arisoy ES, Correa AG, Wagner ML, Kaplan SL. Hepatosplenic cat-scratch disease in children: selected clinical features and treatment. Clin Infect Dis. 1999;28(4):778–84.

13. Wright CA, Hesseling AC, Bamford C, Burgess SM, Warren R, Marais BJ. Fine-needle aspiration biopsy: a first-line diagnostic procedure in pediatric tuberculosis suspects with peripheral lymphadenopathy? Int J Tuberc Lung Dis. 2009;13(11):1373–9.
14. Cruz AT, Starke JR. Pediatric tuberculosis. Pediatr Rev. 2010;31(1):13–26.
15. Marais BJ, Wright CA, Schaaf HS, et al. Tuberculous lymphadenitis as a cause of persistent cervical lymphadenopathy in children from a tuberculosis-endemic area. Pediatr Infect Dis J. 2006;25(2):142–6.
16. American Thoracic Society, Centers for Disease Control and Prevention, Infectious Diseases Society of America. Treatment of tuberculosis. MMWR. 2003;52:1–88.
17. Lindeboom JA, Kuijper EJ, van Bruijnesteijn CES, Lindeboom R, Prins JM. Surgical excision versus antibiotic treatment for nontuberculous mycobacterial cervicofacial lymphadenitis in children: a multicenter, randomized controlled trial. Clin Infect Dis. 2007;44(8):1057–64.
18. Zimmermann P, Tebruegge M, Curtis N, Ritz N. The management of non-tuberculous cervicofacial lymphadenitis in children: a systematic review and meta-analysis. J Infect. 2015;71(1):9–18.
19. Griffith DE, Aksamit T, Brown-Elliott BA, et al. An official ATS/IDSA statement: diagnosis, treatment, and prevention of nontuberculous mycobacterial disease. Am J Respir Crit Care Med. 2007;175(4):367–416.
20. Zeharia A, Eidlitz-Markus T, Haimi-Cohen Y, Samra Z, Kaufman L, Amir J. Management of nontuberculous mycobacteria-induced cervical lymphadenitis with observation alone. Pediatr Infect Dis J. 2008;27:920–2.
21. Penn R, Steehler M, Sokohl A, Harley E. Nontuberculuous mycobacterial cervicofacial lymphadenitis—a review and proposed classification system. Int J Pediatr Otorhinolaryngol. 2011;75:1599–603.
22. Kraus M, Benharroch D, Kaplan D, et al. Mycobacterial cervical lymphadenitis: the histological features of nontuberculous mycobacterial infection. Histopathology. 1999;35(6):534–8.
23. Carvalho AC, Codecasa L, Pinsi G, et al. Differential diagnosis of cervical mycobacterial lymphadenitis in children. Pediatr Infect Dis J. 2010;29(7):629–33.
24. Wong VK, Turmezei TD, Weston VC. Actinomycosis. BMJ. 2011;343:d6099.
25. Ambrosioni J, Lew D, Garbino J. Nocardiosis: updated clinical review and experience at a tertiary center. Infection. 2010;38(2):89–97.
26. Soldes OS, Younger JG, Hirschl RB. Predictors of malignancy in childhood peripheral lymphadenopathy. J Pediatr Surg. 1999;34(10):1447–52.
27. Ratcliffe L, Thomas S, Beeching NJ, Phillips-Howard PA, Taegtmeyer M. Acute presentations of HIV are still missed in low prevalence areas. Postgrad Med J. 2011;87(1025):170–4.
28. Weber IB, Turabelidze G, Patrick S, et al. Clinical recognition and management of tularemia in Missouri: a retrospective records review of 121 cases. Clin Infect Dis. 2012;55(10):1283–90.
29. Shen MW. Diagnostic and therapeutic challenges of childhood brucellosis in a nonendemic country. Pediatrics. 2008;121(5):e1178–83.
30. Satterwhite CL, Torrone E, Meites E, et al. Sexually transmitted infections among US women and men: prevalence and incidence estimates, 2008. Sex Transm Dis. 2013;40(3):187–93.
31. Centers for Disease Control and Prevention. Congenital syphilis—United States, 2003–2008. MMWR. 2010;59(14):413–7.
32. Zaki SA, Shanbag P. Clinical manifestations of dengue and leptospirosis in children in Mumbai: an observational study. Infection. 2010;38(4):285–91.
33. Esposito S, Bosis S, Sabatini C, Tagliaferri L, Principi N. *Borrelia burgdorferi* infection and Lyme disease in children. Int J Infect Dis. 2013;17(3):e153–8.
34. Schneider E, Whitmore S, Glynn KM, et al. Revised surveillance case definitions for HIV infection among adults, adolescents, and children aged 18 months and for HIV infection and AIDS among children aged 18 months to 13 years—United States, 2008. MMWR Recomm Rep. 2008;57(RR-10):1–12.
35. Brick KE, Drolet BA, Lyon VB, Galbraith SS. Cutaneous and disseminated blastomycosis: a pediatric case series. Pediatr Dermatol. 2013;30(1):23–8.
36. Arnold MG, Arnold JC, Bloom DC, Brewster DF, Thiringer JK. Head and neck manifestations of disseminated coccidioidomycosis. Laryngoscope. 2004;114(4):747–52.
37. Robert-Gangneux F, Dardé ML. Epidemiology of and diagnostic strategies for toxoplasmosis. Clin Microbiol Rev. 2012;25(2):264–96.
38. Layegh P, Moghiman T, Ahmadian Hoseini SA. Children and cutaneous leishmaniasis: a clinical report and review. J Infect Dev Ctries. 2013;7(8):614–7.
39. van de Schoot L, Aronson DC, Behrendt H, Bras J. The role of fine-needle aspiration cytology in children with persistent or suspicious lymphadenopathy. J Pediatr Surg. 2001;36:7–11.
40. Locke R, Comfort R, Kubba H. When does an enlarged cervical lymph node in a child need excision? A systematic review. Int J Pediatr Otorhinolaryngol. 2014;78(3):393–401.
41. Handa U, Mohan H, Bal A. Role of fine needle aspiration cytology in evaluation of paediatric lymphadenopathy. Cytopathology. 2003;14:66–9.
42. Rosenberg T, Nolder A. Pediatric cervical lymphadenopathy. Otolaryngol Clin North Am. 2014;47(5):721–31.

Chapter 14
Neck Abscesses and Deep Neck Infections

Carla M. Giannoni and Judith R. Campbell

Introduction

Almost all structures of the head and neck, including the lymph nodes, muscle, fat, vascular system, salivary glands, thyroid, parathyroid glands, and thymus, can become infected and form an inflammatory lesion or mass. In a review of 445 cases of pediatric cervical masses that were biopsied, inflammatory lesions were identified in 27 % of patients [1]. Although the majority of cervical lesions do not require biopsy, inflammatory lesions are more common in children. Inflammatory neck masses in children are most often due to lymphadenitis and in some instances abscesses form within these lymph nodes leading to suppurative lymphadenitis. This chapter addresses suppurative cervical lymphadenitis of superficial and deep cervical lymph nodes. Lymphadenopathy is a prominent feature of many pediatric infections and inflammatory processes including: viral upper respiratory tract infections, Cat-scratch disease (Bartonella infection), Kawasaki disease, mycobacterial (tuberculosis and nontuberculous) infections, acquired immunodeficiency syndrome, and PFAPA syndrome (periodic fevers associated with aphthous stomatitis, pharyngitis, and cervical adenitis) [2]. Diffuse, bilateral cervical lymphadenopathy is commonly seen in systemic viral illnesses such as mononucleosis. Chapter 13 reviews the practical approach to nonsuppurative infectious lymphadenopathy. Congenital cysts may become infected and may have similar features to suppurative cervical lymphadenitis. Anatomic and clinical features suggestive of an infected congenital cyst are discussed in Chap. 15.

C.M. Giannoni, M.D.
Department of Pediatric Otolaryngology, Baylor College of Medicine, 6701 Fannin Street, CC6400.00, Houston, TX 77030, USA

Texas Children's Hospital, Houston, TX, USA
e-mail: cmgianno@texaschildrens.org

J.R. Campbell, M.D. (✉)
Department of Pediatrics, Section of Infectious Diseases, Baylor College of Medicine, Feigin Center, 1102 Bates, Suite 1120, Houston, TX 77030-2399, USA

Texas Children's Hospital, Houston, TX, USA
e-mail: judithc@bcm.edu; jrcampb1@texaschildrens.org

T.A. Valdez, J.G. Vallejo (eds.), *Infectious Diseases in Pediatric Otolaryngology*,
DOI 10.1007/978-3-319-21744-4_14

Neck abscesses and deep neck infections occur as a result of suppurative lymphadenitis of superficial or deep cervical nodes or arise from specific anatomic sources such as odontogenic infection or vertebral osteomyelitis. Fundamental to the understanding of neck abscesses and deep neck infection is the cervical anatomic spaces and fascial planes of cervical anatomy.

Cervical Anatomy

Understanding cervical anatomy is often divided into the lymphatic drainage pathways with associated nodal echelons and the cervical fascial spaces.

Cervical Lymphatic System

Children have an extensive network of cervical lymph nodes which are classified by location. The triangles of the neck are a convention to describe the location of disease in the lateral cervical region relative to the neck musculature and other structural landmarks. In head and neck malignancies the convention of "levels" is used to describe the location of lymph node involvement; this approach is also helpful in describing infections of cervical lymph nodes. Regardless of the nomenclature used, these different systems strive to describe the nodal group which is affected by a disease process (Table 14.1). This is important because understanding lymphatic drainage patterns often assists in ascertaining the source of infectious process [3]. For example, the drainage of the nasopharynx is to the deep cervical and posterior triangle lymph nodes, drainage from the tonsils is to the jugulodigastric nodes and drainage from the oropharyngeal region is to the submandibular cervical nodes. Thus, in tonsillitis it is most common to see enlarged anterior cervical lymph nodes. The retropharyngeal lymph nodes are more active in children than adults and when these nodes become suppurative a retropharyngeal abscess

Table 14.1 Anatomic location of cervical lymph nodes

Nodal group	Location	Common areas draining to nodal group
Submental	Inferior to chin, superior to hyoid	Lower lip, floor of mouth, apex of tongue
Submandibular	Inferior to mandible, superior to hyoid	Cheek, lower lip, gums, anterior tongue
Jugulodigastric	Upper neck, near angle of mandible and posterior digastric muscle	Tonsils, posterior oral cavity and oropharynx
Deep cervical	Deep to SCM[a] and in proximity to the cervical jugular vein	Tongue, trachea, nasopharynx, nasal cavities, palate, esophagus, other nodes in neck
Post auricular	Posterior to auricle and superior to the insertion of the SCM	Auricle
Occipital	Base of scalp at insertion of trapezius	Scalp
Posterior cervical	Posterior to SCM, anterior to trapezius, superior to supraclavicular nodes	
Supraclavicular	Above clavicle in lower neck posterior to SCM	Thorax and abdomen

[a]*SCM* sternocleidomastoid muscle

forms. Because viral upper respiratory infection (URI) is so common in children secondary bacterial infection of inflamed lymph nodes may progress to suppurative lymphadenitis [2].

Cervical Fascial Spaces

Another important concept in understanding infectious disease in the neck is the facial envelopes or "spaces" of the neck (Table 14.2) [4, 5]. These fascia divide the neck into a collection of spaces. There is a superficial and a deep cervical fascia. The deep cervical fascia contains three layers, the superficial, the middle and the deep layers. The spaces superior to the hyoid are the parapharyngeal, submandibular, parotid, masticator, and peritonsillar spaces. Inferior to the hyoid is the anterior visceral space. Extending the length of the neck are the retropharyngeal, "danger" space, and prevertebral

Table 14.2 Cervical anatomy deep neck spaces

Relation to hyoid	Space	Borders of the fascial envelope	Space contents
Superior to hyoid	**Parapharyngeal** (Prestyloid compartment is anterior and Retrostyloid is posterior)	Base of skull superiorly, deep to the pharyngeal constrictor muscle, pretracheal fascia medially, hyoid bone inferiorly, and laterally the mandible, pterygoid muscles and the superficial cervical fascia	Prestyloid: fat, lymph nodes, connective tissue Retrostyloid: Carotid sheath; IX, X, XII cranial n; lymph nodes lateral to carotid sheath; and cervical sympathetic chain
	Submandibular (Submaxillary portion is above the mylohyoid and Sublingual portion is below)	Mucosa of the floor of mouth and the superficial layer of the deep cervical fascia	Submandibular and sublingual glands, lymph nodes, mylohyoid and digastric m, lingual n, hypoglossal n (cranial n XII)
	Parotid (incomplete space; connects with parapharyngeal space)	Superficial layer of the deep cervical fascia splits to enclose parotid gland (closure is incomplete)	Parotid gland, cranial n VII, lymph nodes
	Masticator (anterior and lateral to the parapharyngeal space)	Superficial layer of the deep cervical fascia splits to enclose the mandible and muscles of mastication	Mandible (dental structures), masseter, temporalis, internal pterygoid, inferior alveolar vessels and nerves, mandibular nerve
	Peritonsillar (bordered by the tonsil, the tonsillar pillars and the superior constrictor muscles)	Not a fascial envelop	Tonsil
Inferior to hyoid	**Visceral vascular** (sometimes referred to as the "highway" of the neck and extends the length of the carotid sheath)	Space within carotid sheath composed of all three layers of deep cervical fascia; connects most neck contents	Carotid a, Jugular v, Vagus n (cranial n X)

(continued)

Table 14.2 (continued)

Relation to hyoid	Space	Borders of the fascial envelope	Space contents
Extend length of neck	**Retropharyngeal** (extends from the skull base to the first or second thoracic vertebra)	Space within the middle layer of the deep cervical fascia and the alar layer of the deep layer of the deep cervical fascia	Retropharyngeal nodes
	"Danger" space (skull base to posterior mediastinum; deep to the Retropharyngeal space)	Space within the alar and prevertebral layers of the deep cervical fascia and the alar division of the deep layer of the deep cervical fascia	Loose connective tissue
	Prevertebral (extends from the skull base to the coccyx; deep to the Danger space)	Space deep to the Danger space, within the prevertebral fascia; posterior to the alar division of the deep layer of the deep cervical fascia	Longus colli m

Key: *a* artery, *v* vein, *m* muscle

spaces. The source of infection as well as presenting signs and symptoms are impacted by the contents of the affected space [4]. Infectious processes can spread easily within the fascial space or envelope in which the disease originates, but can also extend to neighboring spaces as disease progresses. Extension of infection into the spaces that extend the length of the neck can spread disease far beyond its origin and thus cause life-threatening complications.

Clinical Manifestations, Evaluation and Management

Suppurative Cervical Lymphadenitis

Lymphadenitis is seen in association with a variety of pharyngeal, dental, skin or other head and neck infections [6]. Cervical adenitis with abscess formation or suppurative cervical lymphadenitis may develop in some cases of lymphadenopathy. Microorganisms penetrate the skin or mucosal surfaces of the head or neck and are cleared via lymphatic vessels to regional lymph nodes. In the lymph nodes T cell proliferation results node enlargement. In response to invasion of bacterial, viral, mycobacterial or fungal pathogens, additional inflammatory cells, specifically neutrophils, may be recruited to the site of infection. In most instances, disruption of mucosal tissues can result in subsequent invasion by group A streptococcus, other colonizing pathogens or oropharyngeal flora (anaerobes) In other instances pathogens invade the nodal tissue hematogenously, as might be the case with *Staphylococcus aureus*. Cervical lymphadenitis occurs as a result of host inflammatory responses to this invasion. Lymphadenitis may progress to abscess formation as the host defenses attempt to contain the infection. Typically abscess material consist of cellular debris from necrotic tissue, inflammatory cells and microorganisms. The inflammatory cellular infiltrate may form an abscess wall. Although most cervical lymphadenopathy is viral in etiology, suppuration of an inflamed lymph node is suggestive of primary or secondary bacterial infection with abscess formation. These infections are most often due to group A streptococcus and other streptococci, *S. aureus* or anaerobes as outlined in Table 14.3.

The diagnostic evaluation of a child with an inflammatory neck mass, suspected cervical neck abscess, or suspected deep neck infection involves a detailed history, physical examination, laboratory

Table 14.3 Laboratory and diagnostic evaluation

Test	Examples of positive findings	These findings may help diagnose
CBC with differential	Elevated white blood cell count and/or left shift	Infectious lesions
	Atypical lymphocytes	Mononucleosis or malignancy
C-reactive protein	Elevated	Non-specific but helpful for following response to therapy; if normal, consider non-inflammatory mass
Sedimentation rate	Elevated	Non-specific but helpful for following response to therapy
		If normal, consider non-inflammatory mass
Rapid Strep or throat culture	Positive for Streptococcus pyogenes or group A Streptococcus	Strep throat and adenitis
Rapid influenza test	Positive	Acute influenza adenitis, but does not rule our secondary bacterial adenitis
Rapid adenovirus test	Positive	Acute adenoviral adenitis but does not rule out secondary bacterial adenitis
Cat scratch serology	Elevated *Bartonella henselae* or *B. quintana* titers	Cat Scratch disease
EBV serology	Elevated EBV VCA IgM	Acute mononucleosis syndrome
CMV serology	Elevated CMV IgM	Acute mononucleosis syndrome
Tuberculin skin test	Induration and erythema	Tuberculosis or non-tuberculous mycobacterial infection (see Chap. 13)
Interferon gamma release assay (IGRA)	Positive	Tuberculosis (see Chap. 13)

studies and if indicated, diagnostic imaging. Helpful historical data includes the age of the child, the duration of illness and mass, the specific associated symptoms involving the upper respiratory tract, and the presence of any symptoms suggestive of a systemic process [7]. Furthermore it is helpful to determine if there has been a change in size or consistency (firm vs. soft) of the mass, presence of fever, recent upper respiratory infection. An exposure history is important to determine if the child has had any animal contact, specifically with kittens or cats, close contact with anyone at risk for tuberculosis, or household members with recurrent boils or soft tissue infection as might be present in cases of methicillin resistant *S. aureus* (MRSA).

The physical inspection of the neck should include the dimensions and location (midline or lateral) of the mass. If the lesion is lateral then it is further described by nodal group or "level" as outlined in Table 14.1. The presence of an overlying discoloration, sinus or fistula, tenderness, palpable consistency (i.e. soft or firm), and its mobility, including the direction of mobility is also important. Tender lesions are commonly inflammatory and a soft or fluctuant consistency is suggestive of either an infected cyst or an abscess. Careful inspection of nasal passages, pharynx, and oral cavity (including teeth and gums) should be performed to determine a possible source of lymphadenitis. The presence of tonsillar exudate is not diagnostic of bacterial infection and can be present in viral (i.e. EBV or adenovirus) infection (Fig. 14.1). Likewise, the absence of exudate does not exclude infection due to group A streptococcus. Careful examination of the scalp and skin should be performed looking for evidence of infected bites, impetigo, or a papule as may be seen in cat scratch disease.

The remainder of the physical examination may provide additional clues as to the etiology of an inflammatory neck mass or a systemic illness. For instance, an enlarged spleen is often associated with mononucleosis and a conjunctivitis and rash may be present in children with adenovirus or Kawasaki disease. A scarlatiniform rash or diffuse erythroderma may be consistent with group A streptococcal infection.

Following a thorough history and physical examination additional diagnostic studies and ancillary laboratory testing may be needed prior to surgical intervention. In specific infections (i.e.

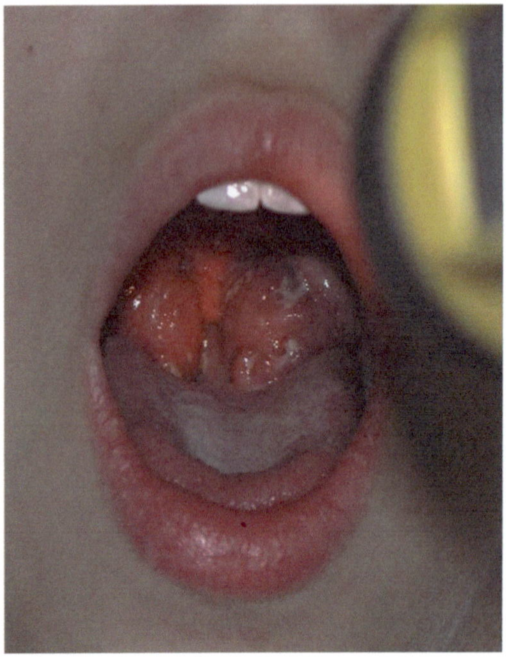

Fig. 14.1 Exudative pharyngitis with EBV infection

Table 14.4 Diagnostic imaging

Test	Examples of positive findings	Comments
Lateral neck ultrasound	Node enlargement, hypoechoic center suggestive of abscess	No radiation or sedation
		Less specific anatomic information
Computed tomography with contrast	Node enlargement, phlegmon, defined abscess, contiguous inflammation	Radiation, sedation for small children
Magnetic Resonance imaging with contrast	Node enlargement, phlegmon, defined abscess, contiguous inflammation, vascular extension or thrombosis	Sedation for small children

Table 14.5 Microbiology and treatment of lateral neck abscesses

Site of source infection	Common microbiology	Recommended empiric treatment (when culture data is not available)
Cervical lymphadenitis	Streptococcus pyogenes, other streptococci	Penicillin, Nafcillin or first generation cephalosporin cefazolin
	Staphylococcus aureus, including	Clindamycin or vancomycin in areas with high prevalence of MRSA
	Methicillin resistant Staphylococcus aureus	Penicillin or ampicillin
	Group B Streptococcus (GBS) in young infants less than 90 days of age	
Odontogenic structures	Viridans and other streptococci, Staphylococcus spp., Peptostreptococcus spp., Bacteroides spp., anaerobes	Penicillin G+metronidazole
		Clindamycin
Lateral neck, source unknown	Streptococci and Staphylococci including MRSA anaerobes	Penicillin, Nafcillin or first generation cephalosporin cefazolin
		Clindamycin or vancomycin in areas with high prevalence of MRSA

tuberculosis) this may prevent unnecessary surgery. Table 14.4 summarizes diagnostic and laboratory testing that may be useful in evaluating a child with neck abscess or deep neck infection.

Diagnostic imaging can help evaluate the presence of suppuration in cervical lymphadenitis and may localize a defined abscess within and inflammatory mass. Ultrasound can be helpful in differentiating cellulitic processes from more evolved abscesses. Contrast enhanced CT can provide additional information about the extent of disease, the presence of a mature abscess collection and with an MRI extent of potential vascular complications or spread of disease to adjacent vascular structures can be detected. Diagnostic imaging may include: lateral neck radiograph, chest radiograph, CT scan, and MRI (Table 14.5) and is often performed prior to surgical intervention and if there is concern for deep neck infection.

Microbiology and Antimicrobial Therapy

Depending on the characteristics of the mass and stability of the patient, empiric antimicrobial therapy is initiated as further diagnostic evaluation is performed. Medical treatment for suspected bacterial lymphadenitis generally begins with empiric antibiotic therapy directed at common organisms, *Staphylococcus aureus* and Group A streptococci (Table 14.3). Suppurative lymphadenitis even with small abscesses may respond with medical therapy alone.

Surgical Intervention

Surgical intervention is performed for either diagnostic and or therapeutic indications. Diagnostic aspiration or incision and drainage should be considered in patients that are not responding to empiric antimicrobial therapy or in patients who may have an abscess due to unusual organisms, (i.e. immunocompromised host). Surgical treatment, usually incision and drainage, is required when lymphadenitis becomes suppurative and develops a significant abscess. Fluctuance and tense, discolored overlying skin may become evident on physical exam in palpable lymphadenopathy. Retrospective reviews of cervical lymphadenitis with abscess formation that required surgical drainage have suggested that young age (<4 years), fluctuance, large abscess (>4 cm) within the node, multiple ED visits for same problem and failure to improve while on appropriate antibiotics are features of cases that subsequently require surgical drainage [8, 9]. Needle aspiration for diagnosis and culture should be considered in cases of suspected *M. tuberculosis* and Bartonella infections as incision and drainage may result in a persistent draining cervical fistula. If atypical mycobacteria infection is suspected, excision rather than simple drainage to eradicate the diseased nodes is preferred (discussed in Chap. 13). Biopsy may be indicated when there are systemic symptoms such as weight loss and night sweats, or when there are other symptoms to suggest malignancy such as loss of cranial nerve function [2]. Biopsy of abscess wall in cases where malignancy is suspected can be performed by fine-needle aspiration [9], if available at your facility, or by open incisional or excisional biopsy. Surgical specimens should be processed for aerobic, anaerobic, mycobacterial and fungal stains and cultures as well as histopathology. Antimicrobial therapy then should be modified based on the culture and susceptibility results and the clinical course of the patient. Duration of therapy is dictated by the clinical course of the patient but generally is 10–14 days following abscess drainage provided the patient is afebrile and clinically improved. In many instances of suppurative cervical lymphadenitis, once the patient is afebrile and oral intake is adequate, antibiotic therapy can be changed to an equivalent oral agent to complete the antibiotic course.

Deep Neck Space Infections

Deep neck space infections either involve the deep cervical chain (Table 14.1) or other deep neck spaces (Table 14.2). Deep neck space infections are potentially life threatening because of critical structures in these areas or the potential to disseminate beyond the neck to the mediastinum. Deep neck

Table 14.6 Signs and symptoms of deep neck infections

Site of infection (space)	Common signs and symptoms	Special considerations
Submandibular, Submaxillary portion	Sore throat	Less likely to cause airway impairment than sublingual compartment infection
	Trismus	
	Swelling, edema, erythema inferior to the mandible	
Submandibular, Sublingual portion	Swelling under chin	"Ludwig's angina"—infection in sublingual component of space
	Fullness in floor of mouth	Risk for airway compromise
	Swelling of tongue base with airway compromise	Commonly odontogenic source
Parotid	Sore throat	Risk factors: decreased salivary flow (due to medications or dehydration), immune compromise, poor oral hygiene. May be due to parotid duct obstruction with salivary stone
	Trismus	
	Swelling, edema, erythema in parotid region	
	Tenderness of parotid gland	
	Purulence at parotid duct	
Masticator	Sore throat	Usually odontogenic source
	Trismus	
	Swelling, edema, erythema over lateral mandible ramus	
Peritonsillar	Sore throat	Usual source: Tonsillitis (bacterial and viral, such as EBV)
	Trismus	(See Chap. 10 for detailed information.)
	Odynophagia	
	Fever	
	Fullness at anterior tonsillar pillar	
	Deviation of uvula to unaffected side	
Parapharyngeal	Sore throat	Wide range of source infections: pharyngitis, tonsillitis, parotitis, otitis/mastoiditis, and odontogenic infections
	Trismus	Extension into Visceral vascular space is an extremely serious complication (see below)
	Neck pain	
	Odynophagia	
	High fevers	
	May impact airway	
Retropharyngeal	Sore throat	Usual source: Retropharyngeal lymphadenitis or pharyngeal trauma
	Trismus	May use lateral soft tissue radiograph as screening tool
	Neck pain	Extension into Danger space is an extremely serious complication (see below)
	Odynophagia	
	Lateral fullness behind tonsil (stops at midline)	
	Airway compromise (esp. young children)	

(continued)

Table 14.6 (continued)

Site of infection (space)	Common signs and symptoms	Special considerations
Visceral vascular (carotid sheath/Lincoln's highway)	(See parapharyngeal above)	Source: parapharyngeal infections
	No characteristic signs/symptoms	Complications: Suppurative thrombophlebitis, carotid artery aneurysm, erosion and rupture.
	Fever/Sepsis	Extension into mediastinum possible
	Neck pain or Torticollis	
"Danger" space	(See retropharyngeal above)	Source: retropharyngeal infections
	Fever	Complications: extension into mediastinum with mediastinitis, pleural effusion and empyema
	Sepsis	
Prevertebral	Neck pain	Usual source: cervical spine disease or local instrumentation of trachea or esophagus
	Fever	May result from hematogenous source
	Fullness in posterior oropharynx (crosses midline) dysphagia	
	Neurologic symptoms (cervical root pain, neuropathy, etc.)	

space infections can be associated with airway compromise, necrotizing fasciitis and spread disease into the thorax. Odontogenic infections can be an especially dangerous source of these infections.

When compared to suppurative lymphadenitis, the signs and symptoms of deep neck space infections may be more subtle on physical examination thus a high index of suspicion must be maintained when evaluation children with fever with neck pain or torticollis. The clinical features of a palpable mass with associated erythema and edema may be absent, yet trismus, torticollis, and odynophagia in addition to sore throat or neck pain are common with certain deep neck space infections. In some instances there are no localizing signs or symptoms but severe systemic illness associated with a history of poor dentition, preceding sore throat or rapidly progressive systemic signs of sepsis as is common in Lemierre's disease or necrotizing fasciitis. Understanding the important anatomic structures contained in specific neck spaces (Table 14.2) can help determine the affected site and or source of such infection; for example cranial neuropathies can provide localizing information. Characteristic symptoms associated with infections in the deep cervical spaces are outlined in Table 14.6 [5, 10].

When evaluating a child for suspected deep neck infection one must first assess the patency of the airway. Given the smaller airway in young children if there is any respiratory distress the airway must first be secured. Presence of airway obstruction clearly changes the management algorithm: if the airway is compromised the airway must be assessed and the obstruction resolved or bypassed prior to further evaluation into the etiology and treatment of the mass. This may require intubation or tracheostomy. Certain deep neck space infections, such as sublingual space infections, are more likely to develop airway distress due to the location of infection. Patients with sepsis may require intensive care management and airway control due to development of septic shock.

A detailed history and physical examination, much like that described above for suppurative lymphadenitis, should be performed with additional details depending on the suspected site. History of retropharyngeal trauma, odontogenic infection, or underlying medical conditions should be considered in patients undergoing evaluation for deep neck space infection. Diagnostic and ancillary laboratory studies are similar to cervical adenitis as summarized in Table 14.4. Given that deep neck infections are often associated with sepsis, blood cultures for aerobic and anaerobic pathogens should be performed. Other features of sepsis, such as coagulopathy, should be included in the diagnostic evaluation.

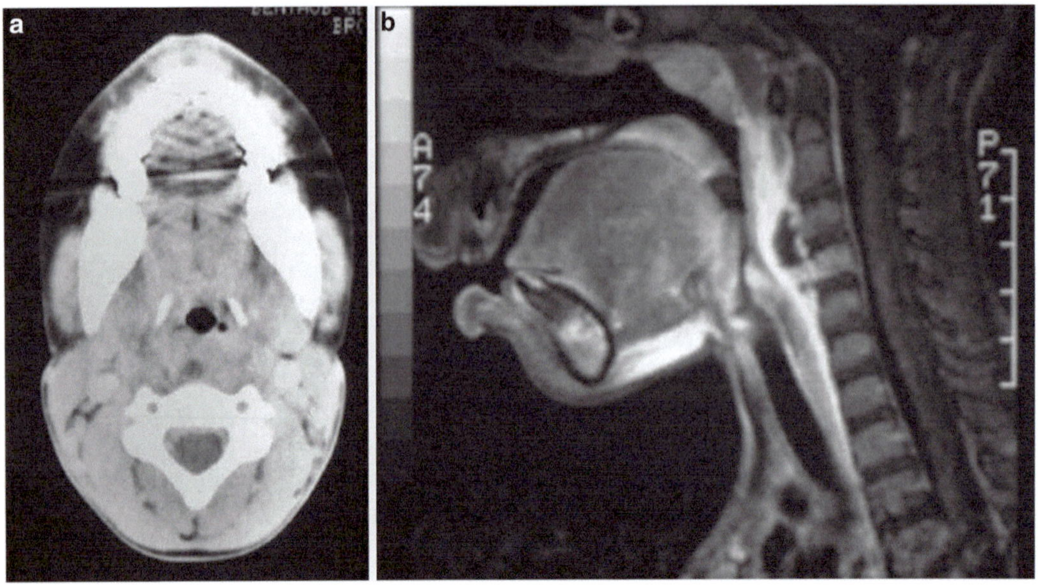

Fig. 14.2 (**a**) 5-year-old who presented with fever and torticollis for 7 days. CT of the neck revealed a prevertebral abscess. (**b**) 5-year-old who presented with fever and torticollis for 7 days. MRI shows prevertebral abscess and C4 osteomyelitis. The abscess was drained and cultures grew MRSA

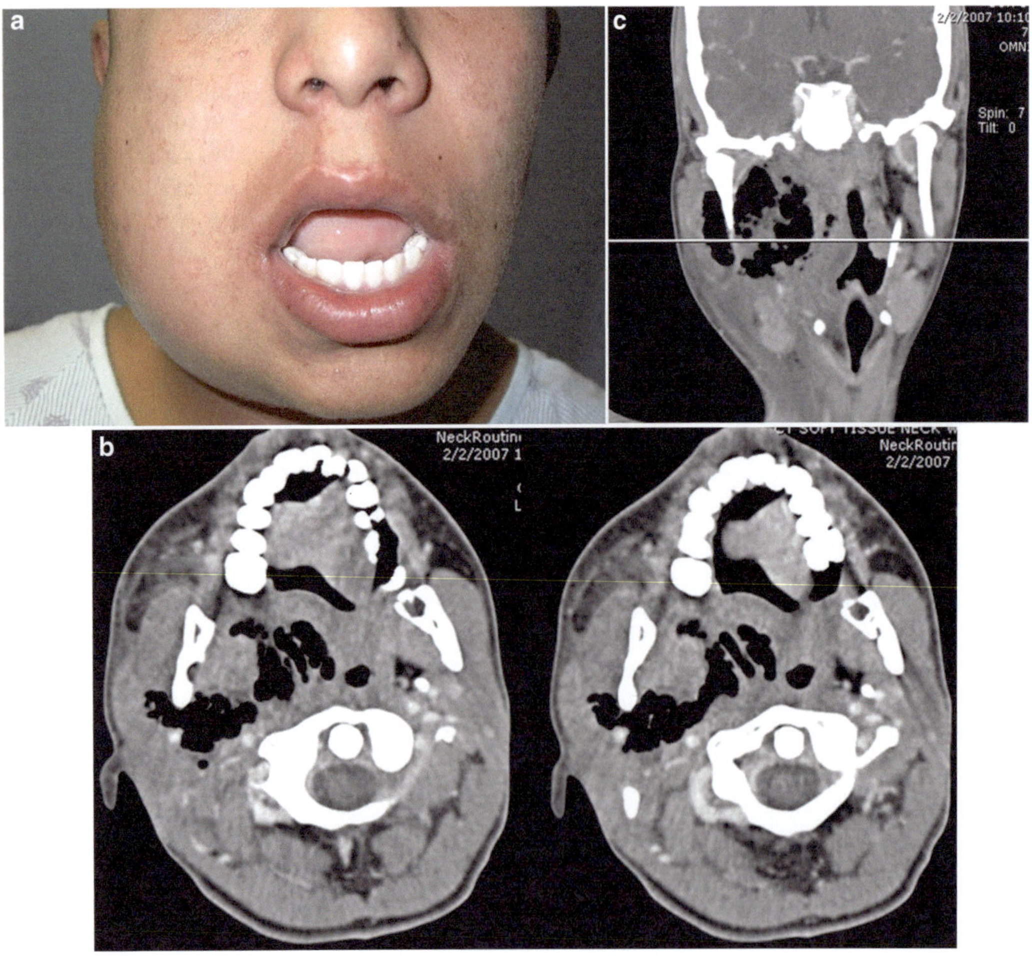

Table 14.7 Microbiology and treatment of deep neck abscesses which may be polymicrobial

Site of source infection	Common microbiology	Recommended empiric treatment (when culture data is not available)
Acute suppurative lymphadenitis	Streptococcus pyogenes (group A streptococci), other streptococci	Penicillin, Nafcillin or first generation cephalosporin cefazolin
	Staphylococcus aureus, including Methicillin resistant Staphylococcus aureus	Clindamycin or vancomycin in areas with high prevalence of MRSA
Odontogenic structures	Viridans and other streptococci, Staphylococcus spp., Peptostreptococcus spp., Bacteroides spp., anaerobes	Penicillin G + metronidazole
		Clindamycin
Tonsillitis or Parapharyngeal trauma	Group A streptococcus, other Streptococci, Staphylococcus aureus	Penicillin, Nafcillin or first generation cephalosporin cefazolin
	Fusobacteria, Prevotella, other oral anaerobes	Clindamycin or vancomycin in areas with high prevalence of MRSA
		Clindamycin or metronidazole
Sialadenitis (parotid or submandibular)	Staphylococcus aureus, including MRSA	Nafcillin, clindamycin, vancomycin
	Haemophilus influenzae, anaerobes	Second or third generation cephalosporin
		Metronidazole
Otitis/Sinusitis	Streptococcus pneumoniae, Haemophilus influenzae, S. aureus, including MRSA, Fusobacterium, Prevotella, other anaerobes	Third generation cephalosporin, vancomycin, metronidazole
Deep neck, source unknown	Often odontogenic source: Viridans and other streptococci, Staphylococcus aureus Peptostreptococcus spp., Fusobacterium, Prevotella, Bacteroides spp., other anaerobes	Penicillin metronidazole

The deep structures of the neck are not easily examined therefore the evaluation of a patient with a suspected deep neck space infection often requires diagnostic imaging such as a computed tomography (CT) with contrast given the severity of these infections. Plain radiographs can be useful screening tools in a few situations, most notably for detecting retropharyngeal edema associated with retropharyngeal or parapharyngeal infections before committing a patient to a CT scan. The evaluation may also include magnetic resonance imaging (MRI) when vascular complications are suspected or additional information about the extent of soft tissue involvement is needed.

CT or MRI may be extended to the chest if there is concern for mediastinal extension or if suspicion for septic pulmonary emboli as in Lemierre's disease. Figures 14.2 and 14.3 illustrate the clinical spectrum of deep neck infections and the value of diagnostic imaging to define the extent and spread of such infections.

Deep neck infections, unlike lateral cervical nodal abscesses, may not be palpable. Retrospective and observational prospective reports have provided general guidance on evaluation of children with suspected deep neck infection [11]. Unless a defined abscess is detected on initial imaging empiric parenteral antibiotic therapy with antimicrobial therapy directed at likely pathogens with the understanding that deep neck infections are often polymicrobial (Table 14.7) [12]. Identifying the suspected source of infection can help direct medical management. Surgical intervention is usually considered

Fig. 14.3 (**a**) 14-year-old with 5 day history of fever, chills, jaw pain, progressive trismus and dysphagia. (**b**) Odontogenic infection associated with a deep neck space infection. A 3×0.7 cm fluid collection medial to the body of the mandible with a large collection of air in the adjacent floor of the mouth and right deep masticator space extending to the right parapharyngeal, retropharyngeal, parotid and submandibular spaces. Cultures of the abscess grew MRSA, *Streptococcus constellatus* and *Gamella morbillorum*. (**c**) There was also lateral deviation and narrowing of the airway

when the infectious process has evolved into a localized abscess collection, however some authors have suggested predictors of successful treatment with antibiotics alone [13]. Decision to proceed with surgical treatment, usually drainage via an open incision but occasionally a needle localized approach, depends on the size of the abscess, the patient's symptoms, and the presence of complications. The surgical approach is determined by the location of the abscess and the important surrounding structures. In an prospective, observational study of deep neck infections in children, Saluja et al noted that this clinical entity is challenging to diagnose and treat even with a practice guideline and criteria for CT interpretation [11]. Of 111 children being evaluated for deep neck infection with a

Table 14.8 Complications of deep neck space infections

Complication	Special notes
Airway distress	Especially with sublingual space infections (Ludwig's Angina)
	When patient exhibits dyspnea, airway evaluation is necessary, possibly including flexible nasopharyngoscopy, to determine if airway control is needed prior to evaluation of infection
Mediastinitis +/– empyema	Present with chest pain, dyspnea
	Widened mediastinum on CXR may suggest pericardial effusion and risk for cardiac tamponade
	Usually polymicrobial infections
Jugular vein suppurative thrombophlebitis (Lemierre's syndrome)	Maybe a source of septic pulmonary emboli
Deep vein thrombosis	Anticoagulation in some cases
Carotid artery aneurysm +/– erosion +/– rupture	Small "herald" bleeds may precede carotid rupture
Necrotizing fasciitis	Toxic appearance of patient
	Requires index of suspicion
	Usually anaerobic infection, commonly odontogenic source
	Requires surgical debridement
Cranial neuropathies	Requires index of suspicion to consider deep neck space infection when patient presents with acute cranial neuropathy

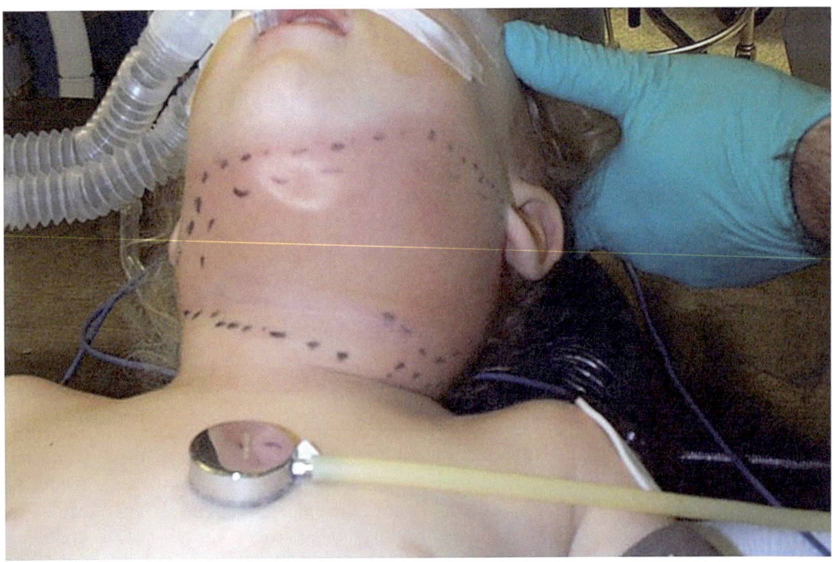

Fig. 14.4 Necrotizing fasciitis due to suppurative lymphadenitis

clinical practice guideline, 75 % had two or more CT scans as this disease process was in evolution prior to surgical drainage and clinical signs. Laboratory values and initial imaging often showed phlegmon and not abscess. Repeat imaging illustrated the maturing of abscess in 39 children and in 29 of those (74 %) frank pus was noted at surgery [11]. Those with an abscess noted on initial imaging, 85 % had purulent material drained at surgery. As noted by others, younger age and elevated WBC seemed to be associated with those with purulent material noted as time of incision and drainage.

Complicated Infections and Complications

Deep neck space infections are feared because of the potential for further spread of infection and resultant complications (Table 14.8) such as sepsis, mediastinitis, empyema, suppurative thrombophlebitis, septic pulmonary emboli, necrotizing fasciitis (Fig. 14.4), carotid artery pseudoaneurysm and cranial neuropathies [4]. The majority of deep neck infections and their complications in adults are due to odontogenic infections, [14, 15] however, in children retropharyngeal and parapharyngeal suppurative lymphadenitis is the leading cause in children [16–18].

References

1. Torsiglieri Jr AJ, Tom LW, Ross 3rd AJ, Wetmore RF, Handler SD, Potsic WP. Pediatric neck masses: guidelines for evaluation. Int J Pediatr Otorhinolaryngol. 1988;16(3):199–210.
2. Rosenfeld R. Cervical adenopathy. In: Bluestone CD, Stool SE, Kenna MA, editors. Pediatric otolaryngology, vol. 2. Philadelphia: W.B. Saunders; 1996.
3. Clary R, Lusk R. Neck masses. In: Bluestone CD, Stool SE, Kenna MA, editors. Pediatric otolaryngology, vol. 2. Philadelphia: W.B. Saunders; 1996.
4. Aynechi BB, Har-El G. Deep neck infections. In: Johnson JT, Rosen C, editors. Bailey's Head and Neck Surgery—Otolaryngology. 5th ed. Philadelphia: Elsevier; 2013. p. 794–813.
5. Chow A. Deep neck space infections. UpToDate 2014.
6. Nash M, Sobol SM. Neck masses. In: Frank LE, Sobol SM, editors. Essentials of otolaryngology. 2nd ed. New York: Raven Press; 1988. p. 314–5.
7. Wiatrak B. Clinical evaluation of the neck. In: Wetmore RF, Muntz HR, McGill TJ, editors. Pediatric otolaryngology: principles and practice pathways. New York: Thieme; 2000.
8. Sauer MW, Sharma S, Hirsh DA, et al. Acute neck infections in children: who is likely to undergo surgical drainage? Am J Emerg Med. 2013;31:906–9.
9. Liu ES, Bernstein JM, Sculerati N, Wu HC. Fine needle aspiration biopsy of pediatric head and neck masses. Int J Pediatr Otorhinolaryngol. 2001;60(2):135–40.
10. Hotaling AJ. Deep Neck Infections: Recognition, Evaluation, and Therapy. In: Cotton R, Myer C, editors. Practical Pediatric Otolaryngology. Philadelphia: Lippincott-Raven; 2000. p. 711–25.
11. Saluja S, Brietzke SE, Egan KK, et al. A prospective study of 113 deep neck infections managed using a clinical practice guideline. Laryngoscope. 2013;123:3211–8.
12. Brook I. Anaerobic bacteria in the upper respiratory tract and head and neck infections: microbiology and treatment. Anaerobe. 2012;18(2):214–20.
13. Bolton M, Wang W, Hahn A. Predictors for successful treatment of pediatric deep neck infections using antimicrobials alone. Pediatr Infect Dis J. 2013;32:1034–6.
14. Flynn TR, Shanti RM, Levi MH, et al. Severe odontogenic infections, part 1: prospective report. J Oral Maxillofac Surg. 2006;64:1093–103.
15. Flynn TR, Shanti RM, Hayes C. Severe odontogenic infections, part 2: prospective outcomes study. J Oral Maxillofac Surg. 2006;64:1104–13.
16. Crisaru-Soen G, Komisar O, Aizenstein O, et al. Retropharyngeal and parapharyngeal abscess in children—epidemiology, clinical features and treatment. Int J Pediatr Otorhinolaryngol. 2010;74:1016–20.
17. Neff L, Newland J, Sykes KJ, et al. Microbiology and antimicrobial treatment of pediatric cervical lymphadenitis requiring surgical intervention. Int J Pediatr Otorhinolaryngol. 2013;77:817–20.
18. Georger E, Gauthier A, Brugel L, et al. Acute cervical lymphadenitis and infections of the retropharyngeal and parapharyngeal spaces in children. BMC Ear Nose Throat Disord. 2014;14.

Chapter 15
Infected Congenital Neck Lesions

Valerie Cote and Claire Bocchini

Introduction

Congenital neck lesions are defined as any cervical cysts, sinuses or fistulae that are present at birth and are the result of a failure of obliteration of normal developmental structures. They can present early in life or through adulthood, usually as an asymptomatic neck mass, but also frequently as infectious processes. While some deep neck infections of congenital origin have characteristic patterns of presentation and can be recognized at the time of the initial infection, many can be hard to distinguish from suppurative lymphadenitis or infections that have spread along fascial planes of the neck from common head and neck sources. Specific clinical and radiological characteristics therefore must be called into play to establish the correct diagnosis for any deep neck infection. This is of upmost importance as the management may differ between a simple infectious versus infected congenital origin. If the diagnosis of an infected congenital neck lesion is initially missed and the lesion is improperly treated, it will have a high likelihood of recurrence, which can lead to additional inflammation and scarring making future surgical management difficult with a higher risk of surgical complications.

The most commonly encountered congenital neck lesions with a potential for infection include thyroglossal duct cysts, branchial cleft anomalies, dermoid cysts, preauricular sinuses, laryngoceles and thymic cysts. Congenital vascular malformations such as lymphatic malformations can also present as deep neck infections and should be included in the differential diagnosis. This chapter aims to cover the embryology, clinical presentation, diagnostic imaging, microbiology and therapeutic approaches of each of these congenital pathologies.

V. Cote, M.D., C.M., F.A.A.P., F.R.C.S.C. (✉)
Division of Pediatric Otolaryngology, University of Connecticut School of Medicine, Farmington, Hartford, CT, USA

Connecticut Children's Medical Center, 282 Washington Street, 2L, Hartford, CT 06106, USA
e-mail: vcote@connecticutchildrens.org

C. Bocchini, M.D.
Department of Pediatrics, Section of Infectious Diseases, Baylor College of Medicine, 1102 Bates St., Suite 1150, Houston, TX 77030, USA

Texas Children's Hospital, Houston, TX, USA
e-mail: cb135591@bcm.edu

T.A. Valdez, J.G. Vallejo (eds.), *Infectious Diseases in Pediatric Otolaryngology*,
DOI 10.1007/978-3-319-21744-4_15

Thyroglossal Duct Cysts

Thyroglossal duct cysts (TGDC) rank as the most common congenital cervical anomaly and the second most common neck mass found in children after inflammatory masses [1, 2]. Their prevalence in the general population is estimated at around 7 % [1]. While many remain asymptomatic, some authors have reported the rate of infection within TGDC at 40 %, making them the most frequently encountered infected congenital neck lesions [3].

Embryology

The thyroid gland forms from the fusion of the median thyroid anlage to the lateral thyroid anlage between the third and fifth weeks of embryonal development. The median thyroid anlage comprises most of the gland and develops from an endodermal diverticulum located between the anterior and posterior muscle complexes of the tongue, which then descends into the neck from the base of the tongue, leaving behind an elongated duct. The lateral thyroid anlage comprise the thyroid C cells and are derived mostly from the fourth branchial pouches. As the thyroid descends into the neck, its pathway encounters a rudimentary hyoid bone and either passes through or anterior to it. Once the thyroid gland takes its final pretracheal position inferior to the cricoid cartilage, the so-called thyroglossal duct obliterates, leaving two remnants at its ends: the foramen cecum proximally and the pyramidal lobe of the thyroid distally. If the mesodermal anlage of the hyoid bone forms before the duct has completed its obliteration, a cyst persists [1]. However, any part of the duct that fails to obliterate completely can form a cyst, and a meta-analysis by Allard in 1982 found that 60 % of the TGDC were found between the hyoid and the thyroid cartilage, 24 % were suprahyoid, 13 % were suprasternal and 2 % were intralingual [3, 4]. The remnant has also been described within the thyroid gland itself [5]. In addition, some thyroid glands fail to completely descend and thyroid tissue remains within the TGDC and can represent the only functional thyroid tissue in certain patients.

Clinical Presentation

Most TGDC present during childhood, with more than half becoming clinically significant before age 10 years [6]. The most classic presentation is that of a painless midline cystic neck mass at the level of the hyoid bone, which moves with tongue protrusion and swallowing (Fig. 15.1). Some variants can be observed at various levels of the neck and a TGDC can occasionally present as a lateral cystic neck mass. TGDC are lined with ductal epithelium, but as they can also contain solid thyroid tissue, they can present as malignancy in 1 % of cases. The most common malignancy is well-differentiated papillary thyroid carcinoma in over 80 % of cases [7].

TGDC frequently become infected, usually causing a painful erythematous swelling or mass found in the midline or occasionally just left of the midline of the neck [3, 8, 9]. The mass can be associated with regional lymphadenopathy. While most patients lack fever, chills, or signs of systemic disease, abscesses frequently occur [10, 11]. TGDC have a tendency for getting recurrently infected and abscesses will commonly drain to the anterior neck, either spontaneously or via a previous site of surgical drainage. Patients with TGDC will complain of various symptoms including dysphagia, cough, airway obstruction, or a foul taste in the mouth if the TGDC spontaneously drains at the level of the foramen cecum [2, 3]. Complications of TGDC include deep neck infections, which can include

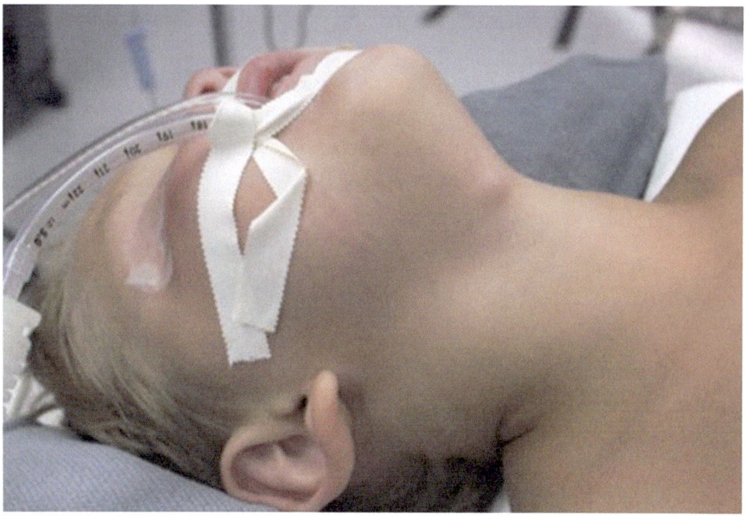

Fig. 15.1 Thyroglossal cysts typically present as midline neck masses at the level of the hyoid bone. (Reprinted from Seminars in Pediatric Surgery, Vol.15, Foley DS, Fallat ME, Thyroglossal duct and other congenital midline cervical anomalies, pp. 70–5, Copyright (2006) with permission from Elsevier.)

extension of the lesion posterior to the hyoid bone with involvement of the preepiglottic space [12]. In rare cases this can result in airway compromise and death [10]. Extension of the infection into the mediastinum, lungs, and visceral vascular space has also been reported [12, 13].

Diagnosis

While a complete history and physical examination can suffice in the workup of a TGDC, imaging is frequently required to confirm the diagnosis. When an infected TGDC is suspected, a contrasted computerized tomography (CT) or magnetic resonance imaging (MRI) of the neck is recommended to define the anatomy and evaluate the extent of the infection.

A comprehensive workup for a TGDC may also include a neck ultrasound and a TSH level. If a midline solid mass or elevated TSH levels are found, a scintiscan can be helpful in the diagnosis of a median ectopic thyroid. Some have advocated that a scintiscan should be performed on any patient with a TGDC, but the radiation exposure and the low yield of positive results mean that a more targeted approach is clinically sound.

Microbiology

TGDC infections occur as a result of accumulation of secretions from the thyroglossal duct epithelial cells. This accumulation leads to dilation of the duct and development of the cystic structure. Low oxygen tension within the cyst and lack of drainage of the cyst secretions leads to bacterial overgrowth. As the cyst is usually connected to the mouth floor, organisms that are frequently identified in infected TGDC are primarily oropharyngeal flora, including streptococcal species and oral anaerobes such as *Prevotella*, *Porphyromonas* spp, *Bacteriodes* spp and *Peptostreptococcus* spp [3, 10, 14–16]. Skin flora including *Staphylococcus aureus* and *Streptococcus pyogenes* are also frequently identified [3, 10, 15–17]. Additional organisms that have been identified in the literature include *Haemophilus influenzae* [18], *Streptococcus pneumoniae* and *Neisseria meningitidis* [19]. Group B streptococcus was reported in an infant with an infected TGDC [20]. A very unusual TGDC infection with coccidioidomycosis has also been reported [21].

Therapeutic Approaches

Empirical antimicrobial therapy should include coverage for oropharyngeal flora. Options include clindamycin or the combination of ampicillin or amoxicillin plus a betalactamase inhibitor (i.e., ampicillin/sulbactam for IV therapy or amoxicillin/clavulanate for PO therapy). Rarely, patients will have severe or life-threatening infections and then most experts recommend ensuring adequate empirical coverage for methicillin-resistant *S. aureus* such as with vancomycin as part of the regimen while culture results are pending.

The route of antibiotic administration depends on the severity of the infection. Intravenous therapy is recommended for toxic-appearing children, children who are unable to tolerate oral therapy, or children who are at risk of respiratory compromise due to the location or severity of the infection. Oral therapy can be considered for children with only minor infections or in children who are clinically improved after initial intravenous therapy.

Definitive antimicrobial therapy should be directed by culture and susceptibility results. Therefore needle aspiration of an acutely infected cyst early in the course of treatment is optimal. Purulent material should be sent for gram stain and aerobic culture, anaerobic culture, fungal culture, mycobacteria culture, and histopathology review to optimize the opportunity to identify the causative organism(s) responsible for the infection as well as to differentiate a TGDC from other congenital neck lesions [10]. Findings on histopathology review that are consistent with (but not specific for) the diagnosis of TGDC include colloid, macrophages, lymphocytes, neutrophils, and ciliated columnar cells [22].

Given that TGDC are a source of chronic inflammation, they are at risk for infection, and they may become malignant, elective surgical excision is the treatment of choice. Complete excision of the entire thyroglossal duct, including the central portion of the hyoid bone and a core of tissue from the muscle at the base of tongue, is paramount to a successful surgery and significantly reduces the risk of postoperative infection and recurrence. A core excision at the base of tongue is recommended since it has been demonstrated that the duct splits into ductules at that level for many patients with a TGDC. Incomplete resections can lead to recurrences in as many as 70 % of cases [2, 6].

The management of infected TGDC differs from standard neck abscesses. Given the need to subsequently operate on any diagnosed TGDC, a more conservative approach including antimicrobial therapy and needle aspiration is recommended. Most patients respond adequately to this approach. Children with progressive induration or airway compromise, or who are critically ill, may require emergent incision and drainage, but this should be avoided if possible to prevent seeding of ductal cells. Other children with fluctuant abscesses not amenable to antimicrobial therapy alone should undergo complete surgical excision when clinically feasible. Complete surgical excision is generally preferred over incision and drainage, as incision and drainage procedures have been associated with a higher risk of recurrence and can obscure landmarks and damage tissue planes therefore making it more difficult to excise the congenital lesion in the future [2, 15].

Children who are treated with antimicrobial therapy alone should undergo surgical removal of the TGDC and the entire length of the tract after the inflammation has completely resolved (usually approximately 6 weeks after completing antimicrobial therapy). Timing of this surgery can occasionally be challenging given that recurrent inflammation and infection of TGDC is common. Sistrunk procedures done on previously incised and drained TGDC should remove all of the operated skin and

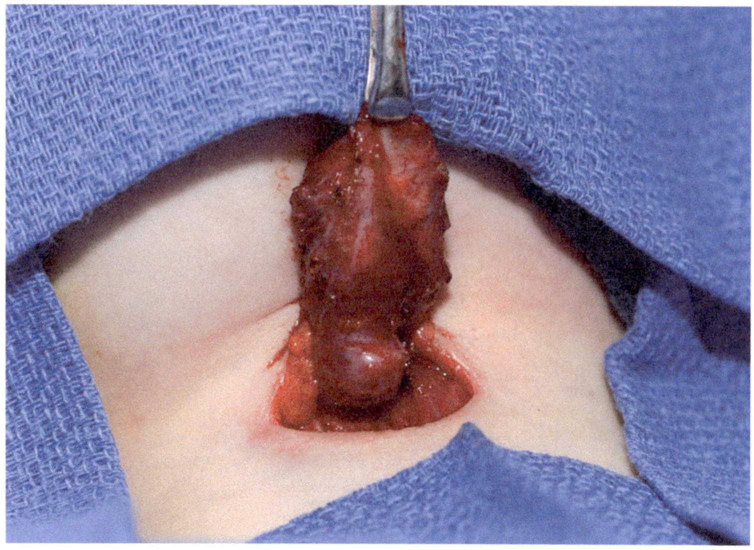

Fig. 15.2 Infected thyroglossal duct cyst in situ with a large walled-off abscess inferiorly in the neck

subcutaneous tissue via an elliptical excision [2]. Figure 15.2 presents an infected thyroglossal duct cyst specimen in situ with a walled-off abscess inferiorly.

Controversy exists regarding the management of median ectopic thyroids. Treatment options include medical treatment with suppressive doses of exogenous thyroid hormone or full resection with postoperative thyroid replacement [2]. Given the need to administer thyroid hormone in both cases and the small but present risk of malignancy in exogenous tissue over a patient's lifetime, many clinicians choose the surgical path for their patients.

Branchial Cleft Cysts, Sinuses and Fistulae

Branchial arch anomalies rank as the second most common congenital cervical anomaly found in children, at 30 % of all congenital head and neck lesions [23]. They comprise cysts, sinuses and fistulae from the first, second, third and fourth branchial arch. Second branchial arch anomalies represent 95 % of all branchial cleft malformations, followed by first, third and fourth branchial arch anomalies [1, 23].

General Branchial Embryology

Branchial arches which will form the head and neck structures start developing at 4 weeks of embryonal development as an external arch covered with ectoderm, an internal pouch covered with foregut endoderm and a midlayer of mesodermal tissue comprising a dominant artery, a nerve, a cartilage rod and muscle [2, 23] (Fig. 15.3). Four out of the six arches are well-defined and form into the structures of the head and neck. Branchial anomalies are remnants of these arches and clefts that fail to regress or obliterate normally [23]. Because the second, third and fourth branchial arches all exit at the cervical sinus of His, a failure of these structures to regress usually ends up in a similar external opening in the neck. However, each type of branchial arch anomaly has a distinct internal course and precise knowledge of its anatomy is crucial during surgical resection to avoid iatrogenic injury to important neck structures and to avoid recurrences [23].

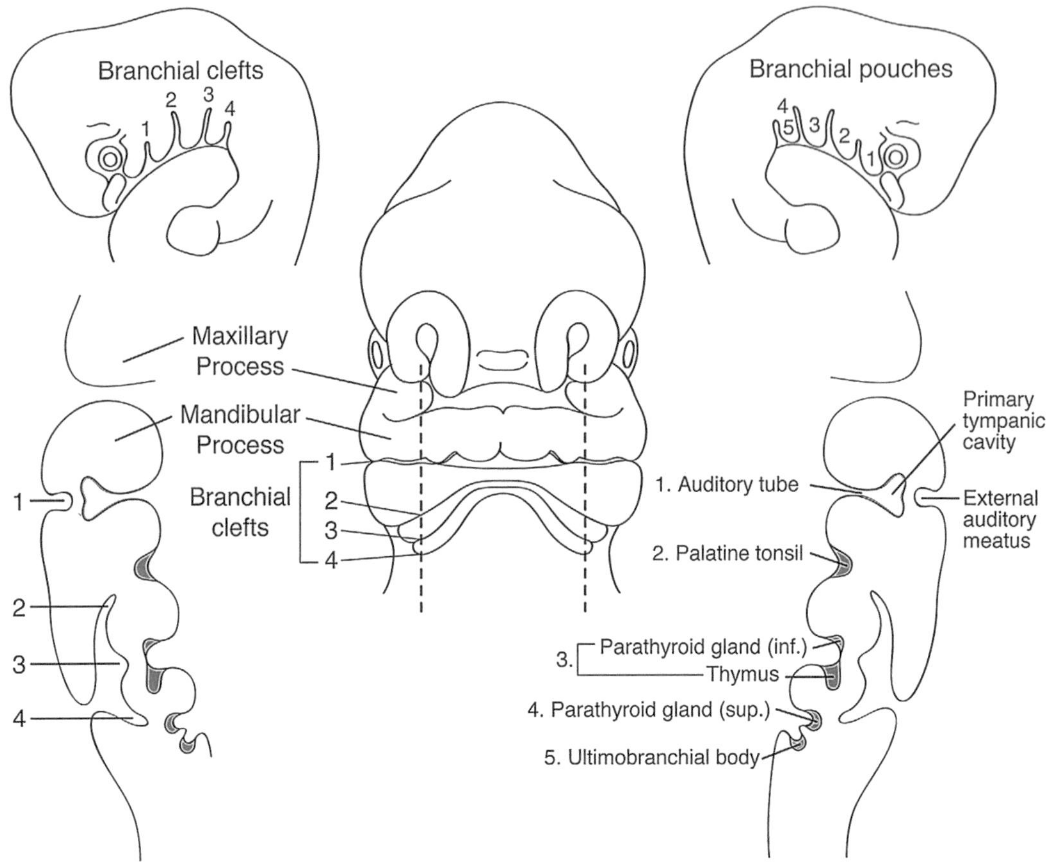

Fig. 15.3 Diagram of the branchial embryology of a 5-week embryo showing how important head and neck structures are derived from branchial clefts and pouches. (Reprinted from Seminars in Pediatric Surgery, Vol. 15, Waldhausen JH, Branchial cleft and arch anomalies in children, pp. 64–9, Copyright (2006) with permission from Elsevier.)

Branchial cysts are usually lined with ciliated and columnar respiratory epithelium, while tracts contain squamous epithelium. In addition, cysts can contain lymphoid tissue and cholesterol crystals within the mucous fluid. Squamous cell carcinoma can be found in branchial cleft lesions, especially in adulthood, although their incidence is extremely rare.

General Clinical Presentation

Infection is very common within branchial anomalies. About 20 % of them have been infected at least once by the time they are excised [24]. Patients with branchial cleft cysts can present with a history of a nontender mass in the neck that appears to fluctuate in size with upper respiratory tract infections [12]. Infected branchial cysts can progress to form abscesses or rupture spontaneously to form draining sinus tracts. Occasionally, internal spontaneous drainage occurs into the pharynx or external auditory meatus. Infants and children with infected branchial cysts can present with respiratory compromise or difficulty swallowing if the cysts enlarge enough to compromise the upper airway or digestive tract [10, 23, 25]. Additional complications include deep neck infections such as parapharyngeal abscesses and mediastinitis [26].

General Microbiology

The microbiology of infected branchial cleft cysts is similar to the microbiology of infected TGDC lesions. Oropharyngeal flora (including streptococcal species and anaerobes such as *Eikenella corrodens*, *Bacteroides* species, and *Actinomyces odontolyticus*), skin pathogens (such as *S. aureus* and *S. pyogenes*), and occasionally middle ear/upper respiratory pathogens (such as *H. influenzae* and *S. pneumoniae*) or gram negative enterics (such as *Klebsiella, Escherichia coli, Pseudomonas aeruginosa, Citrobacter,* and *Proteus*) are identified [27, 28]. More unusual organisms such as fungal, mycobacterial, and even parasitic organisms have been reported [28].

General Therapeutic Considerations

Empirical therapy should include the combination of ampicillin or amoxicillin plus a betalactamase inhibitor or clindamycin. For severe or life-threatening infections, broad-spectrum intravenous therapy is recommended, including empirical coverage for methicillin-resistant *S. aureus* such as with vancomycin plus ampicillin/sulbactam or piperacillin/tazobactam.

Definitive antimicrobial therapy should be directed by culture and susceptibility results. Therefore needle aspiration early in the course of treatment is optimal, and material obtained should be sent for gram stain and aerobic culture, anaerobic culture, fungal culture, mycobacteria culture, and histopathology review.

Surgical excision is recommended as the definitive treatment for all types of branchial anomalies, although specific considerations are detailed below. In order to prevent infections and scarring, early excision might be best, although waiting until the child is 2 or 3 years old might be optimal to minimize surgical and anesthetic risks. All acute infections should be primarily treated with antibiotics and needle aspiration, avoiding incision and drainage as much as possible to prevent field scarring [23]. Further surgical approaches are described below for individual branchial cleft types.

First Branchial Arch Anomalies

Embryology

The first branchial arch is also called the mandibular arch and forms the mandible, a portion of the maxillary process of the upper jaw and portions of the inner ear. The cleft and pouch form the external auditory canal, the Eustachian tube, the middle ear cavity and the mastoid air cells [23]. First branchial anomalies have a close relationship to the facial nerve and they can course deep, between branches or superficial to it. They are usually deep to the superficial lobe of the parotid gland (Fig. 15.4).

Clinical Presentation

A first branchial sinus or fistula can open at the level of the external auditory canal, the middle ear cleft, the postauricular region or the angle of the mandible [29]. First branchial cleft anomalies can be classified according to a few existing systems, the most commonly used being the Arnot and Work classification [30, 31] (Table 15.1).

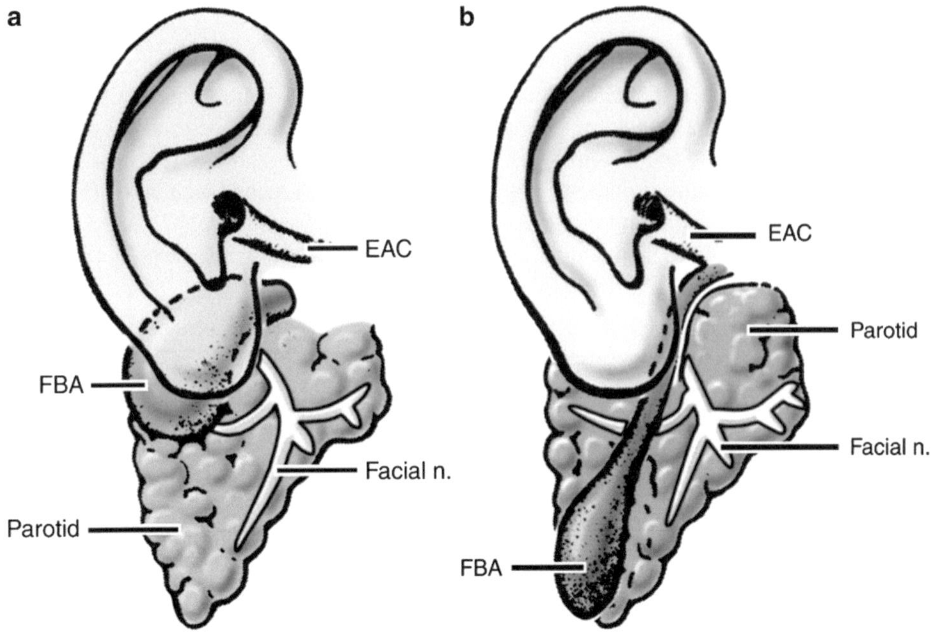

Fig. 15.4 Type 1 (**a**) and 2 (**b**) first branchial cleft anomalies (FBA) according to the Work classification. In type 1 anomalies, the opening of the cyst does not connect to the external auditory canal (EAC). In type 2 anomalies, the opening of the cyst connects to the EAC and is located within the deep lobe of the parotid gland (Reprinted from Neuroimaging Clin N Am, Vol 10, Mukherji SK, Fatterpekar G, Castillo M, et al. Imaging of congenital anomalies of the branchial apparatus, pp. 75–93, Copyright (2000), with permission from Elsevier.)

Table 15.1 Classification of first branchial cleft malformations

Type	Origin	Description
I	Cystic mass of purely ectodermal origin	Duplication of the membranous external auditory canal which courses lateral to the facial nerve
II	Cyst, sinus and/or fistula of ectodermal and mesodermal origin	Lesion may be found in a preauricular, postauricular, infraauricular or angle of the mandible location and it courses medial to the facial nerve

Source: Data from Arnot [30] and Work [31]

Many first arch anomalies are confused with preauricular sinuses and are therefore inadequately treated, with recurring infections preceding surgical excision. Symptoms include the presence of a chronically draining pit at the angle of the mandible, which turns into purulent drainage and submandibular adenitis if the tract becomes infected. Inflamed tracts within the parotid gland can present as a rapidly expanding mass, while tracts connecting to the external auditory canal or tympanic membrane can present with mucous or purulent otorrhea [23]. Complications from infections of a first branchial cleft cyst include damage to the parotid gland and/or facial nerve.

Diagnosis

First branchial cleft cysts are diagnosed clinically, but a contrasted CT or MRI can be very useful in determining the type of lesion and the depth of parotid extension, if it is suspected.

Therapeutic Approaches

Most first branchial cleft tracts lie superficial to the facial nerve, although some investigators have shown that sinuses more often lie superficial to the facial nerve while fistulae are more likely to pass deep to it. The tract is also more likely to be deep to the facial nerve in patients who are less than 6 months at the age of presentation. The safest approach to first branchial cleft cysts and tracts is therefore a conservative superficial parotidectomy with the use of a facial nerve monitor [29]. Involved skin and cartilage from the external auditory canal should also be excised. If the tract extends into the middle ear, this should be excised as well. Incomplete excisions are unfortunately common given the complex course of first branchial anomalies [23].

Second Branchial Arch Anomalies

Embryology

The second branchial arch is also called the hyoid arch and it forms portions of the hyoid bone. The pouch becomes the palatine tonsil and supratonsillar fossa [23]. As such, a fistulous second branchial arch anomaly can connect the tonsillar fossa to the anterior neck.

Clinical Presentation

A diagnosis of branchial cleft cyst is probable when a unilocular, nontranslucent cystic swelling is found in the deep anterior portion of the sternocleidomastoid muscle [12]. A fine needle aspirate containing mature squamous cell and cholesterol crystals is diagnostic [12]. Second cleft anomalies also usually present as a draining cyst of fistula at the lower anterior border of the sternocleidomastoid muscle, which can increase in size with upper respiratory tract infections. Contrary to many other congenital lesions of the head and neck, cysts are most commonly found in adults between the third and fifth decade of life. Fistulae are more easily diagnosed in infancy and childhood, as they are associated with chronic drainage. Infected tracts and cysts can lead to respiratory distress, torticollis and dysphagia [23].

Diagnosis

In order to differentiate second branchial cleft anomalies from masses such as macrocystic lymphatic malformations, lymphadenopathy, plunging ranula and others, an array of diagnostic imaging methods may be necessary, such as ultrasound, CT and MRI. The mass will usually appear as round and sharply demarcated with a thin to imperceptible wall and on ultrasound, a posterior acoustic enhancement is demonstrated in 70 % of cases. A "notch sign", which is an extension of the cyst between the internal and external carotid artery, just above the carotid bifurcation, is pathognomonic on CT scan [32].

Therapeutic Approaches

Second branchial arch anomalies can be excised via a transverse cervical approach, with the addition of a step-ladder approach to visualize the proximal portion of the tract as it enters the superior pharynx.

Third and Fourth Branchial Arch Anomalies

Embryology

The third branchial pouch divides into the inferior parathyroid gland from its dorsal component and the thymus from its ventral component [33]. The fourth branchial pouch forms the superior parathyroid gland by combining the dorsal portion of its caudal pharyngeal complex to the rudimentary fifth pouch. It is thought that it contributes to thyroid development and to the thymus gland as well [34]. The pharynx is formed from a combination of the third and fourth branchial cleft pouches.

Some controversy exists regarding third and fourth branchial pouch anomalies [33]. Some authors define third and fourth branchial anomalies based on the type of tissue that is contained within a cyst, while others define them based on the location of the internal opening of the sinus [23]. For both third and fourth branchial anomalies, the internal opening is at the pyriform sinus; the former opens at the base and the latter, at the apex. They both are more common in the left side of the neck, possibly due to the differential development of the arch vasculature. The course of each anomaly is theoretically predictable, with third arch anomalies passing deep to the internal carotid artery and glossopharyngeal nerve, entering the thyroid membrane above the internal branch of the superior laryngeal nerve and entering the pharynx at the pyriform sinus. Fourth arch anomalies should pass deep to the internal carotid artery, loop around the vessel associated with each side (subclavian artery on the right and aortic arch on the left), ascend to the level of the hypoglossal nerve and descend along the anterior border of the sternocleidomastoid muscle to enter the pharynx at the level of the pyriform apex beneath the superior laryngeal nerve.

Clinical Presentation

Third and fourth branchial cleft cysts generally present in a similar fashion as second branchial cleft cysts, although recurrent neck infections are an even more common presentation, usually after upper respiratory tract infections [33]. In addition, neonates can have airway compromise from large third and fourth branchial cysts [34]. Third branchial anomalies can rarely cause hypoglossal nerve palsy if they become infected. Fourth branchial anomalies are intimately associated with the thyroid gland and infections can manifest with suppurative thyroiditis [23]. In fact, as the thyroid is largely resistant to infection (given its extensive blood supply and lymphatics, strong capsule that protects it from surrounding structures, and high iodine content), any patient with acute or recurrent infectious thyroiditis should be evaluated for an underlying lower brachial cleft abnormality [35, 36] (Fig. 15.5). Skin openings for fourth branchial anomalies are thought to only result from infection and fistulous formations or inadequate surgery.

Diagnosis

Aside from a thorough history, physical examination and neck imaging, upper airway endoscopy and contrast studies can sometimes help in the diagnosis of third and fourth branchial cleft anomalies and rule out thyroiditis or suppurative lymphadenitis. These studies also help in sorting out the differential diagnosis, which includes infected neck nodes, hemangiomas, thyroid cysts, ectopic thyroid gland and cervical thymic cysts [37]. Neck imaging can be done by ultrasonography or contrasted CT or MRI, although CT seems to be best at demonstrating fistulae [23]. Upper airway endoscopy is used to identify the opening into the pyriform sinus and many authors suggest that all suspected cases must undergo direct laryngoscopic examination. Barium esophagram, if performed at least 6 weeks away from an acute infection, can demonstrate a sinus tract in the vast majority of cases [37] (Fig. 15.6).

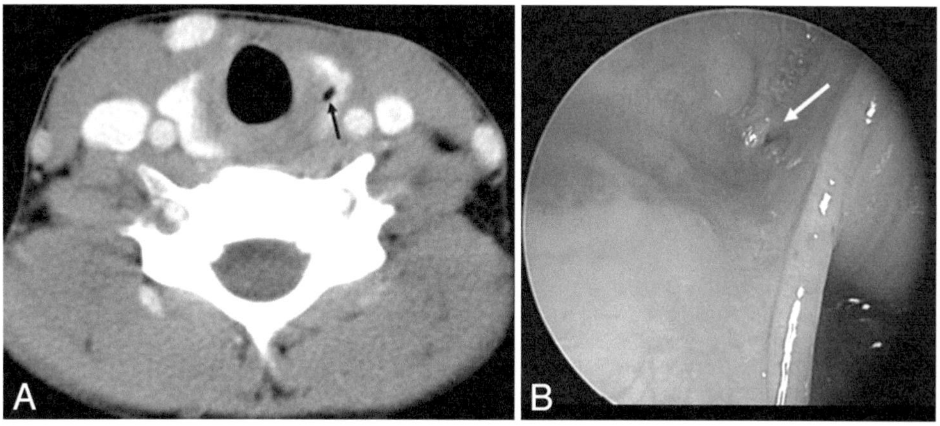

Fig. 15.5 (**a**) Contrast-enhanced axial CT scan at the level of the thyroid gland which is showing a fourth branchial sinus tract remnant within the left lobe of the thyroid (*black arrow*). (**b**) The opening of the sinus tract at the apex of the pyriform sinus can be seen on this pharyngoscopy image (*white arrow*) (From Thomas B, Shroff M, Forte V, et al. Revisiting Imaging Features and the Embryologic Basis of Third and Fourth Branchial Anomalies. AJNR Am J Neuroradiol 2010; 31(4):755–60. Republished with permission.)

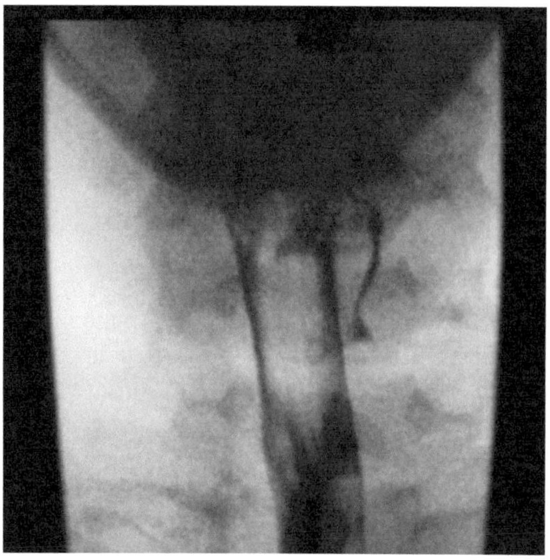

Fig. 15.6 Barium swallow demonstrating a left pyriform sinus tract (Reprinted from the International Journal of Pediatric Otolaryngology, Vol. 68, Pereira KD, Losh GD, Oliver D, et al., Management of Anomalies of the Third and Fourth Branchial Pouches, pp. 43–50, Copyright (2004), with permission from Elsevier.)

Therapeutic Approaches

Infected lesions should be managed by intravenous antibiotics with avoidance of incision and drainage as much as possible, as this can alter anatomic planes and complicate subsequent surgical excision [37]. Transverse cervical excision is usually the best and most definitive approach to treating non-infected third and fourth branchial arch anomalies. Chemo-cauterization of the internal opening has also been used, although there are no long-term results of the technique [23, 37]. An ipsilateral hemithyroidectomy must also be performed at the time of removal of fourth arch anomalies in order to remove the entire tract, which should be followed in its entirety, sometimes going through the thyroid cartilage itself via an oblique thyrotomy above the cricothyroid joint [34]. In all cases, closure of the pyriform sinus is key to preventing recurrence [34]. The rate of recurrence after surgical excision is around 15 %.

Dermoid Cysts

Dermoid cysts are superficial and have no connection with the oropharynx, and therefore infection of dermoid cysts is rare. Cysts can become enlarged with the accumulation of sebaceous material and can rupture secondary to this enlargement or due to trauma. Ruptured cysts can cause a granulomatous inflammation of the surrounding skin and/or soft tissue and need to be differentiated from other cervical neck cysts [14].

Embryology

Dermoid cysts are inclusion cysts that are lined by ectoderm with skin appendages (i.e. hair follicles or sebaceous glands) in their wall. They are germ cell lesions that contain epithelial and endodermal elements from entrapment along embryonal median and paramedian fusion planes [2].

Clinical Presentation

Dermoid cysts are usually painless lesions that grow slowly over time. Twenty percent of head and neck dermoids present in the cervical region. Occasionally, a dermoid cyst can mimic a TGDC, as it can be in close approximation to the hyoid bone and move with swallowing or tongue protrusion [2]. Enlargement of a dermoid cyst due to infection can cause pain with movement of the tongue. If the swelling increases enough, infected dermoid cysts can cause difficulties with feeding or even respiratory compromise.

Diagnosis

A history and physical examination can be supplemented with an ultrasound to aid in confirming the diagnosis of a dermoid cyst. They can appear on ultrasound with both solid and cystic components and they can also contain calcifications. On CT, the appearance of multiple hypoattenuating fat nodules can be pathognomonic of dermoid cysts. MRI can also be helpful in establishing the differential diagnosis of any given mass.

Microbiology

Infection of dermoid cysts is usually secondary to skin flora. Still, it is recommended to perform needle aspiration for cultures and histopathology review as infected dermoid cysts can be difficult to distinguish from TGDC by physical exam alone.

Therapeutic Approaches

Empirical antimicrobial therapy for infected dermoid cysts should target *S. aureus* and *S. pyogenes*. Dermoid cysts that are symptomatic, ruptured or need a definitive diagnosis should undergo full excision. A simple excision is sufficient in most cases, but in the rare cases where the dermoid cyst seems close or attached to the hyoid bone, a Sistrunk procedure should be performed to avoid an incomplete excision of an atypical TGDC [2].

Preauricular Sinuses

Preauricular sinuses are fairly common congenital anomalies of the head and neck and are present in approximately 1 % of the population worldwide, with their incidence varying greatly between different regions of the globe [38].

Embryology

The auricle develops from the six auditory hillocks of His of the first and second branchial arches during the sixth week of gestation. Preauricular sinuses are thought to either develop from a defective fusion of the hillocks, an incomplete closure of the dorsal part of the first pharyngeal groove or from an ectodermal folding [38]. The tract usually connects to the perichondrium of the auricular cartilage in its deepest portion.

Clinical Presentation

Preauricular sinuses are more commonly known as ear pits and can usually be found at the anterior margin of the ascending limb of the helix of the ear [38]. They are more common on the right side, although they can be bilateral in up to 50 % of cases [38, 39]. They can be asymptomatic or intermittently drain mucoid fluid or whitish debris. Infections are common and usually present with edema, erythema and pain in the preauricular area, and there will usually be purulent drainage coming from the pit.

Preauricular sinuses can be either sporadic or inherited as an autosomal dominant pattern with reduced penetrance and variable expression [38]. They are rarely associated with syndromes such as the branchio-oto-renal syndrome.

Preauricular sinuses are usually lined with stratified squamous epithelium with hyperkeratosis and parakeratosis and may contain sebaceous glands, sweat glands and hair follicles [38]. Granulation tissue can replace the lining of repeatedly infected preauricular sinuses.

Diagnosis

The only workup necessary for patients with preauricular sinuses is a thorough history and physical exam. In patients for whom a syndrome is suspected, an audiogram should be ordered. A renal ultrasound has been proposed to be reserved for children with preauricular sinuses and one of the following features: another malformation or dysmorphic feature, a family history of deafness, auricular and/or renal malformations, or a maternal history of gestational diabetes [38].

Microbiology

The most common etiology of infections of preauricular pits, sinuses, and cysts is *S. aureus* [40].

Therapeutic Approaches

Treatment of infected lesions should include warm soaks, drainage of fluctuant abscesses (with purulent material sent for cultures), and anti-staphylococcal therapy such as cephalexin, clindamycin, or TMP/SMX. Ultimately, patients will require surgical excision to prevent recurrence of infection, but most experts recommend waiting until after the acute infection has resolved [40].

Completely asymptomatic preauricular sinuses may be observed, but many advocate their complete excision if they are draining or after any infection. It is advised to treat any infection first with proper antibiotic coverage and plan excision in a quiescent phase. However, some preauricular sinuses become chronically infected and a wide local excision may need to be planned. In some cases of acute infection that does not respond to antibiotics, an incision and drainage may be necessary, but this increases the risk of recurrence [41]. Recurrence rate when the excision is performed in a non-infected preauricular sinus has been found in one series of patients at 8.2 %, while it is at 15.8 % when the site is infected at the time of surgery [41].

The sinus tract is usually found lateral, superior and posterior to the facial nerve and the parotid gland. Injection of the tract with methylene blue can be performed to help identify its course, especially in cases where the preauricular sinuses have been repeatedly infected and are encased in scar tissue. A lacrimal probe can also help and when used with dye injection, there is a decrease in the risk of recurrence [41]. Helical crus cartilage adherent to the deepest portion of the preauricular sinus must be excised with the tract in order to avoid recurrence. The risk of recurrence is more than fourfold higher if this is not performed [41].

Thymic Cysts

Cervical thymic cysts are rare congenital lesions that usually present in the first decade of life. They represent less than 1 % of all cervical neck masses in children [42].

Embryology

The thymus develops from the ventrolateral aspect of the third branchial pouches during the sixth week of embryonal development. Thymic cysts come from ectopic thymic tissue, which results from failure of descent of the thymic anlage from either side of the neck into the mediastinum [43]. Investigators have described two varieties of thymic cysts, thymopharyngeal duct cysts and cysts arising from the degeneration of Hassall's corpuscles within remnants of ectopic thymic tissue [43, 44].

Thymic cysts can be lined by cuboidal, squamous, stratified squamous or respiratory epithelium, fibrocartilaginous tissue, foreign body corpuscles and Hassall's corpuscles. They usually contain cholesterol clefts.

Clinical Presentation

Thymic cysts are more common in males and usually present as asymptomatic, unilocular or multilocular lateral cystic neck mass near the thoracic inlet. They are more common on the left side of the neck. Thymic cysts can be slow-growing, although some investigators have reported that up to 87 %

of children with thymic cysts present after an upper respiratory tract infection [45]. Larger thymic cysts can compress neck structures and can present with pain, dysphagia, dyspnea, stridor and hoarseness [44]. Airway compromise has been reported at the time of initial presentation [43, 45]. Infections within thymic cysts have been reported in neonates, with rapid enlargement causing life-threatening airway compromise [43].

About a third to half of thymic cysts can have a mediastinal extension [43, 44]. A large number of thymic cysts get misdiagnosed as branchial cleft cysts or lymphatic malformations.

Untreated thymic cyst can be at risk for long-term thymic carcinoma [46] and myasthenia gravis (especially mediastinal thymic cysts).

Diagnosis

Imaging by contrast MRI is strongly recommended for any children suspected to have a thymic cyst, in order to demonstrate the extent of the cyst in the neck and the mediastinum. MRI also helps in planning for surgical resection and differentiating the cyst from branchial cleft cysts and lymphatic malformations, although many cases remain uncertain until a final pathology specimen is obtained [43].

Microbiology

The microbiology of infected congenital thymic cysts is similar to the microbiology of infected TGDC or branchial cleft cysts. Oropharyngeal flora (including oral streptococcal organisms and anaerobes), skin pathogens such as *S. aureus* and *S. pyogenes*, and upper respiratory pathogens like *H. influenzae* and *S. pneumoniae* have been reported [43, 47]. Group B Streptococcus has also been reported in a neonate [43].

Therapeutic Approaches

Empirical antimicrobial therapy should be the same as what is recommended for infected TGDC and branchial cleft cysts. Needle aspiration early in the course of treatment is optimal, and definitive antimicrobial therapy should be directed by culture and susceptibility results. In cases that do not respond to initial therapy or in complicated cysts with airway compromise, an incision and drainage might be necessary with planned resection once the inflammation has subsided. Surgical excision can be challenging due to the close relation of thymic cysts to the carotid sheath (Fig. 15.7).

Laryngocele

Congenital cysts of the larynx are very rare phenomena, but they frequently lead to airway obstruction from their size, their location and their tendency to be inflamed or get infected. Laryngoceles are the most common type of cyst within this category.

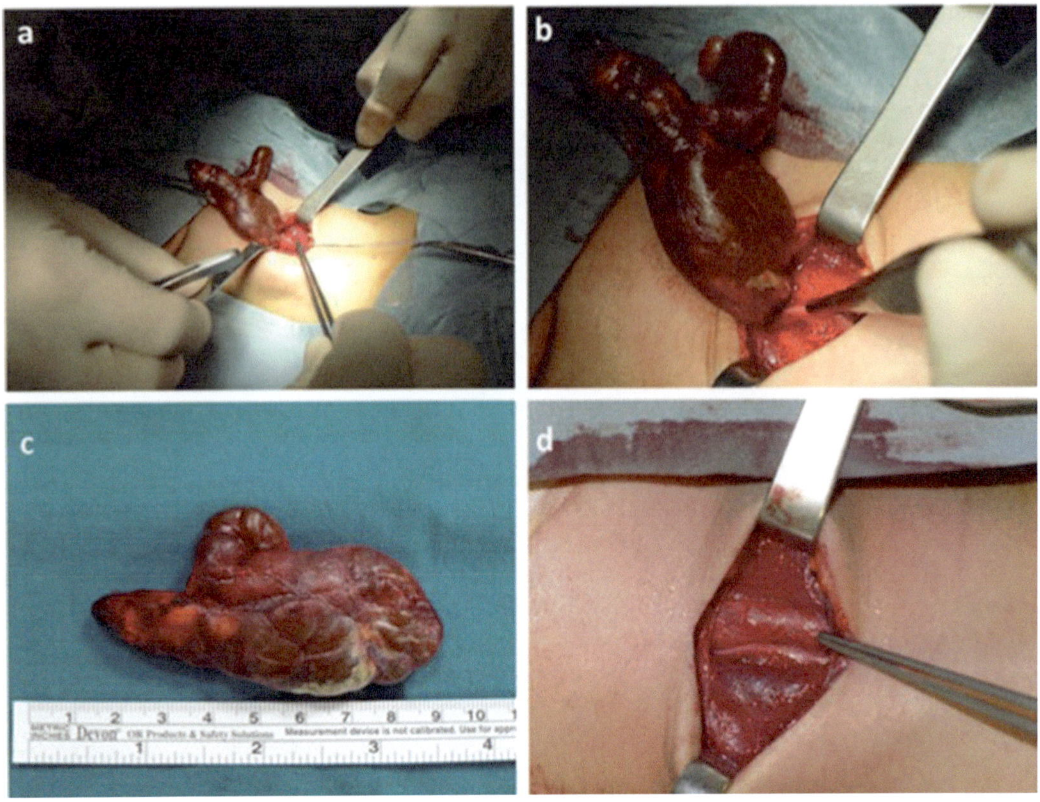

Fig. 15.7 Surgical excision of a thymic cyst showing (**a–b**) dissection from the neurovascular bundle, (**c**) the thymic cyst specimen, (**d**) the carotid artery, vagus nerve and internal jugular vein in situ after specimen removal (From Betti M, Hoseini NH, Martin A, et al. Cervical Thymic Cyst in Childhood: A Case Report. Fetal Pediatr Pathol 2015; 34(1):65–9. Reprinted with kind permission of Springer Science+Business Media.)

Embryology

Laryngocele are thought to originate from the blockage of the saccular duct/failure to recanalize during embryogenesis, leading to accumulation of fluid with progression through the thyrohyoid membrane and other pathways of least resistance in the larynx like the cricothyroid membrane and paratracheal region [48, 49].

Laryngoceles are usually of endodermal and mesodermal origin with respiratory lining and seromucinous glands found in specimen and as such, many refer to them as laryngeal duplication cysts that follow similar patterns as bronchogenic cysts [48]. However, some have specified that this term only applies to cysts that kept a connection to the glottis or ventricle.

Clinical Presentation

Laryngoceles typically will present themselves with stridor, dyspnea, hoarseness and dysphagia [48]. Occasionally the opening of a laryngocele can become blocked and predispose patients to an infection at the side of the neck over the thyroid membrane. When the laryngocele becomes infected, a laryngopyocele is formed. This has been described as very rare, and only approximately 40 cases have been reported in the literature [50]. Symptoms of a laryngopyocele include fever, chills, toxic appearance, rapidly expanding painful neck mass, stridor, difficulty breathing, hoarseness, dysphagia, and odynophagia [50–53]. Airway obstruction requiring emergent tracheostomy has been reported [50]. Additional complications include contiguous spread into the neighboring tissues or spontaneous rupture with inhalation of the purulent material and respiratory compromise.

Diagnosis

The preferred diagnostic method is usually a CT scan or MRI of the neck, followed by confirmation and direct visualization via direct laryngoscopy.

Microbiology

Organisms that have been isolated from laryngopyoceles include oropharyngeal flora, *S. aureus*, *S. pyogenes*, *Escherichia coli*, and *Pseudomonas aeruginosa* [51, 54]. Laryngeal tuberculosis has also been described in patients with infected laryngoceles [53].

Therapeutic Approaches

Broad-spectrum intravenous antibiotics and endoscopic surgical drainage are both important aspects of treatment for a laryngopyocele. Purulent material should be sent for Gram stain and aerobic culture, anaerobic culture, fungal culture, and mycobacteria culture. Intravenous therapy in toxic-appearing patients could include piperacillin/tazobactam plus vancomycin. Definitive therapy includes complete surgical excision—which can be done immediately after endoscopic drainage or at a later time [50].

Surgical excision by an external approach is the appropriate approach to laryngoceles. A midline thyroidotomy converted to a laryngofissure as needed for exposure or a lateral cervical approach to the thyrohyoid membrane have both been described as effective approaches. However, other approaches have been described as well including the use of CO_2 laser to incise the cyst and ablate its lining, or simple unroofing with a 3-day intubation period postoperatively. Cysts tend to recur when treated with more conservative methods [49].

Lymphatic malformations

Over 50 % of the lymphatic malformations (LM) occur in the head and neck region. They represent about 5 % of benign pediatric tumors.

Embryology

Lymphatic malformations result in the abnormal embryogenesis of the lymphatic system. Lymphatic tissue gets sequestered during the formation of lymphaticovenous sacs, which then fails to communicate with the remainder of the lymphatic system and results in cystic spaces of various sizes [55].

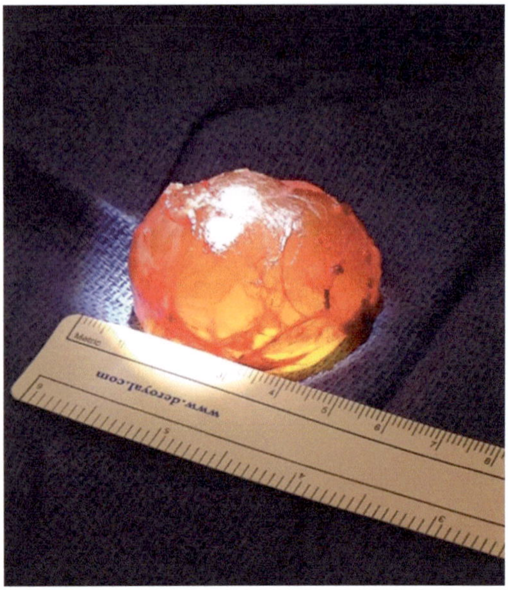

Fig. 15.8 Macrocystic lymphatic malformation status post excision from the neck

Table 15.2 Lymphatic malformation staging system

Stage	Location
I	Unilateral infrahyoid
II	Unilateral suprahyoid
III	Unilateral infrahyoid and suprahyoid
IV	Bilateral suprahyoid
V	Bilateral infrahyoid and suprahyoid

Source: Data from De Serres [56]

LMs are made of endothelial-lined channels and cystic spaces with associated inflammation and accumulation of fluid. They usually contain lymphocytes (Fig. 15.8 depicts a macrocystic lymphatic malformation post-surgical excision).

Clinical Presentation

LM are usually present at birth, although trauma or infections can make them grow bigger and to a clinically significant level. They most commonly present in the neck or in the oral cavity within the tongue and buccal mucosa [55]. Depending on their size, they can impair breathing, eating and speech. Cysts equal or larger than 2 cm are classified as macrocystic (previously called cystic hygromas), whereas cysts smaller than 2 cm are considered microcystic. Mixed lesions contain both.

The de Serres [56] staging system is the most commonly used classification system to predict prognosis and surgical outcome for lymphatic malformations (Table 15.2).

It has been reported that up to 16 % of patients with cervicofacial LM present with an acute infection and that up to 70 % of patients with large cervicofacial LM have an infectious complication [57–59]. Infections of LM usually present with rapid enlargement of the lesion. Bacterial infections are associated with increased erythema, warmth, tenderness, and systemic signs such as fever [15, 40]. Children with bacterial infections of LM can become bacteremic and present with sepsis.

Systemic viral infections or upper respiratory infections can also result in significant expansion of the malformation. Local complications of infection can include respiratory compromise, especially in infants with large malformations, and mediastinal extension [40, 60].

Diagnosis

Ultrasound is very useful as a primary imaging method, as it assesses for internal blood flow, while CT and MRI will delineate the extension and show the lesion's relation to the neck structures. LM will usually have internal septations and no internal blood flow.

Microbiology

LM can become infected through multiple mechanisms. Spontaneous lymphatic leakage from the skin can occur and is associated with cellulitis secondary to skin pathogens such as *S. aureus* and *S. pyogenes*. LM are also commonly infected with oropharyngeal flora—especially in children with poor oral hygiene. Middle ear pathogens can also cause infection of LM, so children should be treated promptly for middle ear infections.

Therapeutic Approaches

Empirical antibiotic therapy should include coverage for oropharyngeal, upper respiratory, and skin flora. Options include clindamycin or amoxicillin/clavulanate plus an anti-staphylococcal agent. For severe or life-threatening infections most experts recommend broad-spectrum empirical coverage such as vancomycin and piperacillin-tazobactam.

While aspiration and drainage can be used as a temporizing measure in life-threatening situations, this procedure is generally avoided due to the high risk of introducing a new infectious process or persistent drainage.

Treatment options include observation, aspiration, ablation, sclerotherapy and surgery. Spontaneous regression is rare and only occurs in 4–6 % of cases. Indications for treatment include recurrent infections, cosmetic disfigurement or compression of local structures [55]. Aspiration can temporarily reduce the size of the lesion, but it can lead to infection and internal hemorrhage. Ablation is mostly used for superficial lesions and most commonly consists of laser treatments, although radiofrequency ablation has also been used.

Sclerotherapy is particularly effective in macrocystic malformations. Agents used in the United States include alcohol, sodium tetradecyl sulfate (STS), doxycycline and bleomycin. Picibanil (OK-432) is commonly used in Europe, but it is not approved in the United States. Sclerosants appear to induce inflammation within the cavity and fibrin and collagen get deposited, which eventually leads to involution of the LM [61]. Concerns over sclerotherapy include the potential for the agent to enter the bloodstream or postsclerosis inflammation causing airway or vascular compromise [62]. Post-sclerotherapy infection and fever can also occur. Surgery can be considered for all types of LM, although there is a high risk of complications in extensive LM and other alternatives should be sought for these patients. Reported complication rate with surgery varied from 17 % in stage I lesions to 100 % in stage V lesions [56]. Overall, a recent systematic review of surgery vs. sclerotherapy was unable to establish the superiority of one treatment over another [62]. LM persistence is common after any treatment, especially in higher staged LMs [62].

Conclusion

Children with recurrent neck infections should be fully evaluated for a congenital neck lesion. These lesions frequently present when they are inflamed or infected. The most common organisms isolated from these lesions include oropharyngeal pathogens, (aerobic and anaerobic), upper respiratory tract organisms, and skin flora. More unusual organisms can occasionally be identified, so it is frequently recommended that children undergo needle aspiration and that studies are sent for gram stain and aerobic culture, anaerobic culture, fungal culture, and mycobacteria culture when clinically feasible. Antimicrobial therapy should be targeted based on culture results. Optimally patients should undergo definitive surgical correction of the congenital lesion after the acute infection subsides.

References

1. Acierno SP, Waldhausen JHT. Congenital cervical cysts, sinuses and fistulae. Otolaryngol Clin North Am. 2007;40(1):161–76; vii–viii.
2. LaRiviere CA, Waldhausen JHT. Congenital cervical cysts, sinuses, and fistulae in pediatric surgery. Surg Clin North Am. 2012;92(3):583–97. viii.
3. Brousseau VJ, Solares CAA, Xu M, Krakovitz P, Koltai PJ. Thyroglossal duct cysts: presentation and management in children versus adults. Int J Pediatr Otorhinolaryngol. 2003;67(12):1285–90.
4. Allard RH. The thyroglossal cyst. Head Neck Surg. 1982;5(2):134–46.
5. Pérez-Martínez A, Bento-Bravo L, Martínez-Bermejo MA, Conde-Cortes J, de Miguel-Medina C. An intra-thyroid thyroglossal duct cyst. Eur J Pediatr Surg. 2005;15(6):428–30.
6. Enepekides DJ. Management of congenital anomalies of the neck. Facial Plast Surg Clin North Am. 2001;9(1):131–45.
7. Weiss SD, Orlich CC. Primary papillary carcinoma of a thyroglossal duct cyst: report of a case and literature review. Br J Surg. 1991;78(1):87–9.
8. Brereton RJ, Symonds E. Thyroglossal cysts in children. Br J Surg. 1978;65(7):507–8.
9. Geller KA, Cohen D, Koempel JA. Thyroglossal duct cyst and sinuses: a 20-year Los Angeles experience and lessons learned. Int J Pediatr Otorhinolaryngol. 2014;78(2):264–7.
10. Al-Dajani N, Wootton SH. Cervical lymphadenitis, suppurative parotitis, thyroiditis, and infected cysts. Infect Dis Clin North Am. 2007;21(2):523–41. 2.
11. Mohan PS, Chokshi RA, Moser RL, Razvi SA. Thyroglossal duct cysts: a consideration in adults. Am Surg. 2005;71(6):508–11.
12. Nour YA, Hassan MH, Gaafar A, Eldaly A. Deep neck infections of congenital causes. Otolaryngol Head Neck Surg. 2011;144(3):365–71.
13. Boscolo-Rizzo P, Marchiori C, Zanetti F, Vaglia A, Da Mosto MC. Conservative management of deep neck abscesses in adults: the importance of CECT findings. Otolaryngol Head Neck Surg. 2006;135(6):894–9.
14. Foley DS, Fallat ME. Thyroglossal duct and other congenital midline cervical anomalies. Semin Pediatr Surg. 2006;15(2):70–5.
15. Brook I. Microbiology and management of infected neck cysts. J Oral Maxillofac Surg. 2005;63(3):392–5.
16. Brook I. Microbiology of abscesses of the head and neck in children. Ann Otol Rhinol Laryngol. 1987;96(4):429–33.
17. Kottmeier PK, Rosenthal S, Minkowitz S. Retropharyngeal abscess secondary to thyroglossal cyst. Am J Dis Child. 1965;109:160–1.
18. Rogers KB, Zinnemann K, Foster WP. The isolation and identification of Haemophilus spp, from unusual lesions in children. J Clin Pathol. 1960;13:519–24.
19. Gupta R, Levent F, Healy CM, Edwards MS. Unusual soft tissue manifestations of Neisseria meningitidis infections. Clin Pediatr (Phila). 2008;47(4):400–3.
20. Baker CJ. Group B, streptococcal cellulitis-adenitis in infants. Am J Dis Child. 1982;136(7):631–3.
21. Nelson JJ, Hall DA, Wolf GT, Prince ME. An unusual thyroglossal duct cyst infection with coccidioidomycosis. J Otolaryngol. 2007;36(1):69–71.
22. Shahin A, Burroughs FH, Kirby JP, Ali SZ. Thyroglossal duct cyst: a cytopathologic study of 26 cases. Diagn Cytopathol. 2005;33(6):365–9.
23. Waldhausen JHT. Branchial cleft and arch anomalies in children. Semin Pediatr Surg. 2006;15(2):64–9.

24. Roback SA, Telander RL. Thyroglossal duct cysts and branchial cleft anomalies. Semin Pediatr Surg. 1994;3(3):142–6.
25. Mandell DL. Head and neck anomalies related to the branchial apparatus. Otolaryngol Clin North Am. 2000;33(6):1309–32.
26. Chang L, Chi H, Chiu N-C, Huang F-Y, Lee K-S. Deep neck infections in different age groups of children. J Microbiol Immunol Infect. 2010;43(1):47–52.
27. Montgomery GL, Ballantine TV, Kleiman MB, Wright JC, Reynolds J. Ruptured branchial cleft cyst presenting as acute thyroid infection. Clin Pediatr (Phila). 1982;21(6):380–3.
28. Nicoucar K, Giger R, Pope HG, Jaecklin T, Dulguerov P. Management of congenital fourth branchial arch anomalies: a review and analysis of published cases. J Pediatr Surg. 2009;44(7):1432–9.
29. D'Souza AR, Uppal HS, De R, Zeitoun H. Updating concepts of first branchial cleft defects: a literature review. Int J Pediatr Otorhinolaryngol. 2002;62(2):103–9.
30. Arnot RS. Defects of the first branchial cleft. S Afr J Surg. 1971;9(2):93–8.
31. Work WP. Newer concepts of first branchial cleft defects. Laryngoscope. 1972;82(9):1581–93.
32. Second branchial cleft cyst. Radiology reference article at Radiopaedia.org. http://radiopaedia.org/articles/second-branchial-cleft-cyst. Accessed 20 Nov 2014.
33. Thomas B, Shroff M, Forte V, Blaser S, James A. Revisiting imaging features and the embryologic basis of third and fourth branchial anomalies. AJNR Am J Neuroradiol. 2010;31(4):755–60.
34. Pereira KD, Losh GG, Oliver D, Poole MD. Management of anomalies of the third and fourth branchial pouches. Int J Pediatr Otorhinolaryngol. 2004;68(1):43–50.
35. Madana J, Yolmo D, Kalaiarasi R, Gopalakrishnan S, Saxena SK, Krishnapriya S. Recurrent neck infection with branchial arch fistula in children. Int J Pediatr Otorhinolaryngol. 2011;75(9):1181–5.
36. Yolmo D, Madana J, Kalaiarasi R, Gopalakrishnan S, Kiruba Shankar M, Krishnapriya S. Retrospective case review of pyriform sinus fistulae of third branchial arch origin commonly presenting as acute suppurative thyroiditis in children. J Laryngol Otol. 2012;126(7):737–42.
37. Carta F, Sionis S, Mascia L, Puxeddu R. Fourth branchial cleft anomaly: management strategy in acute presentation. Int J Pediatr Otorhinolaryngol. 2014;78(9):1480–4.
38. Scheinfeld NS, Silverberg NB, Weinberg JM, Nozad V. The preauricular sinus: a review of its clinical presentation, treatment, and associations. Pediatr Dermatol. 2004;21(3):191–6.
39. Paulozzi LJ, Lary JM. Laterality patterns in infants with external birth defects. Teratology. 1999;60(5):265–71.
40. Brown RL, Azizkhan RG. Pediatric head and neck lesions. Pediatr Clin North Am. 1998;45(4):889–905.
41. Gur E, Yeung A, Al-Azzawi M, Thomson H. The excised preauricular sinus in 14 years of experience: is there a problem? Plast Reconstr Surg. 1998;102(5):1405–8.
42. Hsieh Y-Y, Hsueh S, Hsueh C, Lin J-N, Luo C-C, Lai J-Y, et al. Pathological analysis of congenital cervical cysts in children: 20 years of experience at Chang Gung Memorial Hospital. Chang Gung Med J. 2003;26(2):107–13.
43. Billings KR, Rollins NK, Timmons C, Biavati MJ. Infected neonatal cervical thymic cyst. Otolaryngol Head Neck Surg. 2000;123(5):651–4.
44. Shenoy V, Kamath MP, Hegde MC, Rao Aroor R, Maller VV. Cervical thymic cyst: a rare differential diagnosis in lateral neck swelling. Case Rep Otolaryngol. 2013;2013:350502.
45. Wagner CW, Vinocur CD, Weintraub WH, Golladay ES. Respiratory complications in cervical thymic cysts. J Pediatr Surg. 1988;23(7):657–60.
46. Yamashita S, Yamazaki H, Kato T, Yokota T, Matsumoto N, Matsukura S. Thymic carcinoma which developed in a thymic cyst. Intern Med. 1996;35(3):215–8.
47. Youngson GG, Ein SH, Geddie WR, Cutz E. Infected thymic cyst: an unusual cause of respiratory distress in a child. Pediatr Pulmonol. 1987;3(4):276–9.
48. Saha D, Sinha R, Pai RR, Kumar A, Chakraborti S. Laryngeal cysts in infants and children—a pathologist's perspective (with review of literature). Int J Pediatr Otorhinolaryngol. 2013;77(7):1112–7.
49. Forte V, Fuoco G, James A. A new classification system for congenital laryngeal cysts. Laryngoscope. 2004;114(6):1123–7.
50. Vasileiadis I, Kapetanakis S, Petousis A, Stavrianaki A, Fiska A, Karakostas E. Internal laryngopyocele as a cause of acute airway obstruction: an extremely rare case and review of the literature. Acta Otorhinolaryngol Ital. 2012;32(1):58–62.
51. Cassano L, Lombardo P, Marchese-Ragona R, Pastore A, Marchese RR. Laryngopyocele: three new clinical cases and review of the literature. Eur Arch Otorhinolaryngol. 2000;257(9):507–11.
52. Illum P, Nehen AM. Laryngopyocele with a report of three cases. J Laryngol Otol. 1980;94(2):211–8.
53. Porter PW, Vilensky JA. The laryngeal saccule: clinical significance. Clin Anat. 2012;25(5):647–9.
54. Altamar-Ríos J, Morales RO. Laryngocele and pyolaryngocele. An Otorrinolaringol Ibero Am. 1992;19(4):393–9.
55. Colbert SD, Seager L, Haider F, Evans BT, Anand R, Brennan PA. Lymphatic malformations of the head and neck-current concepts in management. Br J Oral Maxillofac Surg. 2013;51(2):98–102.

56. De Serres LM, Sie KC, Richardson MA. Lymphatic malformations of the head and neck. A proposal for staging. Arch Otolaryngol Head Neck Surg. 1995;121(5):577–82.
57. Padwa BL, Hayward PG, Ferraro NF, Mulliken JB. Cervicofacial lymphatic malformation: clinical course, surgical intervention, and pathogenesis of skeletal hypertrophy. Plast Reconstr Surg. 1995;95(6):951–60.
58. Charabi B, Bretlau P, Bille M, Holmelund M. Cystic hygroma of the head and neck—a long-term follow-up of 44 cases. Acta Otolaryngol Suppl. 2000;543:248–50.
59. Raveh E, de Jong AL, Taylor GP, Forte V. Prognostic factors in the treatment of lymphatic malformations. Arch Otolaryngol Head Neck Surg. 1997;123(10):1061–5.
60. Burezq H, Williams B, Chitte SA. Management of cystic hygromas: 30 year experience. J Craniofac Surg. 2006;17(4):815–8.
61. Jamal N, Ahmed S, Miller T, Bent J, Brook A, Parikh S, et al. Doxycycline sclerotherapy for pediatric head and neck macrocystic lymphatic malformations: a case series and review of the literature. Int J Pediatr Otorhinolaryngol. 2012;76(8):1127–31.
62. Adams MT, Saltzman B, Perkins JA. Head and neck lymphatic malformation treatment: a systematic review. Otolaryngol Head Neck Surg. 2012;147(4):627–39.

Part V
Other Conditions

Chapter 16
PFAPA: Periodic Fever, Aphthous Stomatitis, Pharyngitis, and Cervical Adenitis

Katherine R. Kavanagh and Henry M. Feder Jr.

In 1987, Marshall and colleagues described a new periodic fever syndrome in children, which was characterized by recurring self-limited high fevers [1]. These fevers were frequently associated with pharyngitis. Throat cultures were negative and antibiotic therapy or antibiotic prophylaxis was ineffective at controlling symptoms or halting the fever. This syndrome was later named PFAPA—**P**eriodic **F**ever, **A**phthous stomatitis, **P**haryngitis, and cervical **A**denitis. In 1989, Abramson and colleagues reported that tonsillectomy resolved this periodic episodes of fever in four patients [2]. Fever and pharyngitis are common in children and usually associated with infectious etiologies. Periodic fevers in children are unusual but when they occur they can be distressing to parents and challenging to pediatric clinicians. The cause of PFAPA is unknown and diagnosis is based on recognizing the clinical syndrome. Laboratory testing is not usually helpful except to rule-out other periodic fever syndromes.

Signs and Symptoms of PFAPA

A number of studies have described the symptoms, diagnostic criteria, and long-term follow up data for cohorts of patients with PFAPA [1–6]. The criteria for the diagnosis of PFAPA include the following: recurring fevers usually starting before 5 years of age, at least one constitutional symptom associated with most of the fevers (aphthous ulcers, cervical lymphadenitis, and pharyngitis), absence of neutropenia, no symptoms between episodes, and normal growth and development [3–5]. About half

K.R. Kavanagh, M.D. (✉)
Department of Otolaryngology, Connecticut Children's Medical Center, 282 Washington, Hartford, CT 06119, USA
e-mail: kkavana@connecticutchildrens.org

H.M. Feder Jr., M.D.
Department of Pediatrics and Family Medicine, University of Connecticut Medical Center, 263 Farmington Ave, Farmington, CT 06030, USA
e-mail: hfeder@connecticutchildrens.org;
feder@uchc.edu

T.A. Valdez, J.G. Vallejo (eds.), *Infectious Diseases in Pediatric Otolaryngology*,
DOI 10.1007/978-3-319-21744-4_16

Table 16.1 PFAPA compared with other periodic fever syndromes

	PFAPA	Familial Mediterranean fever	Hyper IgD	Systemic onset juvenile rheumatoid arthritis
Onset at <5 years of age	Common	Unusual	Common	Common
Length of fever episode	4 days	2 days	4 days	>30 days
Interval between fever episodes	2–8 weeks	Not periodic	Not periodic	Hectic quotidian
Associated symptoms	Aphthous stomatitis, pharyngitis, adenitis	Painful pleuritis, peritonitis	Arthralgias, abdominal pain, diarrhea, splenomegaly, rashes	Rash, generalized lymphadenopathy, hepatosplenomegaly, arthritis
Ethnic, geographic	None	Mediterranean	Dutch	None
Special laboratory test results	None	Gene analysis	Elevated serum IgD concentration	None
Sequelae	None	Amyloidosis	None	Symmetric polyarthritis

Source: Reprinted from The Journal of Pediatrics, Thomas KT, Feder HM, Lawton AR, Edwards KM, Periodic Fever Syndrome in Children, Vol. 135(1), pp. 15–21, Copyright (1999), with permission from Elsevier

of the patients with PFAPA have a prodrome beginning 6–24 h before the onset of fever. The prodrome is usually characterized by fatigue and loss of appetite but other symptoms include headache, irritability, abdominal pain and aphthous stomatitis. With or without a prodrome a PFAPA episode begins with a sudden spike of fever (usually greater than 38.9 °C). The fever then lasts 2–6 days (mean = 4.8 days) and may be associated with aphthous ulcers, cervical lymphadenitis, and pharyngitis [4]. These episodes occur on a fairly regular schedule, typically at an interval between 2 and 8 weeks (mean = 28 days). Some families may plan vacations during a time when they don't expect a fever [6]. A hallmark of the syndrome is the complete lack of inter-current symptoms in otherwise healthy, normal developing children and that when the subject gets sick all the other family members remain well.

Apart from the previously described diagnostic criteria, other etiologies may need to be excluded to make the diagnosis of PFAPA [7]. Patients with PFAPA should not have arthritis, rash, or neutropenia [6]. Blood testing including CBC may show an elevated WBC with a left shift. The ESR and CRP are generally elevated during the acute febrile episode. All laboratory values are normal during the inter-current afebrile periods. Alternative diagnoses to consider include Behcet's syndrome, Familial Mediterranean Fever, cyclic neutropenia, Crohn's disease, hyper IgD syndrome, and juvenile inflammatory arthritis [8]. Table 16.1 delineates differences between these diagnoses to aid the clinician in ruling out alternative entities [4]. In one study, the clinical characteristics of 105 children with PFAPA were reviewed over a 10 year period [6]. The results showed diverse ancestry and a male predominance (62 %). In this large group of patients, fevers began at 3 years of age (range 3 months to 12 years), had an average episode length of 4.8 days, and showed an average interval between episodes of 28 days. Of these 105 patients with PFAPA, aphthous stomatitis was present in 38 %, pharyngitis was present in 85 %, and cervical adenitis was present in 72 %. Parents reported a prodrome beginning 4–48 h prior to the fever in the majority of patients. During febrile episodes WBC counts (as high as 30,500 cells/mm^3 with a left shift), ESRs, and CRPs were frequently elevated versus when the subjects were well these tests were normal. Laboratory testing to rule out definable causes of recurrent fevers included a CBC at the onset of the febrile episode to exclude neutropenia ANA, rheumatoid factor, and quantitative immunoglobulins (IgG, IgA, IgM, IgE, and IgD).

The etiology of PFAPA has not been defined. Theories ranging from infectious to genetic to immune mediated have been proposed. Many investigators have postulated an infectious trigger (like a minor viral exposure) followed by dysregulation of immune mediators (e.g. cytokines). In three large studies, only three siblings have been diagnosed with PFAPA [4, 6, 9]. Thus, an inherited genetic defect or a contagious infectious disease would be unlikely culprits as the cause of PFAPA. Stojanov and colleagues (2011) analyzed blood samples from PFAPA patients during febrile episodes and found that complement and IL-1 were up regulated suggesting that PFAPA was an up regulation defect of innate immunity [10]. They postulated that a simple trigger (like an asymptomatic or mildly symptomatic viral infection) causes a PFAPA flare and this flare is followed by a period of time that the dysregulated immune response cannot be activated again.

Management and Outcomes

Patients with PFAPA have an excellent prognosis. In the initial study of 94 PFAPA patients the fevers resolved in about 5 years (or after about 60 episodes) in 40 % of patients (34 of 83) [4]. In a later study, PFAPA resolved spontaneously in about 3 years [6]. Both medical and surgical options for management of PFAPA patients have been reported. Over 90 % of patients with PFAPA will dramatically become afebrile after 1 mg/kg dose of prednisolone. In a study of 105 patients, 74 patients used prednisolonefor at least one PFAPA episode. Fifty-eight had their fevers resolve with one dose, 13 needed two doses, and one needed three doses spaced 12 h apart. Half the patients given prednisolone had the interval between episodes initially shorten by 7–14 days. However, over time of using prednisone the interval between febrile episodes returned to the baseline interval. Prednisolone (or prednisone) effectively aborts individual episodes of PFAPA but does not change the long-term outcomes of PFAPA. Since there are no laboratory tests available to establish the diagnosis of PFAPA, a dramatic resolution of fever with one or two doses of prednisolone is strong evidence that PFAPA is the diagnosis. In our personal experience (unpublished data), with febrile non-specific viral infections and asthma exacerbations, fever may persist following the first few doses of steroids. The use of prednisolone or prednisone relieves the fever and pharyngitis (but usually not the aphthous ulcers and adenitis) usually in a matter of hours. This response may be useful in distinguishing attacks of PFAPA from familial Mediterranean fever (FMF) or other hereditary autoinflammatory periodic fever syndromes.

Cimetidine is another medical therapy that has been successful in PFAPA (with 7 of 26 PFAPA patients having the syndrome resolve with cimetidine for 6–12 months) [6, 11]. Cimetidine is an H_2 antagonist used to decrease gastric acid that also has very slight immune modulating properties including effects on CD8 cells, interferon gamma, neutrophils, eosinophils, and lysosomal enzyme, and inhibitory factors. It is not known why cimetidine works in some PFAPA patients and not in others, although the immune modulating properties are suspected to bethe cause for the patients in whom cimetidine halts the fever episodes [6, 11].

Tonsillectomy with or without adenoidectomy has been shown to be curative in some patients with PFAPA. Multiple studies have noted an association between removal of the tonsils and resolution of PFAPA symptoms. In a prospective, long-term study by Licameli et al., 99 of 102 patients had complete resolution of symptoms after tonsillectomy with an average follow up of 43 months [9]. A recent Cochrane review (2014) analyzed two randomized controlled trials from 2007 and determined that tonsillectomy can be highly effective for resolution of PFAPA symptoms [12]. A meta-analysis comparing medical with surgical treatment of PFAPA found that tonsillectomy with or without adenoidectomy was the most effective for resolution of symptoms [13]. However, the risks of surgery including hemorrhage and dehydration must be weighed against the burden of disease when considering tonsillectomy.

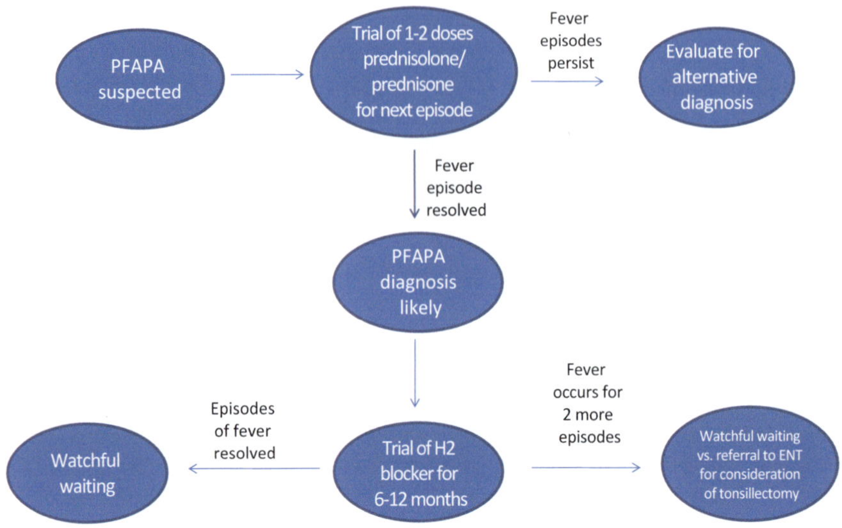

Fig. 16.1 An algorithmic approach to the diagnosis and management of PFAPA

Conclusion

The diagnosis of PFAPA is usually made by the typical history and the response of the episodes to one or two doses of steroids. Trying an H_2 blocker to see if this resolves the illness is a reasonable next step. If the subject gets two typical fevers while taking the H_2 blocker, than this therapy has failed. The choice of waiting and watching versus tonsillectomy has to be made on patient by patient basis by the ENT physician and the family (Fig. 16.1).

References

1. Marshall GS, Edwards KM, Butler J, Lawton AR. Syndrome of periodic fever, pharyngitis, and aphthous stomatitis. J Pediatr. 1987;110:43–6.
2. Abramson JS, Givner LB, Thompson JN. Possible role of tonsillectomy and adenoidectomy in children with recurrent fever and tonsillopharyngitis. Pediatr Infect Dis J. 1989;8:119–20.
3. Feder HM, Bialecki CA. Periodic fever associated with aphthous stomatitis, pharyngitis and cervical adenitis. Pediatr Infect Dis J. 1989;8(3):186–7.
4. Thomas KT, Feder HM, Lawton AR, Edwards KM. Periodic fever syndrome in children. J Pediatr. 1999;135(1):15–21.
5. Wurster VM, Carlucci JG, Feder HM, Edwards KM. Long-term follow-up of children with periodic fever, aphthous stomatitis, pharyngitis, and cervical adenitis syndrome. J Pediatr. 2011;159:958–64.
6. Feder HM, Salazar JC. A clinical review of 105 patients with PFAPA (a periodic fever syndrome). Acta Paediatr. 2010;99:178–84.
7. Caorsi R, Pelagatti MA, Federici S, Finetti M, Martini A, Gattorno M. Periodic fever, apthous stomatitis, pharyngitis, and adenitis syndrome. Curr Opin Rheumatol. 2010;22:579–84.
8. Long S. Syndrome of periodic fever, aphthous stomatitis, pharyngitis, and adenitis (PFAPA)-what it isn't. What is it? J Pediatr. 1999;135(1):1–5.
9. Licameli G, Lawton M, Kenna M, Dedeoglu F. Long-term surgical outcomes of Adenotonsillectomy for PFAPA syndrome. Arch Otolaryngol Head Neck Surg. 2010;138(10):902–6.
10. Stojanov S, Lapidus S, Chitkara P, et al. Periodic fever, aphthous stomatitis, pharyngitis, and adenitis (PFAPA) is a disorder of innate immunity and Th1 activation responsive to IL-1 blockade. Proc Natl Acad Sci U S A. 2011;108:7148–53.

11. Feder HM. Cimetidine treatment for periodic fever associated with aphthous stomatitis, pharyngitis and cervical adenitis. Pediatr Infect Dis J. 1992;11:318–21.
12. Burton MJ, Pollard AJ, Ramsden JD, Chong LY, Venekamp RP. Tonsillectomy for periodic fever, aphthous stomatitis and cervical adenitis syndrome (PFAPA). Cochrane Database Syst Rev. 2014;9, CD008669.
13. Peridis S, Pilgrim G, Koudoumnakis E, Athanasopoulos I, Houlakis M, Parpounas K. PFAPA syndrome in children: a meta-analysis on surgical versus medical treatment. Int J Pediatr Otorhinolaryngol. 2010;74:1203–8.

Index

T. Valdez, J. Vallejo (eds.), *Infectious Diseases in Pediatric Otolaryngology*,
DOI 10.1007/978-3-319-21744-4